Marijuana and Madness

Psychiatry and Neurobiology

This book provides a comprehensive and up-to-date overview of the psychiatry and neuroscience of *Cannabis sativa* (marijuana), with particular emphasis on psychotic disorders. It outlines the very latest developments in our understanding of the human cannabinoid system, and links this knowledge to clinical and epidemiological facts about the impact of cannabis on mental health. Clinically focused chapters review not only the direct psychomimetic properties of cannabis, but also the impact consumption has on the courses of evolving or established mental illness such as schizophrenia. A number of controversial issues are critically explored, including whether a discrete 'cannabis psychosis' exists, and whether cannabis can actually cause schizophrenia. Effects of cannabis on mood, notably depression, are reviewed, as are its effects on cognition. This book will be of interest to all members of the mental health team, as well as to neuroscientists and those involved in drug and alcohol research.

David Castle is Professor at the Mental Health Research Institute and University of Melbourne, Melbourne, Australia.

Robin Murray is Professor at the Maudsley Hospital and Institute of Psychiatry, London.

Marijuana and Madness

Psychiatry and Neurobiology

Edited by

David Castle
Mental Health Research Institute and University of Melbourne, Australia

Robin Murray
Maudsley Hospital and Institute of Psychiatry, London, UK

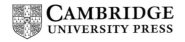
CAMBRIDGE
UNIVERSITY PRESS

PUBLISHED BY THE PRESS SYNDICATE OF THE UNIVERSITY OF CAMBRIDGE
The Pitt Building, Trumpington Street, Cambridge, United Kingdom

CAMBRIDGE UNIVERSITY PRESS
The Edinburgh Building, Cambridge CB2 2RU, UK
40 West 20th Street, New York, NY 10011–4211, USA
477 Williamstown Road, Port Melbourne, VIC 3207, Australia
Ruiz de Alarcón 13, 28014 Madrid, Spain
Dock House, The Waterfront, Cape Town 8001, South Africa

http://www.cambridge.org

First published 2004
Reprinted 2005

Printed in the United Kingdom at the University Press, Cambridge

Typefaces Minion 10.5/14pt. and Formata   *System* LATEX 2_ε [TB]

A catalogue record for this book is available from the British Library

Library of Congress Cataloguing in Publication data
Marijuana and madness : psychiatry and neurobiology / edited by David Castle and Robin Murray.
   p.   cm.
Includes bibliographical references and index.
ISBN 0 521 81940 7 (hardback)
1. Marijuana – Physiological effect.   2. Marijuana – Psychological aspects.   3. Marijuana abuse –
Complications.   4. Psychoses – Etiology.   5. Schizophrenia – Etiology.   I. Castle, David J.   II. Murray,
Robin, MD, M Phil, MRCP, MRC Psych.
[DNLM: 1. Marijuana smoking – psychology.   2. Marijuana smoking – adverse effects.
3. Mental disorders – complications. WM 276 M33485 2004]
RC568.C2M375   2004
615′.7827 – dc22   2003055906

ISBN 0 521 81940 7 hardback

This book is dedicated to the memory of Frances Rix Ames, whose belief in the potential medical and environmental benefits of marijuana was never obscured by the smoke of political rhetoric.

Contents

Just take tiny bits from each paragraph! chapter

vii

Contributors

Louise Arseneault, Ph.D.
Social, Genetic and Developmental
  Psychiatry
Research Centre
Institute of Psychiatry
King's College
London
UK

Mary Cannon M.D. Ph.D. M.R.C.Psych.
Division of Psychological Medicine
Institute of Psychiatry
King's College
London
UK

**David J. Castle M.B.Ch.B. M.Sc. M.D.
DLSHTM M.R.C.Psych. FRANZCP**
Mental Health Research Institute
University of Melbourne
155 Oak Street
Parkville VIC 3052
Australia

Hyun-Sang Cho M.D.
Department of Psychiatry
Yale University School of Medicine
Psychiatry Service 116A
VA Connecticut Healthcare
  System
950 Campbell Avenue
West Haven CT 06516
USA

Carolyn Coffey B.Sc. Grad. Dip. Epi.
Centre for Adolescent Health
Murdoch Children's Research Institute
2 Gatehouse Street
Parkville VIC 3052
Australia

David Copolov
Mental Health Research Institute
University of Melbourne
155 Oak Street
Parkville VIC 3052
Australia

Brian Dean
Mental Health Research Institute
University of Melbourne
155 Oak Street
Parkville VIC 3052
Australia

**Louisa Degenhardt Ph.D.
M.Psychol.(Clinical)**
National Drug and Alcohol
  Research Centre
University of NSW
Sydney NSW 2052
Australia

Lieuwe de Haan
Academic Medical Center
University of Amsterdam
Amsterdam
The Netherlands

D. Cyril D'Souza M.D.
Department of Psychiatry
Yale University School of Medicine
Psychiatry Service 116A
VA Connecticut Healthcare System
950 Campbell Avenue
West Haven CT 06516
USA

Wayne Hall Ph.D.
Office of Public Policy and Ethics
Institute for Molecular Bioscience
University of Queensland
St Lucia QLD 4072
Australia

Lumir Hanuš Ph.D.
Medical Faculty
Department of Medicinal Chemistry and
   Natural Products
The Hebrew University of Jerusalem
Ein Kerem Campus
Jerusalem 91120
Israel

Leslie Iversen Ph.D. F.R.S.
University of Oxford
Department of Pharmacology
South Parks Road
Oxford OX1 3QT
UK

**Wynne James R.N. Dip.N.(Lond.)
B.Sc.(Hons)**
Manager
Next Step Specialist Drug and Alcohol
   Services
26 Dugdale Street
Warwick WA 6024
Australia

John H. Krystal M.D.
Department of Psychiatry
Yale University School of Medicine
Psychiatry Service 116A
VA Connecticut Healthcare System
950 Campbell Avenue
West Haven CT 06516
USA

Don Linszen
Academic Medical Centre
University of Amsterdam
Amsterdam
The Netherlands

Michael Lynskey Ph.D.
Missouri Alcoholism Research Center
Department of Psychiatry
Washington University School of Medicine
40 N. Kingshighway, Suite One
St Louis MO 63108
USA

Raphael Mechoulam, Ph.D.
Medical Faculty
Department of Medicinal Chemistry and
   Natural Products
The Hebrew University of Jerusalem
Ein Kerem Campus
Jerusalem 91120
Israel

Robin Murray M.D. D.Sc. F.R.C.Psych.
Division of Psychological Medicine
Institute of Psychiatry
King's College
London
UK

George Patton M.D. FRANZCP
Centre for Adolescent Health
Murdoch Children's Research Institute
2 Gatehouse Street
Parkville VIC 3052
Australia

Edward B. Perry M.D.
Department of Psychiatry
Yale University School of
   Medicine
Psychiatry Service 116A
VA Connecticut Healthcare System
950 Campbell Avenue
West Haven CT 06516
USA

Bart Peters
Academic Medical Center
University of Amsterdam
Amsterdam
The Netherlands

Harrison G. Pope, Jr M.D. M.P.H.
Biological Psychiatry Laboratory
McLean Hospital/Harvard Medical
  School
115 Mill Street
Belmont MA 02478
USA

Nadia Solowij B.Sc. M.A. Ph.D.
Illawarra Institute for Mental Health
Department of Psychology
University of Wollongong
Wollongong NSW 2522
Australia

Catherine Spencer B.Psych. M.Psych.
c/o Mental Health Research Institute
University of Melbourne
155 Oak Street
Parkville VIC 3052
Australia

Suresh Sundram
Mental Health Research Institute
University of Melbourne
155 Oak Street
Parkville VIC 3052
Australia

Hélène Verdoux M.D. Ph.D.
University Department
Hôpital Charles Perrens
121 rue de la Béchade
33076 Bordeaux Cedex
France

John Witton
National Addiction Centre
Institute of Psychiatry
King's College
London
UK

Deborah Yurgelun-Todd Ph.D.
Cognitive Neuroimaging Laboratory
McLean Hospital/Harvard Medical School
115 Mill Street
Belmont MA 02478
USA

Foreword

Research on the relationship between cannabis and mental health is a vivid illustration of the fact that the pace at which new scientific insights are embraced by the community is determined in an idiosyncratic, non-linear fashion. In 1987, a landmark study by Andreasson in the *Lancet* presented credible confirmation of the classic clinical observation that use of cannabis was associated with onset of psychosis. One would have expected that the link between one of the most widely used psychotropic drugs and one of the most devastating of mental illnesses would have resulted in an animated public health discussion. In actual fact, nothing happened very much. In the ensuing 15 years, however, the cumulative weight of a range of clinical, epidemiological and basic science investigations became such that by 2003 both the scientific and public health communities have gradually become aware of the potential significance of cannabis use.

Therefore, if ever a book was timely and topical, it is this one. The editors have done a remarkable job in bringing together the views of the principal experts in the field from around the world, providing a balanced summary of all the evidence that relates the use of cannabis to mental health outcomes. It includes a comprehensive overview of studies of the direct psychotropic effects of cannabis whilst in other chapters this evidence is elegantly linked to the possible neurobiological mechanisms underlying cannabis-induced mental states. The authors go on to address the question, at the population level, of whether widespread use of cannabis in many societies is associated with the onset of psychiatric disorders and, if so, whether this is because individuals with mental health problems use cannabis to help them feel better or whether use of cannabis increases the risk of onset of mental health problems. Furthermore, it addresses the question whether some individuals are more vulnerable than others to the effects of cannabis on mental health. The book includes an analysis of why some people with mental health problems would use cannabis, how it affects the course of their illness and how treatment should be tailored to take into account dysfunctional use of cannabis.

The scientific information contained in this book not only serves clinicians, it will also help to inform public health discussions on if and how cannabis use should be regulated. Are the numerous coffee shops in the cities of the Netherlands where many young people gather on a daily basis a great good or should they be restricted? Is the rising proportion of people using cannabis a source of concern or does it show that we have learned to use the drug recreationally? In summary, does cannabis do more harm than good? Whatever the pre-existing opinion of the person when taking up this book, it is unlikely to be the same after.

Jim van Os
Professor of Psychiatric Epidemiology
Maastricht University, the Netherlands

Preface

Cannabis sativa (marijuana) has been used by humans for centuries, largely for its psychological effects. Currently, it is the most widely used illicit substance in the world, and there is heated public debate about whether it should be legalized, or at least decriminalized, in a number of countries. There is also considerable public and commercial interest in its medicinal properties, and in hemp as an environmentally friendly plant with numerous potential uses. This discussion needs to be informed by a consideration of the effects of cannabis on the human brain, notably its effects on cognition, and its potential to cause psychotic symptoms, particularly in vulnerable individuals. Recent advances in our understanding of the human cannabinoid system, and methodologically robust epidemiological, clinical and experimental studies of the effects of cannabis in humans, allow us to understand better how cannabis exerts both its beneficial and its adverse effects.

It has been known for many years that people who suffer psychotic illness are far more likely to consume cannabis than the general population, and there has been much dispute about the reasons for this. Unfortunately, until recently there were relatively few data available to inform this debate. The situation has changed greatly over the last decade with the publication of new basic and clinical studies. Therefore, this book provides a comprehensive and up-to-date overview of the psychiatry and neurobiology of cannabis, with particular emphasis on psychotic disorders. It outlines the very latest developments in our understanding of the human cannabinoid system, and links this knowledge to established and emerging clinical and epidemiological facts about the impact of cannabis on mental health. The clinically focused chapters review not only the direct psychomimetic properties of cannabis, but also the impact consumption has on the course of evolving and established mental illnesses such as schizophrenia.

The expert contributors explore a number of controversial issues, including whether a discrete 'cannabis psychosis' exists, and whether cannabis can actually *cause* schizophrenia. Effects of cannabis on mood, notably depression, are reviewed, with particular attention paid to recent prospective studies. The impact of cannabis on cognition (both in the short- and long-term) is covered in some detail, with a careful weighing of the evidence for and against any long-term adverse effects. There are chapters on some of the 'cutting-edge' aspects of neurobiological cannabis research, including studies of the cannabinoid system in schizophrenia, the effect of cannabis CB_1-receptor blockade on the psychomimetic effects of cannabis and cannabis–dopamine interactions.

We believe that this book provides a timely and comprehensive update on the psychiatry and neurobiology of *C. sativa*, by international experts in the field. We anticipate that the book will be of interest to those working in the mental health and drug and alcohol fields, as well as to psychopharmacologists and neuroscientists, and also to many consumers of cannabis.

The cannabinoid system: from the point of view of a chemist

Raphael Mechoulam and Lumir Hanuš

Hebrew University Medical Faculty, Jerusalem, Israel

This book is about cannabis (marijuana) and psychotic illnesses; more specifically, it outlines how our increasing understanding of cannabis itself, the effects of
cannabis on the brain and psychic functions and of the cannabinoid system can
inform our understanding of the relationships between cannabis and psychosis.
This chapter serves as an introduction to this topic, with a brief historical overview
of the psychic effects of cannabis, followed by an exposition on the cannabinoid
system.

Cannabis and mental illness

J. J. Moreau, the first nineteenth-century psychiatrist with an interest in psychopharmacology, described in great detail his experiments with hashish (Moreau, 1973). He
took the drug himself and asked his students to follow his example. He also administered it to his patients. By modern standards the doses used were enormously high.
The effects on one of his assistants, who swallowed 16 g of an extract – presumably
containing several hundred milligrams of tetrahydrocannabinol (THC), which we
know today to be the major psychotropic principal of cannabis – were intense agitation, incoherence, delirium and hallucinations. On the basis of numerous such
experiments, Moreau declared that 'there is not a single, elementary manifestation
of mental illness that cannot be found in the mental changes caused by hashish,
from simple manic excitement to frenzied delirium, from the feeblest impulse, the
simplest fixation, the merest injury to the senses, to the most irresistible drive,
the wildest delirium, the most varied disorders of feelings'. He considered hashish
intoxication to be a model of endogenous psychoses, which could offer an insight
into the nature of psychiatric diseases. Some of the effects described by Moreau –
obsessive ideas, irresistible impulses, persecutory delusions and many others – are

Marijuana and Madness: Psychiatry and Neurobiology, ed. D. Castle and R. Murray. Published by Cambridge
University Press. © Cambridge University Press 2004.

certainly seen in psychiatric patients, but any relationship of the physiological and biochemical basis of cannabis action to that of mental disease is still questionable.

About the same time O'Shaughnessy in India experimented with charas – the local brand of cannabis – as a therapeutic drug (O'Shaugnessy, 1841; 1843). He administered small doses of charas to dogs and 'three kids'. The dogs 'became stupid and sleepy', 'assumed a look of utter and helpless drunkenness', and 'lost all power of the hinder extremities'. As to the kids, 'In one no effect was produced; in the second there was much heaviness and some inability to move; in the third a marked alteration of countenance was conspicuous, but no further effect.' In none of these, or several other experiments, was pain or any degree of convulsive movement observed. These experiments apparently convinced O'Shaugnessy that 'no hesitation could be felt as to the perfect safety of giving the resin of hemp an extensive trial in the cases in which its apparent powers promised the greatest degree of utility', and clinical trials were initiated.

Ethanol extracts (tincture) of cannabis resin were administered to patients with rheumatism, tetanus, rabies, infantile convulsions, cholera and delirium tremens. These diseases were chosen in order to confirm well-established local medical traditions. In the case of rheumatism two out of three cases were 'much relieved . . . They were discharged quite cured in three days after'. In both cases the huge doses caused side-effects such as catalepsy or uncontrollable behaviour, which today would be considered unacceptable. Further trials with lower doses gave closely analogous effects: 'alleviation of pain in most – remarkable increase of appetite in all – unequivocal aphrodisia, and great mental cheerfulness. The disposition developed was uniform in all'. O'Shaughnessy also noted that cannabis was a potent antivomiting agent. This property was rediscovered about 120 years later; no credit has been given to O'Shaugnessy in any of the numerous contemporary publications on this topic.

The reports by O'Shaugnessy were received with considerable interest. Gradually Indian hemp became an accepted drug in therapy, originally in England and later, to a limited extent, in other European countries and in North America (Mechoulam, 1986). Cannabis was used in a variety of conditions – mostly in pain and inflammation – but its use in psychiatric cases appears to have been minimal.

Donovan (1845) confirmed many of O'Shaughnessy's observations, in particular the potent anti-inflammatory effects. He also observed the effect of causing hunger and suggested its use in anorexia. However, he does not seem to have done any work in this direction.

Russell Reynolds recorded that cannabis is 'absolutely successful for months, without any increasing dose, in cases of senile insomnia'. In mania cannabis was 'worse than useless'. He found no effect in depression (Reynolds, 1890).

Numerous nineteenth-century physicians, mainly in the UK, confirmed the anti-inflammatory effects of Indian cannabis. Good results were also seen with persistent headaches and as calmatives. The main problem seems to have been the lack of consistency of therapeutic results. It is known today that THC undergoes oxidation with ease. While fresh imported Indian charas was effective initially, it probably lost its potency gradually (Mechoulam, 1986).

Understanding cannabinoid chemistry

A comparison between the chemistry of opium and cannabis, the two major illicit drugs in most of the world, can perhaps explain the lag in research and therapeutic use of these natural products. The active constituent of opium, morphine, was easily identified early in the nineteenth century as it is an alkaloid which forms isolable crystalline salts. It was introduced in medical practice shortly thereafter. By contrast, the active constituent of cannabis, in spite of numerous trials, could not be isolated and identified. We know today that the active THC is present in a mixture of many, chemically closely related, terpeno-phenols which are difficult to separate and purify.

In the late 1930s and early 1940s Roger Adams, in the USA (Adams, 1941–1942), and Alexander Todd, in England (Todd, 1946), made significant progress in cannabinoid chemistry, but the active constituent was not isolated and further research in this field was abandoned. Our group renewed work on cannabis in the early 1960s and, using novel separation techniques, which by then had been developed, we were able to identify in hashish many new cannabinoids, including the major psychotropic constituent, Δ^9-tetrahydrocannabinol (Δ^9-THC: Gaoni and Mechoulam, 1964). Numerous additional cannabinoids were isolated by column chromatography and their structures were elucidated. The major ones were cannabidiol (CBD), cannabinol, cannabigerol and cannabichromene (Mechoulam, 1973; Turner et al., 1980; Fig. 1.1). The rest were exiguous. All the purified compounds were tested in rhesus monkeys (Mechoulam and Edery, 1973). Only Δ^9-THC showed psychotropic activity: the monkeys became sedated, indifferent to the environment, and decline of aggression was noted. The effects were dose-dependent. CBD, cannabigerol and cannabichromene had no THC-like activity. However, cannabinol has some activity and Δ^8-THC, which is a very minor component, parallels Δ^9-THC activity, although it is somewhat less potent. Since 1964 thousands of papers on the chemistry, pharmacology, metabolism and clinical effects of Δ^9-THC and related synthetic compounds have appeared.

A comparison of the somatic and behavioural effect of Δ^9-THC in human subjects and in monkeys has been made (Mechoulam and Edery, 1973). Both species have comparable threshold effective doses (50 μg/kg), dose-dependent effects,

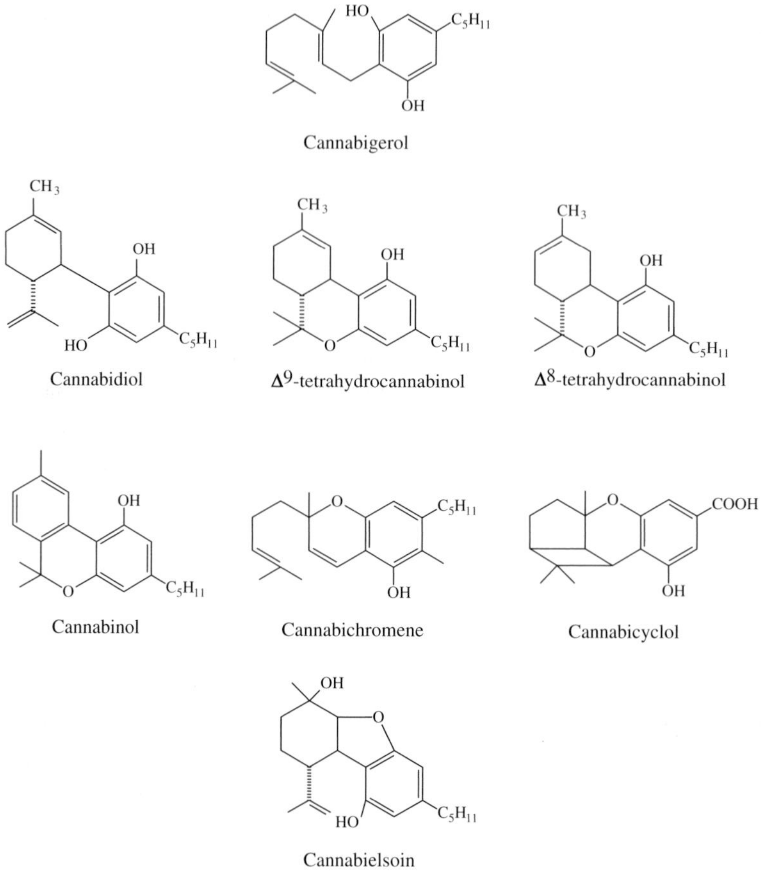

Figure 1.1 Major cannabinoids in marijuana.

impairment of motor coordination and of performance, redness of the conjunctiva, loss of muscle strength, heart rate increase and slow movements. Unfortunately, due to legal–ethical considerations, very little further work on monkeys, either with the plant cannabinoids or with the endogenous cannabinoids (see later), has been done over the last few decades.

Some studies indicate that Δ^9-THC alone accounts for the activity of cannabis. Thus we showed that in rhesus monkeys, Δ^9-THC alone and Δ^9-THC together with several of the major cannabis components (in a ratio found in the crude drug) caused the same effects (Mechoulam *et al.*, 1970). A more recent study in healthy volunteers came to the same conclusion (Wachtel *et al.*, 2002). However, marijuana users insist that smoked cannabis and Δ^9-THC administered orally do not have identical action (Grinspoon and Bakalar, 1997). Smoking is a more efficient and rapid route of administration and maybe this is the main reason for the differences observed; the presence of additional non-psychotropic constituents may also be of importance.

Cannabidiol

Most of the non-psychotropic cannabinoids have only been examined cursorily for their biological effects. However, there is renewed interest in CBD. In view of its putative action in anxiety and schizophrenia (see below), its pharmacological effects are discussed here in some detail.

CBD was first isolated from the cannabis plant in the late 1930s and early 1940s (Todd, 1946). Its structure was elucidated in 1963 (Mechoulam and Shvo, 1963). The chemistry of CBD was recently reviewed (Mechoulam and Hanuš, 2002). No detailed pharmacological work was reported on CBD until the early 1970s, except that it had no THC-like activity in vivo (Mechoulam and Edery, 1973). Then, by a strange coincidence, two groups, at almost the same time, reported that CBD reduces or blocks convulsions produced in animals by a variety of procedures (Carlini et al., 1973; Turkanis et al., 1974). It was also found to enhance the anticonvulsant effects of diphenylhydantoin and phenobarbital. Since then a considerable amount of research has been done in this area (for a review, see Consroe, 1998). The anticonvulsive activity of CBD differs from that of THC. While the effects of THC can be blocked by cannabinoid receptor antagonists (see below), those of CBD are not affected (Wallace et al., 2001). Apparently the anticonvulsive action of CBD is not mediated through these receptors. The research over the last few decades indicates that CBD is inactive in animal models of absence seizures produced by electroshock or chemical shock. However, it is active against cortical focal seizures produced by electrical stimulation or application of convulsant metals, as well as in generalized maximal seizures produced by electroshock (Consroe, 1998).

A double-blind clinical trial with CBD on 15 patients with secondary generalized epilepsy with temporal focus was undertaken in Brazil in 1980. Most of the patients remained essentially free of convulsions or demonstrated partial improvement in their clinical condition (Cunha et al., 1980). This clinical trial has not been repeated since then, presumably due to the large amounts of CBD required (200–300 mg/day).

CBD causes reduction of cytokine production in in vitro assays and in mice (Watzl et al., 1991; Srivastava et al., 1998). These reports led to a recent study on its effect on collagen-induced arthritis in mice, a model of human rheumatoid arthritis (Malfait et al., 2000). CBD was shown to block the progression of the disease. CBD has also been reported to block nausea in a rat model based on conditioned rejection (Parker et al., 2002).

CBD is mildly sedative in mice: its ED_{50} is 4.7 mg/kg, compared to 1.3 mg/kg for chlorpromazine (Pickens, 1981). It also increased the entry ratio (open/total number of entries) in the elevated plus maze test, which is a widely accepted assay for anxiety (Onaivi *et al.*, 1990; Guimaraes *et al.*, 1990).

CBD blocks the anxiety produced by THC, or by a simulated public-speaking test, in normal subjects (Zuardi *et al.*, 1982; 2002). However, the antianxiety effect observed is less than that of diazepam. Carlini and Cunha (1981) also reported that CBD caused longer sleep in insomniacs than those on placebo.

South African cannabis, known as dagga, contains very low levels of CBD (Field and Arndt, 1980) and, not surprisingly, its effects seem to differ considerably from those seen in Europe, America or the Middle East, where users smoke cannabis (marijuana and hashish) with high levels of CBD. Rottanburg *et al.* (1982) have reported that South Africans, after smoking dagga, frequently exhibit psychosis with hypomanic features. While this effect could be due to the high doses apparently consumed, it is also possible that the absence of CBD in dagga could be the reason. This conjecture is supported by more recent work. Zuardi *et al.* (1991) have shown that CBD is active in animal models predictive of antipsychotic activity. On the basis of the positive results observed, a single-case clinical trial was undertaken (Zuardi *et al.*, 1995). A patient with schizophrenia was administered CBD (up to 1.5 g/day). Improvement was noted in all items of a standard rating scale, and was close to the improvement seen with haloperidol. Leweke *et al.* (2000) have reported that while nabilone (a cannabinoid agonist) causes impairment of binocular depth inversion, a visual phenomenon also noted in schizophrenics, CBD reduced this impairment. A clinical trial is in progress evaluating the antipsychotic activity of CBD (Gerth *et al.*, 2002).

Cannabichromene, cannabigerol, cannabinol and the minor plant cannabinoids have not been investigated in any depth and it is quite possible that some of them may have a pharmacological profile close to that of CBD.

The endocannabinoids

Between 1964, when the active principal of cannabis was identified, and the mid-1980s, thousands of papers were published on the biochemistry, pharmacology and clinical effects of Δ^9-THC. Its mechanism of action, however, remained an enigma. Mainly conceptual problems hampered work in this direction. One of these was the presumed lack of stereoselectivity. Compounds acting through a biomolecule – an enzyme, a receptor or a gene – generally show a very high degree of stereoselectivity. This was not initially thought to be the case with cannabinoids. Synthetic $(+)$-Δ^9-THC showed some cannabimimetic activity when compared with that of natural $(-)$-Δ^9-THC. This observation was not compatible with the existence of a specific cannabinoid receptor and hence of a cannabinoid mediator. However, in the mid-1980s it was established that cannabinoid activity is highly stereoselective and that the previous observations resulted from separation problems (Mechoulam et al., 1988; Howlett et al., 1990).

A second conceptual problem was the assumption that the cannabinoids belong to the group of biologically active lipophiles and that their effects should be compared with the chronic effects of anaesthetics at low dose levels. The action of cannabinoids hence could be explained without necessarily postulating the existence of a specific cannabinoid receptor and of an endogenous mediator of cannabinoid action.

The first solid indication that cannabinoids act through receptors was brought forward by Howlett's group. Howlett and Fleming, using the neuroblastoma N18TH2 cell line as a model system, demonstrated that cannabinoids interact with the adenylate cyclase second-messenger pathway in an inhibitory fashion. The level of potency of a variety of cannabinoids to inhibit adenylate cyclase paralleled cannabinoid effects in animal models (Howlett and Fleming, 1984).

This line of research culminated in the discovery in the brain of specific, high-affinity cannabinoid-binding sites, whose distribution is consistent with the pharmacological properties of psychotropic cannabinoids (Devane et al., 1988). Shortly thereafter this cannabinoid receptor, which was designated CB_1, was cloned (Matsuda et al., 1990; Gerard et al., 1991). A peripheral receptor (CB_2) was identified in the spleen (Kaminski et al., 1992; Munro et al., 1993). Surprisingly, the CB_2 receptor has only 44% chemical homology with the CB_1 receptor. (For reviews covering various aspects of the cannabinoid receptors, see Felder and Glass, 1998; Howlett, 1998; Piomelli et al., 2000; Di Marzo et al., 2002; Pertwee and Ross, 2002.)

Anandamide

We assumed that the presence of a specific cannabinoid receptor indicates the existence of endogenous specific cannabinoid ligands that activate these receptors.

In order to isolate the putative endogenous cannabinoids we first synthesized a tritium-labelled probe [^{3}H] HU-243, which binds to the CB_1 receptor (Devane et al., 1992a). To screen for endogenous cannabinoid compounds, we tested the ability of fractions from porcine brain extracts to displace [^{3}H] HU-243 in a ligand-binding assay. All plant or synthetic cannabinoids are lipid-soluble compounds. Hence the procedures employed for the isolation of endogenous ligands by our group were based on the assumption that such constituents are also lipid-soluble, an assumption that ultimately proved to be correct. Porcine brains were extracted with organic solvents, and the extract was chromatographed according to standard protocols for the separation of lipids. We isolated a fraction which eluted mainly as one main peak on gas chromatography-mass spectrometry (GC-MS). This compound represented the first example of a purified brain constituent which exhibited most of the properties of Δ^9-THC (Devane et al., 1992b).

We named the active constituent anandamide, based on the Sanskrit work *ananda*, meaning bliss, and on its chemical nature (Fig. 1.1). This constituent inhibited the specific binding of [^{3}H] HU-243 in a manner typical of competitive ligands with a K_i value of 52 ± 1.8 nmol/l. Surprisingly, this value is almost identical to that of Δ^9-THC in this system ($K_i = 46 \pm 3$ nmol/l; Devane *et al.*, 1992b).

In addition to the specific binding to the cannabinoid receptor it seemed to us of considerable importance to determine the activity of natural anandamide in an additional bioassay. Pertwee *et al.* (1992) had reported that cannabinoids inhibit the twitch response of murine vas deferens (the secretory duct of the testicle) caused by electric current. Indeed, anandamide elicited a concentration-dependent inhibition of the twitch response, decreasing the twitch height by 50% at a concentration of 90 nmol/l (Devane *et al.*, 1992b).

Anandamide also activates VR1 receptor (Di Marzo *et al.*, 2002) and possibly other, not yet well defined receptors (see below).

Arachidonoylglycerol (2-AG)

The identification of a second cannabinoid receptor (CB$_2$) in immune cells led us to look for the presence of additional active endogenous ligands in the gut and later in the spleen, an organ with well established immune functions, again using fractionation guided by a binding assay. The active fraction consisted mainly of three compounds – 2-arachidonoylglycerol (2-AG), 2-palmitoylglycerol (2-palm-G) and 2-linoleoylglycerol (2-lino-G: Mechoulam *et al.*, 1995). The structure of 2-AG is presented in Figure 1.2.

2-AG parallels anandamide in in vitro and in vivo activity, while 2-lino-G and 2-palm-G showed no binding activity to either CB$_1$ or CB$_2$. However, both 2-lino-G and 2-palm-G separately or together (in the ratio present in the spleen) potentiated the apparent binding of 2-AG to CB$_1$ and CB$_2$ (Ben-Shabat *et al.*, 1998). The same type of 'entourage' effect was observed in several in vivo cannabinoid tests (see, for example, Panikashvili *et al.*, 2001). This 'entourage' effect is in part due to inhibition of the enzymatic hydrolysis of 2-AG by cells.

2-AG was later isolated from brain (Sugiura *et al.*, 1995).

Additional endocannabinoids

Besides anandamide, several additional acylethanolamides which bind to the CB$_1$ receptor have been found in porcine brain but biological work with them has been limited (Hanuš *et al.*, 1993). For structures, see Figure 1.2.

Recently two new types of endocannabinoids, noladin ether and virodhamine, were identified (Hanuš *et al.*, 2001; Porter *et al.*, 2002). Noladin ether binds well to the CB$_1$ receptor and weakly to CB$_2$. It causes sedation, hypothermia, intestinal immobility and mild antinociception in mice. Virodhamine is a partial agonist

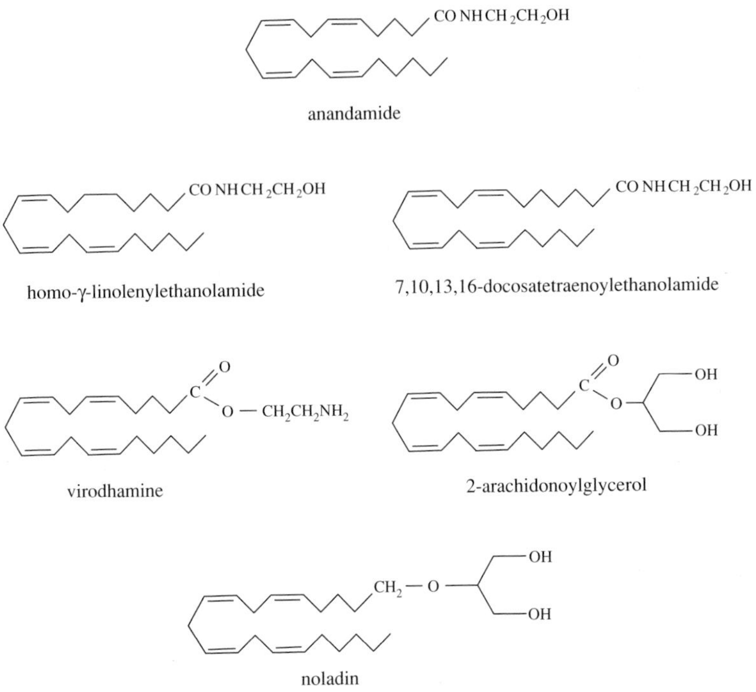

anandamide

homo-γ-linolenylethanolamide

7,10,13,16-docosatetraenoylethanolamide

virodhamine

2-arachidonoylglycerol

noladin

Figure 1.2 Endocannabinoids.

(with in vivo antagonistic activity) at the CB_1 receptor and a full agonist at the peripheral CB_2 receptor.

Both anandamide and 2-AG undergo the whole gamut of enzymatic transformations leading to prostaglandin, thromboxane and leukotriene-type endocannabinoid derivatives (Kozak and Marnett, 2002; van der Stelt et al., 2002). However, it is as yet unknown whether these derivatives are formed in the mammalian body and represent a part of the endocannabinoid system.

Biosynthesis and inactivation of the endocannabinoids

The biosynthesis and metabolism of the endocannabinoids have been discussed in detail in numerous reviews (Mechoulam et al., 1998; Di Marzo et al., 1999; Hillard, 2000; Schmid, 2000; Giuffrida et al., 2001; Sugiura et al., 2002). Hence they are only outlined here (Figs 1.3 and 1.4).

Anandamide is formed following a pathway previously proposed for other fatty-acid ethanolamides, namely the initial formation of N-acylphosphatidylethanolamine (NAPE). Indeed, primary cultures of neurons contain detectable levels of NAPE. The biosynthesis of NAPE itself is stimulated by intracellular levels of calcium and is potentiated by a protein kinase. Enzymatic hydrolysis of NAPE

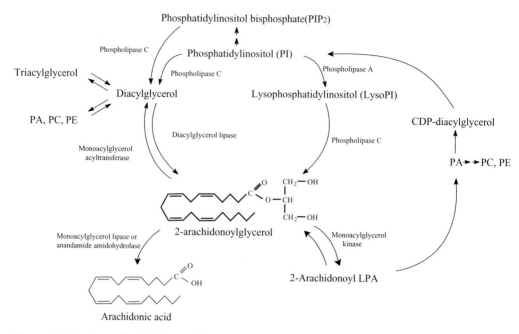

Figure 1.3 Pathways for the biosynthesis and degradation of 2-arachidonoylglycerol (2-AG).

by phospholipase D yields anandamide. This endocannabinoid is not stored in the cells but is formed mainly when needed.

The biosynthesis of 2-AG is also dependent on calcium influx into cells. Enzymatic hydrolysis of diacylglycerol (DAG) seems to be the most important route, although the phospholipase C hydrolysis of phosphatidylcholine or phosphatidyl inositol has also been noted. The intermediacy of DAG, a second messenger associated with stimulation of the activity of protein kinase C, is a further example of the propensity of biological systems for using existing constituents for various purposes (Sugiura *et al.*, 2002).

Anandamide is inactivated in central neurons by both reuptake and enzymatic hydrolysis. Administration of AM-404, an inhibitor of anandamide uptake (Beltramo *et al.*, 1997), indeed causes potentiation of its action. It is not clear whether the uptake of the endocannabinoids is a passive diffusion process or whether carrier proteins are also involved. The reuptake of 2-AG is partly inhibited by other endogenous acylglycerols and is part of the 'entourage' effect (see above). For a recent review on the cellular transport of endocannabinoids and its inhibition, see Fowler and Jacobsson (2002).

Within the cell, anandamide and 2-AG are enzymatically hydrolysed to arachidonic acid and ethanolamine or glycerol respectively. The fatty-acid amide hydrolase (FAAH: Deutsch *et al.*, 2002) which hydrolyses anandamide has been cloned. It also hydrolyses oleamide, a sleep-inducing factor (Boger *et al.*, 1998; Fowler *et al.*,

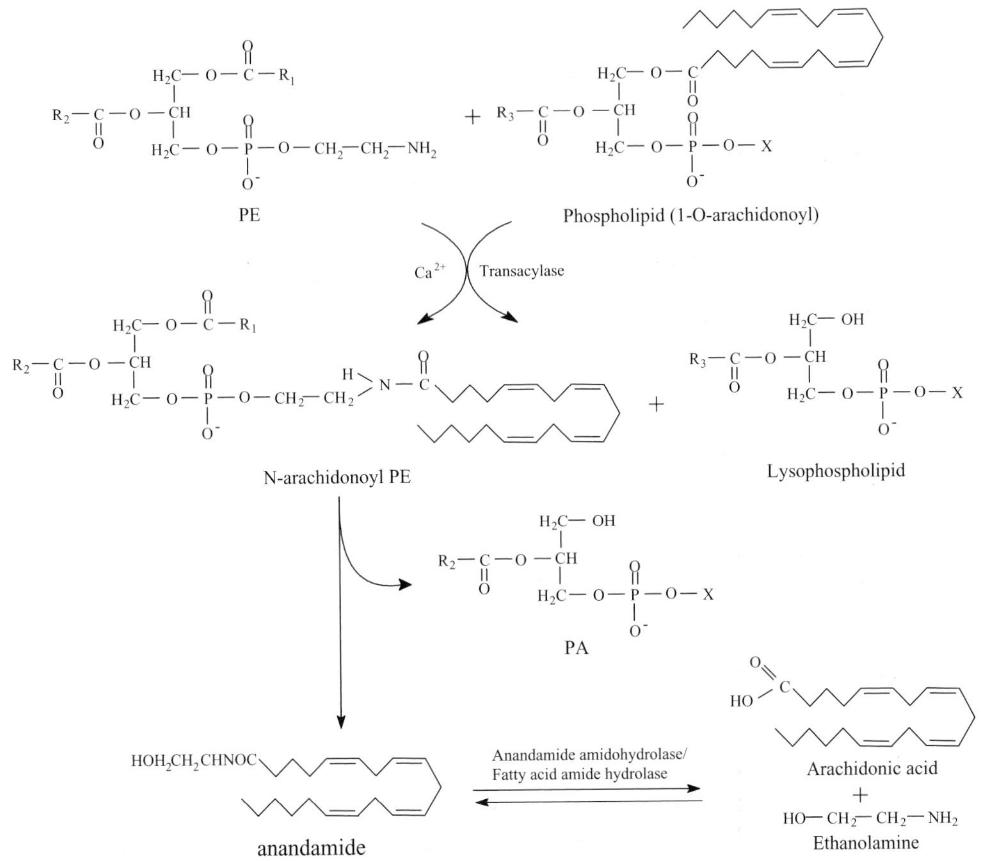

Figure 1.4 Pathways for the biosynthesis and degradation of anandamide.

2001). Surprisingly, FAAH also seems to hydrolyse 2-AG. However, this ester is also broken down in cells which do not contain FAAH, hence lipases can contribute to this reaction.

The detailed pharmacology, biochemistry and molecular biology of Δ^9-THC and of the endocannabinoids are beyond the scope of this chapter. Hundreds of publications have appeared in recent years. The original publication alone describing the identification of anandamide as a major endocannabinoid (Devane et al., 1992b) has been cited about 1100 times. Numerous excellent reviews have been published on specific aspects of the pharmacology and biochemistry of cannabinoids. Some recent ones are those of Kunos et al. (2000), Elphick and Egertova (2001), Schlicker and Kathmann (2001) and Lutz (2002).

Synthetic cannabinoids

Δ^9-THC is not a very potent cannabinoid, either in vitro or in vivo. Much more potent compounds have been synthesized and are widely used in research. HU-210 is apparently the most active cannabinoid used at present. It is up to 800 times more active than Δ^9-THC in mice. For a recent review on HU-210, see Ottani and Giuliani (2001).

The enantiomer (mirror image) of HU-210, namely HU-211, does not bind to the cannabinoid receptors and is not active in animal cannabinoid assays. However, it is an N-methyl-D-aspartate (NMDA) antagonist and an antioxidant. It is at present in phase III clinical trials as a drug in brain trauma (Feigenbaum *et al.*, 1989; Shohami and Mechoulam, 2000; Knoller *et al.*, 2002).

Anandamide, an amide, is rapidly hydrolysed in the body. In order to lower the hydrolysis rate, several analogues have been prepared which, by obstructing the amide bond, reduce the rate of the breakdown. The most widely used compound is metanandamide (Abadji *et al.*, 1994).

Several specific agonists are available. Noladin ether (Hanuš *et al.*, 2001) is essentially specific for the CB_1 receptor, while compounds such as HU-308 (Hanuš *et al.*, 1999) and JWH-133 (Huffman, 2000) are specific for the CB_2 receptor.

Numerous compounds are known which reduce the rate of endocannabinoid uptake into the cell and thus prolong and enhance their activity. These include AM-404 (Beltramo *et al.*, 1997) and several CBD derivatives (Bisogno *et al.*, 2001).

Compounds which block FAAH, the enzyme which hydrolyses anandamide, enhance its activity. Several such compounds are known and widely used (Deutsch *et al.*, 2002).

Specific antagonists for the cannabinoid system have been described: SR-141 716A is specific for the CB_1, and SR-144 528 is specific for the CB_2 receptor (Rinaldi-Carmona *et al.*, 1994; 1998). Two CB_1 antagonists, AM-281 and AM-251, are commercially available (Lan *et al.*, 1999; Pertwee and Ross, 2002).

Quo vadimus?

Where does cannabis research stand today? We do not believe that additional chemical research on the plant material will lead to the discovery of important new constituents. However, work from several groups strongly indicates that additional receptors are present in both the brain and the periphery and these receptors may explain some of the 'non-specific' effects seen with some cannabinoids, particularly anandamide (Wagner *et al.*, 1999; Breivogel *et al.*, 2001; Ford *et al.*, 2002). (For recent reviews, see Di Marzo *et al.*, 2002; Pertwee and Ross, 2002.) It is quite possible that additional endocannabinoids will also be identified, presumably with very specific functions. For example, we have indications that an as-yet unidentified endocannabinoid is involved in hibernation.

As the cannabinoid system is involved in many physiological processes, it is conceivable that the chemistry involved may not be identical in each case. Thus, the endogenous stearoyl ethanolamide has recently been shown to be antiproliferative (Maccarrone *et al.*, 2002), oleamide is a sleep factor (Boger *et al.*, 1998) and palmitoyl ethanolamide is anti-inflammatory (Schmid and Berdyshev, 2002). None of these compounds binds to the CB_1 or CB_2 cannabinoid receptors, but they show some endocannabinoid-like activity.

It is also conceivable that dysregulation of the cannabinoid system, like that of other mediator systems, may lead to specific symptoms or diseases. Indeed, it has been shown that differences in the levels of FAAH, the enzyme that causes hydrolysis of anandamide, may cause spontaneous abortions (Maccarrone *et al.*, 2000). Do dysfunctions of the endocannabinoid system also contribute to the biological basis for psychiatric diseases? This question forms the basis for subsequent chapters in this volume.

REFERENCES

Abadji, V., Lin, S., Taha, G. *et al.* (1994). (*R*)-methanandamide: a chiral novel anandamide possessing higher potency and metabolic stability. *J. Med. Chem*, **37**, 1889–1893.

Adams, R. (1941–1942). Marihuana. *Harvey Lect.*, **37**, 168–197.

Beltramo, M., Stella, N., Calignano, A. *et al.* (1997). Functional role of high-affinity anandamide transport, as revealed by selective inhibition. *Science*, **227**, 1094–1097.

Ben-Shabat, S., Fride, E., Sheskin, T. *et al.* (1998). An entourage effect: inactive endogenous fatty acid glycerol esters enhance 2-arachidonoyl-glycerol cannabinoid activity. *Eur. J. Pharmacol.*, **353**, 23–31.

Bisogno, T., Hanuš, L., De Petrocellis, L. *et al.* (2001). Molecular targets for cannabidiol and its synthetic analogues: effect on vanilloid VR1 receptors and on the cellular uptake and enzymatic hydrolysis of anandamide. *Br. J. Pharmacol.*, **135**, 845–852.

Boger, D. L., Henriksen, S. J. and Cravatt, B. F. (1998). Oleamide: an endogenous sleep-inducing lipid and prototypical member of a new class of biological signaling molecules. *Curr. Pharm. Design*, **4**, 303–314.

Breivogel, C. S., Griffin, G., Di Marzo, V. and Martin, B. R. (2001). Evidence for a new G protein-coupled cannabinoid receptor in mouse brain. *Mol. Pharmacol.*, **60**, 155–163.

Carlini, E. A. and Cunha, J. M. (1981). Hypnotic and antiepileptic effects of cannabidiol. *J. Clin. Pharmacol.*, **21**, 417S–427S.

Carlini, E. A., Leite, J. R., Tanhauser, M. and Bernardi, A. C. (1973). Cannabidiol and *Cannabis sativa* extract protect mice and rats against convulsive agents. *J. Pharm. Pharmacol.*, **25**, 664–665.

Consroe, P. (1998). Brain cannabinoid system as targets for the therapy of neurological disorders. *Neurobiol. Dis.*, **5**, 534–551.

Cunha, J. M., Carlini, E. A., Pereira, A. E. *et al.* (1980). Chronic administration of CBD to healthy volunteers and epileptic patients. *Pharmacologia*, **21**, 175–185.

Deutsch, D. G., Ueda, N. and Yamamoto, S. (2002). The fatty acid amide hydrolase (FAAH). *Prostaglandins Leukot. Essent. Fatty Acids*, **66**, 201–210.

Devane, W. A., Dysarz, F. A. 3rd, Johnson, M. R., Melvin, L. S. and Howlett, A. C. (1988). Determination and characterization of a cannabinoid receptor in rat brain. *Mol. Pharmacol.*, **34**, 605–613.

Devane, W. A., Breuer, A., Sheskin, T. *et al.* (1992a). A novel probe for the cannabinoid receptor. *J. Med. Chem.*, **35**, 2065–2069.

Devane, W. A., Hanuš, L., Breuer, A. *et al.* (1992b). Isolation and structure of a brain constituent that binds to the cannabinoid receptor. *Science*, **258**, 1946–1949.

Di Marzo, V., De Petrocellis, L., Bisogno, T. and Melck, D. (1999). Metabolism of anandamide and 2-arachidonoylglycerol: an historical overview and some recent developments. *Lipids*, **34**, S319–S325.

Di Marzo, V., De Petrocellis, L., Fezza, F., Ligresti, A. and Bisogno, T. (2002). Anandamide receptors. *Prostaglandins Leukot. Essent. Fatty Acids*, **66**, 377–391.

Donovan, M. (1845). On the physical and medicinal qualities of Indian hemp (*Cannabis indica*). *Dublin J. Med. Sci.*, **26**, 368–402.

Elphick, M. R. and Egertova, M. (2001). The neurobiology and evolution of cannabinoid signalling. *Philos. Trans. R. Soc. Lond.*, **356**, 381–408.

Feigenbaum, J. J., Bergman, F., Richmond, S. A. *et al.* (1989). Nonpsychotropic cannabinoid acts as a functional *N*-methyl-D-asparate (NMDA) receptor blocker. *Proc. Natl Acad. Sci. USA*, **86**, 9584–9587.

Felder, C. C. and Glass, M. (1998). Cannabinoid receptors and their endogenous agonists. *Annu. Rev. Pharmacol. Toxicol.*, **38**, 179–200.

Field, B. I. and Arndt, R. R. (1980). Cannabinoid compounds in South African *Cannabis sativa* L. *J. Pharm. Pharmacol.*, **32**, 21–24.

Ford, W. R., Honan, S. A., White, R. and Hiley, C. R. (2002). Evidence of a novel site mediating anandamide-induced negative inotropic and coronary vasodilator responses in rat isolated hearts. *Br. J. Pharmacol.*, **135**, 1191–1198.

Fowler, J. J. and Jacobsson, S. O. P. (2002). Cellular transport of anandamide, 2-arachidonoylglycerol and palmitoylethanolamide – targets for drug development? *Prostaglandin Leukot. Essent. Fatty Acids*, **66**, 193–200.

Fowler, C. J., Jonsson, K. O. and Tiger, G. (2001). Fatty acid amide hydrolase: biochemistry, pharmacology, and therapeutic possibilities for an enzyme hydrolyzing anandamide, 2-arachidonoylglycerol, palmitoylethanolamide, and oleamide. *Biochem. Pharmacol.*, **62**, 517–526.

Gaoni, Y. and Mechoulam, R. (1964). Isolation, structure and partial synthesis of an active constituent of hashish. *J. Am. Chem. Soc.*, **86**, 1646.

Gerard, C. M., Mollereau, C., Vassart, G. and Parmentier, M. (1991). Molecular cloning of a human cannabinoid receptor which is also expressed in testis. *Biochem. J.*, **279** (Pt 1), 129–134.

Gerth, C. W., Schultze-Lutter, F., Mauss, C. *et al.* (2002). The natural cannabinoid cannabidiol in the treatment of acute schizophrenia. *Schizophr. Res. (Suppl.)*, **53**, 192, B113.

Giuffrida, A., Beltramo, M. and Piomelli, D. (2001). Mechanisms of endocannabinoid inactivation: biochemistry and pharmacology. *J. Pharmacol. Exp. Ther.*, **298**, 7–14.

Grinspoon, L. and Bakalar, J. B. (1997). *Marihuana, the Forbidden Medicine*. New Haven, CT: Yale University Press.

Guimaraes, F. S., Chiaretti, T. M., Graeff, F. G. and Zuardi, A. W. (1990). Antianxiety effect of cannabidol in the elevated plus-maze. *Psychopharmacology*, **100**, 558–559.

Hanuš, L., Gopher, A., Almog, S. and Mechoulam, R. (1993). Two new unsaturated fatty acid ethanolamides in brain that bind to the cannabinoid receptor. *J. Med. Chem.*, **36**, 3032–3034.

Hanuš, L., Breuer, A., Tchilibon, S. *et al.* (1999). HU-308: a specific agonist for CB_2, a peripheral cannabinoid receptor. *Proc. Natl Acad. Sci. USA*, **96**, 14228–14233.

Hanuš, L., Abu-Lafi, S., Fride, E. *et al.* (2001). 2-Arachidonyl glyceryl ether, a novel endogenous agonist of the cannabinoid CB_1 receptor. *Proc. Natl Acad. Sci. USA*, **98**, 3662–3665.

Hillard, C. J. (2000). Biochemistry and pharmacology of the endocannabinoids arachidonylethanolamide and 2-arachidonylglycerol. *Prostagladins Other Lipid Mediat.*, **61**, 3–18.

Howlett, A. C. (1998). The CB_1 cannabinoid receptor in the brain. *Neurobiol. Dis.*, **5**, 405–416.

Howlett, A. C. and Fleming, R. M. (1984). Cannabinoid inhibition of adenylate cyclase. Pharmacology of the response in neuroblastoma cell membranes. *Mol. Pharmacol.*, **26**, 532–538.

Howlett, A. C., Champion, T. M., Wilken, G. H. and Mechoulam, R. (1990). Stereochemical effects of 11-OH-Δ^8-tetrahydrocannabinol-dimethylheptyl to inhibit adenylate cyclase and bind to the cannabinoid receptor. *Neuropharmacology*, **29**, 161–165.

Huffman, J. W. (2000). The search for selective ligands for the CB_2 receptor. *Curr. Pharm. Des.*, **6**, 1323–1337.

Kaminski, N. E., Abood, M. E., Kessler, F. K., Martin, B. R. and Schatz, A. R. (1992). Identification of a functionally relevant cannabinoid receptor on mouse spleen cells that is involved in cannabinoid-mediated immune modulation. *Mol. Pharmacol.*, **42**, 736–742.

Knoller, N., Levi, L., Shoshan, I. *et al.* (2002). Dexanabinol (HU-211) in the treatment of severe closed head injury: a randomized, placebo-controlled phase II clinical trial. *Crit. Care Med.*, **30**, 548–554.

Kozak, K. R. and Marnett, L. J. (2002). Oxidative metabolism of endocannabinoids. *Prostaglandins Leukot. Essent. Fatty Acids*, **66**, 211–220.

Kunos, G., Jarai, Z., Varga, K. *et al.* (2000). Cardiovascular effects of endocannabinoids – the plot thickens. *Prostaglandins Other Lipid Mediat.*, **61**, 71–84.

Lan, R., Liu, Q., Fan, P. *et al.* (1999). Structure–activity relationships of pyrazole derivatives as cannabinoid receptor antagonists. *J. Med. Chem.*, **42**, 769–776.

Leweke, F. M., Schneider, U., Radwan, M., Schmidt, E. and Emrich, H. M. (2000). Different effects of nabilone and cannabidiol in binocular depth inversion in man. *Pharmacol. Biochem. Behav.*, **66**, 175–181.

Lutz, B. (2002). Molecular biology of cannabinoid receptors. *Prostaglandin Leukot. Essent. Fatty Acids*, **66**, 123–142.

Maccarrone, M., Valensise, H., Bari, M. *et al.* (2000). Relation between decreased anandamide hydrolase concentrations in human lymphocytes and miscarriage. *Lancet,* **355,** 1326–1329.

Maccarrone, M., Pauselli, R., Rienzo, M. D. and Finazzi-Agro, A. (2002). Binding, degradation and apoptotic activity of stearoylethanolamide in rat C6 glioma cells. *Biochem. J.,* **15,** 137–144.

Malfait, A. M., Gallily, R., Sumariwalla, P. F. *et al.* (2000). The nonpsychoactive cannabis constituent cannabidiol is an oral anti-arthritic therapeutic in murine collagen-induced arthritis. *Proc. Natl Acad. Sci. USA,* **97,** 9561–9566.

Matsuda, L. A., Lolait, S. J., Brownstein, M. J., Young, A. C. and Bonner, T. I. (1990). Structure of a cannabinoid receptor and functional expression of the cloned cDNA. *Nature,* **346,** 561–564.

Mechoulam, R. (1973). Cannabinoid chemistry. In *Marijuana Chemistry, Metabolism, Pharmacology and Clinical Effects,* ed. R. Mechoulam, pp. 1–99. New York: Academic Press.

   (1986). The pharmacohistory of *Cannabis sativa.* In *Cannabinoids as Therapeutic Agents,* pp. 1–19. Boca Raton, FL. CRC Press.

Mechoulam, R. and Edery, H. (1973). Structure–activity relationships in the cannabinoid series. In *Marijuana Chemistry, Metabolism, Pharmacology and Clinical Effects,* ed. R. Mechoulam, pp. 101–136. New York: Academic Press.

Mechoulam, R. and Hanuš, L. (2002). Cannabidiol: an overview of some chemical and pharmacological aspects. Part I. Chemical aspects. *Chem. Phys. Lipids,* **121,** 35–43.

Mechoulam, R. and Shvo, Y. (1963). The structure of cannabidiol. *Tetrahedron,* **19,** 2073–2078.

Mechoulam, R., Shani, A., Edery, H. and Grunfeld, Y. (1970). The chemical basis of hashish activity. *Science,* **169,** 611–612.

Mechoulam, R., Feigenbaum, J. J., Lander, N. *et al.* (1988). Enantiomeric cannabinoids: stereospecificity of psychotropic activity. *Experientia,* **44,** 762–764.

Mechoulam, R., Ben-Shabat, S., Hanuš, L. *et al.* (1995). Identification of an endogenous 2-monoglyceride, present in canine gut, that binds to the peripheral cannabinoid receptors. *Biochem. Pharmacol.,* **50,** 83–90.

Mechoulam, R., Fride, E. and Di Marzo, V. (1998). Endocannabinoids. *Eur. J. Pharmacol.,* **359,** 1–18.

Moreau, J-J. (1973). *Hashish and Mental Illness.* Translated from the French original (1845). New York: Raven Press.

Munro, S., Thomas, K. L. and Abu-Shaar, M. (1993). Molecular characterization of a peripheral receptor for cannabinoids. *Nature,* **365,** 61–65.

Onaivi, E. S., Green, M. R. and Martin, B. R. (1990). Pharmacological characterization of cannabinoids in the elevated plus maze. *J. Pharmacol. Exp. Ther.,* **253,** 1002–1009.

O'Shaugnessy, W. B. (1841). Cannabis. In *The Bengal Dispensatory and Pharmacopoeia,* pp. 579–604. Calcutta: Bishop's College Press.

   (1843). On the *Cannabis indica* or Indian hemp. *Pharmacol. J. Trans.,* **2,** 594–595.

Ottani, A. and Giuliani, D. (2001). HU 210: a potent tool for investigations of the cannabinoid system. *CNS Drug Rev.,* **7,** 131–45.

Panikashvili, D., Simeonidou, C., Ben-Shabat, S. *et al.* (2001). An endogenous cannabinoid (2-AG) is neuroprotective after brain injury. *Nature,* **413,** 527–531.

Parker, L. A., Mechoulam, R. and Schlievert, C. (2002). Cannabidiol, a non-psychoactive component of cannabis, and its dimethylheptyl homolog suppress nausea in an experimental model with rats. *Neuroreport*, **13**, 567–570.

Pertwee, R. G. and Ross, R. A. (2002). Cannabinoid receptors and their ligands. *Prostaglandins Leukot. Essent. Fatty Acids*, **66**, 101–121.

Pertwee, R. G., Stevenson, L. A., Elrick, D. B., Mechoulam, R. and Corbett, A. D. (1992). Inhibitory effects of certain enantiomeric cannabinoids in the mouse vas deferens and the myenteric plexus preparation of guinea-pig small intestine. *Br. J. Pharmacol.*, **105**, 980–984.

Pickens, J. T. (1981). Sedative activity of cannabis in relation to its delta-1-*trans*-tetrahydrocannabinol and cannabidiol content. *Br. J. Pharmacol.*, **72**, 649–656.

Piomelli, D., Giuffrida, A., Calignano, A. and De Fonseca, F. R. (2000). The endocannabinoid system as a target for therapeutic drugs. *Trends Pharmacol. Sci.*, **21**, 218–223.

Porter, A. C., Sauer, J. M., Knierman, M. D. *et al.* (2002). Characterization of a novel endocannabinoid, virodhamine, with antagonist activity at the CB_1 receptor. *J. Pharmacol. Exp. Ther.*, **301**, 1020–1024.

Reynolds, J. R. (1890). Therapeutic uses and toxic effects of *Cannabis indica*. *Lancet*, **1**, 637–638.

Rinaldi-Carmona, M., Barth, F., Heaulme, M. *et al.* (1994). SR141716A, a potent and selective antagonist of the brain cannabinoid receptor. *FEBS Lett.*, **350**, 240–244.

Rinaldi-Carmona, M., Barth, F., Millan, J. *et al.* (1998). SR 144528, the first potent and selective antagonist of the CB_2 cannabinoid receptor. *J. Pharmacol. Exp. Ther.*, **284**, 644–650.

Rottanburg, D., Robins, A. H., Ben-Arie, O., Teggin, A. and Elk, R. (1982). Cannabis-associated psychosis with hypomanic features. *Lancet*, **2**, 1364–1366.

Schlicker, E. and Kathmann, M. (2001). Modulation of transmitter release via presynaptic cannabinoid receptors. *Trends Pharmacol. Sci.*, **22**, 565–572.

Schmid, H. H. (2000). Pathways and mechanisms of *N*-acylethanolamine biosynthesis: can anandamide be generated selectively? *Chem. Phys. Lipids*, **108**, 71–87.

Schmid, H. H. O. and Berdyshev, E. V. (2002). Cannabinoid receptor-inactive *N*-acylethanolamines and other fatty acid amides: metabolism and function. *Prostaglandins Leukot. Essent. Fatty Acids*, **66**, 363–376.

Shohami, E. and Mechoulam, R. (2000). Dexanabinol (HU-211): a non-psychotropic cannabinoid with neuroprotective properties. *Drug Dev. Res.*, **50**, 211–215.

Srivastava, M. D., Srivastava, B. I. and Brouhard, B. (1998). Delta-9-tetrahydrocannabinol and cannabidiol alter cytokine production by human immune cells. *Immunopharmacology*, **40**, 179–185.

Sugiura, T., Kondo, S., Sukagawa, A. *et al.* (1995). 2-Arachidonoylglycerol: a possible endogenous cannabinoid receptor ligand in brain. *Biochem. Biophys. Res. Commun.*, **215**, 89–97.

Sugiura, T., Kobayashi, Y., Oka, S. and Waku K. (2002). Biosynthesis and degradation of anandamide and 2-arachidonoylglycerol and their possible physiological significance. *Prostaglandins Leukot. Essent. Fatty Acids*, **66**, 173–192.

Todd, A. R. (1946). Hashish. *Experientia*, **2**, 55–60.

Turkanis, S. A., Cely, W., Olsen, D. M. and Karler, R. (1974). Anticonvulsant properties of cannabidiol. *Res. Commun. Chem. Pathol. Pharmacol.*, **8**, 231–246.

Turner, C. E., Elsohly, M. A. and Boeren E. G. (1980). Constituents of *Cannabis sativa* L. XVII. A review of the natural constituents. *J. Nat. Prod.*, **43**, 169–234.

van der Stelt, M., van-Kuik, J. A., Bari, M. *et al.* (2002). Oxygenated metabolites of anandamide and 2-arachidonylglycerol: conformational analysis and interaction with cannabinoid receptors, membrane transporter, and fatty acid amide hydrolase. *J. Med. Chem.*, **45**, 3709–3720.

Wachtel, S. R., ElSohly, M. A., Ross, S. A., Ambre, J. and 'de Wit, H. (2002). Comparison of the subjective effects of Δ^9-tetrahydrocannabinol and marijuana in humans. *Psychopharmacology*, **161**, 331–339.

Wagner, J. A., Varga, K., Jarai, Z. and Kunos, G. (1999). Mesenteric vasodilation mediated by endothelial anandamide receptors. *Hypertension*, **33**, 429–434.

Wallace, M. J., Wiley, J. L., Martin, B. R. and DeLorenzo, R. J. (2001). Assessment of the role of CB_1 receptors in cannabinoid anticonvulsant effects. *Eur. J. Pharmacol.*, **28**, 51–57.

Watzl, B., Scuderi, P. and Watson, R. R. (1991). Marijuana components stimulate human peripheral blood mononuclear cell secretion of interferon-gamma and suppress interleukin-1 alpha in vitro. *Int. J. Immunopharmacol.*, **13**, 1091–1097.

Zuardi, A. W., Shirakawa, I., Finkelfarb, E. and Karniol, I. G. (1982). Action of cannabidiol on the anxiety and other effects produced by delta-9-THC in normal subjects. *Psychopharmacology*, **76**, 245–250.

Zuardi, A. W., Rodrigues, J. A. and Cunha, J. M. (1991). Effects of cannabidiol in animal models predictive of antipsychotic activity. *Psychopharmacology*, **104**, 260–264.

Zuardi, A. W., Morais, S. L., Guimaraes, F. S. and Mechoulam, R. (1995). Antipsychotic effect of cannabidiol. *J. Clin. Psychiatry*, **56**, 485–486.

Zuardi, A. W., Guimaraes F. S., Guimaraes, V. M. C. and Del Bel, E. A. (2002). Cannabidiol: possible therapeutic application. In *Cannabis and Cannabinoids*, ed. F. Grotenhermen and E. Russo, pp. 359–369. New York: Haworth Press.

2

How cannabis works in the brain

Leslie Iversen

University of Oxford, UK

Important advances have been made in the past decade in understanding how cannabis affects the brain. As with morphine 20 years earlier, research on the psychopharmacology of a plant-derived drug led to the discovery of a naturally occurring cannabinoid system in the brain, whose functions are only now beginning to be understood. This chapter will review what is known about the interactions of cannabis with the cannabinoid system in the brain and how the drug affects psychomotor, cognitive, perceptual and appetitive functions. There is also speculation on what brain mechanisms may underly the intoxicant effects of cannabis, and a review of its addictive properties.

Cannabinoid receptors

In Chapter 1 the identification of Δ^9-tetrahydrocannabinol (THC) was reviewed as the principal active component in the complex mixture of cannabinoids present in extracts of the plant *Cannabis sativa*, and the discovery of a series of naturally occurring endogenous cannabinoids (endocannabinoids), of which anandamide has so far been most intensively studied, was outlined. A series of synthetic cannabinoids – some of which are more potent and more water-soluble than THC – is also available (Pertwee, 1999) (Fig. 2.1). All of these compounds act as agonists at the CB_1 cannabinoid receptor (Matsuda *et al.*, 1990), which is the only one known to be expressed in the brain. A second cannabinoid receptor, CB_2, is expressed only in peripheral tissues, principally in the immune system (Munro *et al.*, 1993; Felder and Glass, 1998; Pertwee, 1999). THC and the synthetic cannabinoids also act to some extent as agonists at the CB_2 receptor. A series of synthetic drugs is also now available which act as specific antagonists at CB_1 or CB_2 receptors (D'Souza and Kosten, 2001; see also Chapters 9 and 10). One of these compounds, rimonabant

Marijuana and Madness: Psychiatry and Neurobiology, ed. D. Castle and R. Murray. Published by Cambridge University Press. © Cambridge University Press 2004.

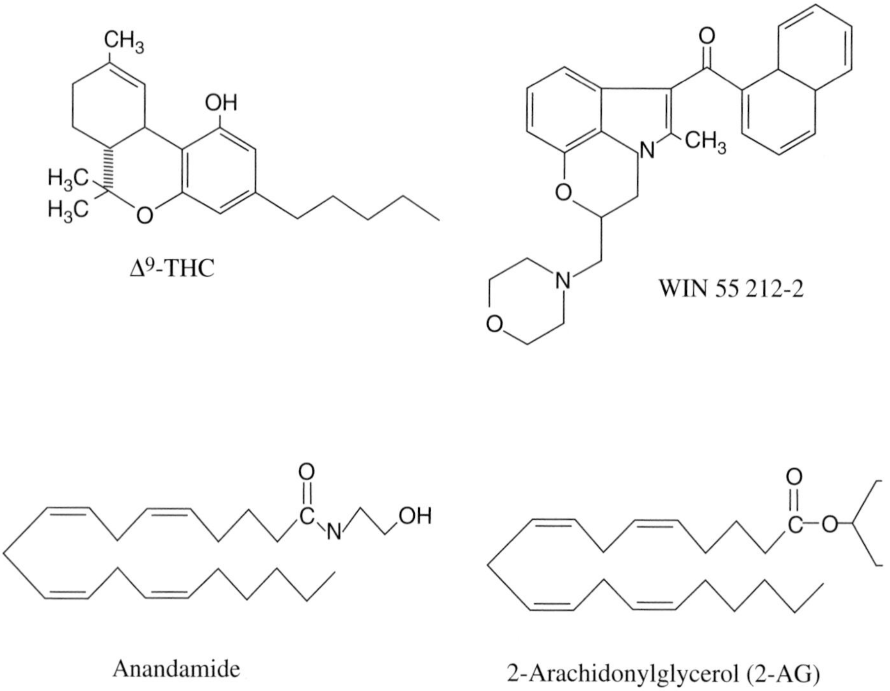

Δ^9-THC

WIN 55 212-2

Anandamide

2-Arachidonylglycerol (2-AG)

Figure 2.1 Chemical structures of Δ^9-tetrahydrocannabinol (THC), the synthetic CB$_1$ receptor agonist WIN 55 212-2 and the endocannabinoids.

(SR141 716A), which acts selectively to block CB$_1$ receptors (Rinaldi-Carmona et al., 1994; Compton et al., 1996), has been widely used in studies of the actions of cannabinoids in the central nervous system (CNS: Fig. 2.2). The availability of the synthetic cannabinoid agonists and antagonists has also been supplemented in recent years by the generation of genetically engineered strains of mice that do not express the CB$_1$ receptor (knockout mice).

Neuroanatomical distribution of CB$_1$ receptors in brain

The distribution of cannabinoid receptors was first mapped in rat brain in auto-radiographic studies, using the radioligand [H^3] CP-55 940, which binds with high affinity to CB$_1$ sites (Herkenham et al., 1991: Fig. 2.3). More recently, antibodies that target the C-terminal or N-terminal regions of the CB$_1$ receptor protein have been used for immunohistochemical mapping studies (Egertová et al., 1998; Pettit et al., 1998; Egertová and Elphick, 2000). Immunohistochemistry provides a superior degree of spatial resolution than autoradiography but the overall pattern of distribution of CB$_1$ receptors revealed by the two approaches is very similar (Elphick and Egertová, 2001).

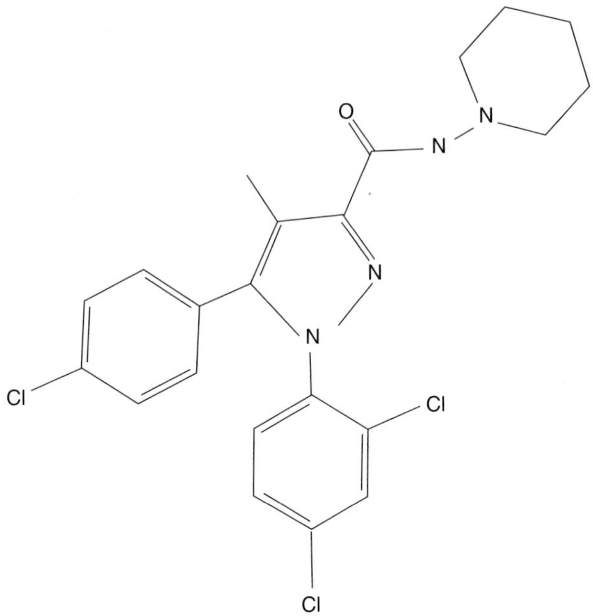

SR141 716A

Figure 2.2   Chemical structure of the CB$_1$-selective antagonist drug rimonabant.

The mapping studies in rat brain showed that CB$_1$ receptors are mainly localized to axons and nerve terminals and are largely absent from the neuronal soma or dendrites. The finding that cannabinoid receptors are predominantly presynaptic rather than postsynaptic is consistent with the postulated role of cannabinoids in modulating neurotransmitter release (see below).

In both animals and humans the cerebral cortex, particularly frontal regions, contains high densities of CB$_1$ receptors. There are also very high densities in the basal ganglia and in the cerebellum (Fig. 2.3). In the limbic forebrain CB$_1$ receptors are found particularly in the hypothalamus and in anterior cingulate cortex. The hippocampus also contains a high density of CB$_1$ receptors. The relative absence of the cannabinoid receptors from brainstem nuclei may account for the low toxicity of cannabinoids when given in overdose.

Effects of cannabinoids on synaptic function

Inhibition of neurotransmitter release

The presynaptic localization of CB$_1$ receptors suggests a role for cannabinoids in modulating the release of neurotransmitters from axon terminals and this has been confirmed by a substantial body of experimental data. Early reports (Gill et al., 1970; Roth, 1978) showed that THC inhibited acetylcholine release from

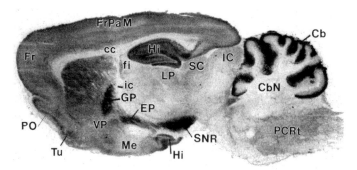

Figure 2.3 Distribution of cannabinoid CB$_1$ receptors in rat brain revealed by an autoradiograph of the binding of radioactively labelled CP-55 940 (a high-affinity agonist ligand) to a sagittal brain section. The brain regions labelled are: Cb, cerebellum; CbN, deep cerebellar nucleus; cc, corpus callosum; EP, entopeduncular nucleus; fi, fimbria hippocampus; Fr, frontal cortex; FrPaM, frontoparietal cortex motor area; GP, globus pallidus; Hi, hippocampus; IC, inferior colliculus; LP, lateral posterior thalamus; Me, medial amygdaloid nucleus; PO, primary olfactory cortex; PCRt, parvocellular reticular nucleus; SC, superior colliculus; SNR, substantia nigra reticulate; Tu, olfactory tubercle; VP, ventroposterior thalamus. (Courtesy of Dr Miles Herkenham, National Institutes of Mental Health, USA.)

electrically stimulated guinea-pig ileum. Similar inhibitory effects of THC and other cannabinoids on the release of a variety of neurotransmitters from CNS neurons have been observed in many subsequent studies (Schlicker and Kathmann, 2001). The neurotransmitters involved include L-glutamate, γ-aminobutyric acid (GABA), noradrenaline (norepinephrine), dopamine, 5-hydroxytryptamine (5-HT) and acetylcholine. The brain regions most often studied in vitro, usually in tissue slice preparations, have been cerebellum, hippocampus or neocortex. Neurotransmitter release has been studied directly in superfused preparations, or indirectly by measuring postsynaptic currents. Although most of these studies involved rat or mouse brain, a few studies have shown similar results using human brain tissue (Katona *et al.*, 2000; Schlicker and Kathmann, 2001). Because THC is only poorly water-soluble, the more soluble synthetic CB$_1$ receptor agonists WIN552 123, HU210 or CP55 940 were most commonly used in these in vitro studies. The specificity of the cannabinoid effects was confirmed by demonstrating that the inhibitory effects of the agonists were completely blocked by the CB$_1$-selective antagonist rimonabant.

Endogenous cannabinoids act as retrograde signal molecules at synapses

Important new insights into the physiological role of cannabinoids emerged from neurophysiological studies published independently by three different research groups in 2001. A phenomenon known as 'depolarization-induced suppression of inhibition' (DSI) has been known to neurophysiologists for some years (Alger and Pitler, 1995). It is a form of fast retrograde signalling from postsynaptic neurons back to inhibitory cells that innervate them, and is particularly prominent in the hippocampus and cerebellum. Three properties of DSI suggested to Wilson and Nicoll (2001) that a cannabinoid mechanism might be involved. First, DSI, like endocannabinoid synthesis, requires Ca^{2+} influx into the postsynaptic neuron (Lenz et al., 1998). Second, DSI is probably presynaptic, since the sensitivity of the postsynaptic cell to GABA is unaffected (Pitler and Alger, 1992). Finally, DSI is blocked by pertussin toxin, which interacts with the Gi/o protein to which the CB_1 receptor is coupled (Pitler and Alger, 1994). Wilson and Nicoll (2001) used slice preparations of rat hippocampus and induced DSI by brief depolarizing steps in the holding potential of voltage-clamped CA1 pyramidal neurons. They found that DSI was completely blocked by the cannabinoid CB_1 receptor antagonists AM251 or rimonabant. DSI could be mimicked by application of the CB_1 receptor agonist WIN552 122, but the continued presence of the agonist prevented DSI by occlusion. Wilson and Nicoll (2001) were also able to show by recording from pairs of nearby CA1 neurons that depolarizing one of these neurons caused DSI to spread and affect adjacent neurons up to 20 μm away. They suggested that the small lipid-soluble, freely diffusible endocannabinoids act as retrograde synaptic signals that can affect axon terminals in a sphere of influence some 40 μm in diameter.

Ohno-Shosaku et al. (2001) came to a similar conclusion using a different experimental paradigm. Recording from pairs of cultured hippocampal neurons with inhibitory synaptic connections, they found that depolarization of the postsynaptic neurons led to DSI in approximately two-thirds of the neuron pairs, and showed that this was due to inhibition of GABA release. Those that exhibited DSI, but not the others, proved to be sensitive to the CB_1 receptor agonist WIN552 122, which mimicked the inhibitory effect of DSI on DSI. Both DSI and the cannabinoid effect could be blocked by the CB_1 receptor antagonists AM-281 or rimonabant.

Further support for the conclusion that a cannabinoid-mediated mechanism underlies DSI came from Varma et al. (2001), who found that DSI was completely absent in hippocampal slices prepared from CB_1 receptor knockout mice (Ledent et al., 1999). Varma et al. (2001) also reported that agonists which stimulate metabotropic glutamate (mGlu) receptors enhanced DSI, whereas the broad-spectrum antagonist of mGlu receptors LY341495 tended to reduce DSI, suggesting that glutamate may also be involved. Interestingly, Varma et al. (2001) found that mGlu agonists failed to have any effect on DSI in the CB_1 knockout animals, suggesting that glutamate acts to enhance the endocannabinoid signal.

Retrograde signalling by endocannabinoids is not restricted to the inhibitory inputs to postsynaptic neurons. Kreitzer and Regehr (2001a) showed that depolarization of rat cerebellar Purkinje cells leads to a transient inhibition of excitatory inputs from parallel fibre and climbing fibre inputs, a phenomenon described as 'depolarization-induced suppression of excitation' or DSE. They found that DSE was triggered by calcium influx into the Purkinje cells, and it could be completely blocked by the CB_1 antagonist AM-251 and mimicked and occluded by the CB_1 receptor agonist WIN55 212-2. Kreitzer and Regehr (2001b) went on to show that inhibitory inputs to rat cerebellar Purkinje cells from basket cells and stellate cells were subject to DSI, and that this was also blocked by AM-251 and occluded by WIN55 212-2. The DSE phenomenon in the cerebellum is also linked to mGlu receptors. Maejima *et al.* (2001) reported that mGlu agonists acting on mouse Purkinje cells mimicked DSE, and the effects could be blocked by CB_1 antagonists.

These findings suggest that endocannabinoids are involved in the rapid modulation of synaptic transmission in the CNS by a retrograde signalling system that can influence synapses in a local region of some 40 μm diameter, causing inhibitory effects on both excitatory and inhibitory neurotransmitter release that persist for tens of seconds. Retrograde cannabinoid signalling has been likened to a 'molecular coincidence detector' activated by the temporal and spatial convergence of multiple neurochemical signals (Gerdeman *et al.*, 2002). This may play an important role in the control of neural circuits, particularly in cerebellum and hippocampus (see below). Exogenously administered THC or other cannabinoids cannot mimic the physiological effects of locally released endocannabinoids. Exogenous cannabinoids cause a long-lasting activation of CB_1 receptors in all brain regions and their overall effect is to cause a persistent inhibition of neurotransmitter release from those nerve terminals which express CB_1 receptors. As a consequence, they temporarily occlude and prevent the phenomena of DSI and DSE.

Effects of cannabinoids on CNS function and psychomotor control

CB_1 receptors are expressed at particularly high densities in the basal ganglia and cerebellum, so it is not surprising that cannabinoids have complex effects on psychomotor function (reviewed by Rodríguez de Fonseca *et al.*, 1998). One of the earliest reports of the effects of cannabis extracts in experimental animals described the awkward swaying and rolling gait caused by the drug in dogs, with periods of intense activity provoked by tactile or auditory stimuli, and followed eventually by catalepsy and sleep (Dixon, 1899). In rodents cannabinoids tend to have a triphasic effect. Thus in rats, low doses of THC (0.2 mg/kg) decreased locomotor activity, while higher doses (1–2 mg/kg) stimulated movements and catalepsy emerged at doses of 2.5 mg/kg (Sañudo-Peña *et al.*, 2000). Similarly, in mice Adams and Martin (1996) described a 'popcorn effect' in animals treated with THC. Groups of mice are sedated by the drug, but will jump in response to auditory or tactile stimuli; as they fall into other animals, these in turn jump, resembling corn popping in a popcorn machine. Interestingly, the CB_1 receptor antagonist rimonabant stimulated loco-motor activity in mice, suggesting that there is tonic activity in the endocannabinoid system that contributes to the control of spontaneous levels of activity (Compton et al., 1996).

These effects of cannabinoids may be due in part to actions at cerebellar or striatal receptors. Patel and Hillard (2001) used tests of specific cerebellar functions to show that cannabinoids caused increased gait width and number of slips on a bar-cross test. DeSanty and Dar (2001) observed rotorod impairments in mice after direct injection of synthetic cannabinoids into the cerebellum. These defects were no longer seen in animals pretreated with cerebellar injections of an antisense oligonucleotide directed to a sequence in the CB_1 receptor.

In human subjects it is also possible to demonstrate that cannabis causes impaired performance in tests of balance (Greenberg et al., 1994), or in tests that require fine psychomotor control, for example tracking a moving point of light on a screen (Manno et al., 1970). Human cannabis users may also seek isolation and remain immobile for long periods.

A number of authors have attempted to combine what is known of the neuro-anatomical distribution of the cannabinoid system and the results of behavioural and electrophysiological studies to speculate on the mechanisms underlying cannabinoid modulation of psychomotor function (Breivogel and Childers, 1998; Sañudo-Peña et al., 2000; Giuffrida and Piomelli, 2000; Elphick and Egertová, 2001). The CB_1 receptor is expressed particularly by the main output cells of the stria-tum, GABAergic medium-spiny projection neurons. The receptor is abundant in regions containing the axon terminals of these cells (globus pallidus, entopedun-cular nucleus and substantia nigra reticulata, and in axon collaterals feeding back to medium-spiny projection neurons in striatum).

CB_1 receptors are also abundant on the terminals of glutamatergic projection neurons from the subthalamic nucleus to globus pallidus, entopeduncular nucleus and substantia nigra reticulata. Cannabinoids might thus be expected to inhibit GABA release in striatum and GABA and glutamate release in the other nuclei. Sañudo-Peña et al. (2000) suggested that the primary role of the endocannabinoid system may be to inhibit tonic release of glutamate in the substantia nigra, regulating levels of basal motor activity. Exogenous cannabinoids also lead to decreased GABA release in substantia nigra which could lead to a disinhibition of the inhibitory nigral input to the thalamocortical pathway, resulting in inhibition of movement. High-frequency activation of cortical inputs to medium-spiny neurons in the striatum leads to long-term depression (LTD) of excitatory synaptic transmission. This form of synaptic plasticity appears to be dependent on cannabinoid signalling; it is absent in CB_1 receptor knockout mice and enhanced by anandamide loading (Gerdeman et al., 2002).

The results of eliminating the expression of CB₁ receptors in knockout mice have yielded conflicting results. The knockout animals studied by Zimmer *et al.* (1999) displayed reduced levels of basal activity – lending support to the hypothesis put forward by Sañudo-Peña *et al.* (2000) that tonic activation of CB$_1$ receptors promotes movement. However, the CB$_1$ knockout animals studied by Ledent *et al.* (1999) showed no change in spontaneous activity, and in some tests they exhibited increased motor activity. This is also in line with the observations of Compton *et al.* (1996) that the CB$_1$ antagonist rimonabant caused an increase in locomotor activity. Clearly there is as yet only a poor understanding of the actions of cannabinoids in the basal ganglia and cerebellum. Interactions with other chemical signalling systems in the brain are likely to be important. Giuffrida *et al.* (1999) showed, for example, that dopamine D2 receptor agonists caused an increase in anandamide synthesis and release in striatum. Deadwyler *et al.* (1995) described the convergence of multiple presynaptic controls on the terminals of granule cells in cerebellum. In addition to the CB$_1$ receptor, these terminals also express high densities of kappa opioid, adenosine A$_1$ and GABA-B receptors, all of which are coupled through a similar Gi/o type G protein to inhibit adenylate cyclase, and all are capable of inhibiting glutamate release. Such complexities are likely to prove the norm.

Cannabinoid mechanisms in the hippocampus and effects on memory

One of the well-established effects of acute intoxication with cannabis in humans is an impairment of short-term memory. The extensive literature on human studies is reviewed by Jones (1978), Miller and Branconnier (1983), Solowij (1998) and Earlywine (2002: see also Chapter 3). Many studies have shown significant effects on short-term memory, particularly when tests were used that depend heavily on attention (Abel, 1971; Mendelson *et al.*, 1976). Animal studies have also found that THC, synthetic cannabinoids and anandamide cause deficits in short-term memory in spatial learning tasks (for review, see Hampson and Deadwyler, 1999). These include delayed matching or non-matching tests in rodents (Mallet and Beninger, 1998; Hampson and Deadwyler, 1999), performance in a radial arm maze (Stiglick and Kalant, 1985; Lichtman and Martin, 1996), and a fixed-ratio food acquisition task in squirrel monkeys (Nakamura-Palacios *et al.*, 2000). The effects of both cannabinoids (Lichtman and Martin, 1996) and anandamide (Mallet and Beninger, 1998) were reversed by rimonabant, indicating that they are mediated by the CB$_1$ receptor.

A likely site for these effects is the hippocampus. Hampson and Deadwyler (1999) claimed that the effects of treatment of rats with cannabinoids on short-term memory in a delayed non-matching to sample test were equivalent to the effects seen after surgical removal of the hippocampus. In each case the animals were unable to segregate information between trials in the task because of disruptions to the processing of sensory information in hippocampal circuits. CB_1 receptors are expressed at high densities in the hippocampus. They are particularly abundant on the terminals of a subset of GABAergic basket cell interneurones which also contain the neuropeptide cholecystokinin (Katona *et al.*, 1999), and this is also the case in human hippocampus (Katona *et al.*, 2000). These are presumably the GABAergic neurons involved in the endocannabinoid-mediated DSI phenomenon described above. The terminals of these cells surround large pyramidal neuron somata in the CA1-CA4 fields. GABAergic neurons in the dentate gyrus also express CB_1 receptors, with terminals concentrated at the boundary of the molecular and granule cell layers (Egertová and Elphick, 2000). In addition, CB_1 receptors are expressed, at a lower level, in the glutamatergic pyramidal cells and their terminals. Cannabinoids can thus inhibit the release of both GABA and glutamate in hippocampal circuits.

The mechanisms underlying synaptic plasticity have been studied more intensely in the hippocampus than in any other brain region. In particular the electrophysiological phenomena of long-term potentiation (LTP) and LTD are thought to be involved in memory formation at glutamatergic synapses in the hippocampus. In contrast to the role of cannabinoids in LTD in striatum, a number of studies have shown that cannabinoids inhibit the induction of both LTP and LTD in hippocampus (for review, see Elphick and Egertová, 2001). Cannabinoids appear to work by reducing glutamate release below the level needed to activate N-methyl-D-aspartate (NMDA) receptors, a requirement for LTP and LTD (Shen *et al.*, 1996; Misner and Sullivan, 1999). Although the actions of cannabinoids in reducing GABA release from hippocampal interneurones might have been expected to increase the level of excitability of hippocampal pyramidal cells, it seems that the cannabinoid-induced reduction in glutamate release predominates. The administration of exogenous cannabinoids is of course wholly unphysiological and cannot mimic the effects of endocannabinoids that are released in discrete local regions in response to particular patterns of afferent inputs. CB_1 receptors are capable of regulating both inhibitory and excitatory neurotransmitter release in the hippocampus and are thus capable of subtle control of synaptic plasticity. The CB_1-containing GABAergic interneurones are thought to control oscillatory electrical activity in the hippocampus in the theta and gamma frequencies, and this plays a role in synchronizing pyramidal cell activity (Hoffman and Lupica, 2000). CB_1 agonists decrease the power of such oscillations in hippocampal slices (Hájos *et al.*, 2000) and may thus influence the synchronous activity of pyramidal cells. The physiological importance of cannabinoid-mediated DSI may be to decrease GABAergic inhibition of these cells and thus facilitate learning when hippocampal inputs are active (Wilson and Nicoll, 2001).

One approach to answering the question of what role the tonic release of endo-cannabinoids may play in hippocampal function has been to examine the effects of CB_1 receptor knockout or the effects of selective CB_1 receptor antagonists. Unfortunately these studies have so far yielded conflicting results. Bohme *et al.* (2000) reported a significant enhancement of LTP in CB_1 knockout mice, and Reibaud *et al.* (1999) found a significant enhancement of memory in such animals. However, tests with the CB_1 antagonist rimonabant showed no effects on LTP (Terranova *et al.*, 1995) or on learning and memory in a spatial learning task (Mallet and Beninger, 1998), although Terranova *et al.* (1996) reported that rimonabant enhanced memory in a short-term olfactory memory test in rats (social recognition test).

A novel role for cannabinoids in the extinction of aversive memories was suggested by the finding that CB_1 receptor knockout mice showed impaired extinction of auditory fear-conditioned tests (Marsicano *et al.*, 2002).

Cannabinoids and the neocortex

Like other intoxicant drugs, cannabis causes profound changes in a variety of higher brain functions. The literature on the acute effects of the drug in human subjects is large, and can only be summarized here: for reviews, see Jones (1978), Solowij (1998), Iversen (2000) and Earleywine (2002). The distribution of CB_1 receptors in the neocortex has been described in detail (Herkenham *et al.*, 1991; Egertová and Elphick, 2000). As in the hippocampus, the majority of cortical interneurones expressing high levels of CB_1 receptor are GABAergic cells which also express cholecystokinin (Marsicano and Lutz, 1999). CB_1-positive terminals are concentrated in layers II–III and layers V–VI, with few in layers I or IV. Despite the obvious importance of the abundant CB_1 receptors in the neocortex there have so far been few electrophysiological studies of their effects on neural activity.

The earlier literature, however, contains several reports of the effects of acute and chronic cannabis use on electroencephalogram (EEG) activity, both in humans and animals (reviewed by Adams and Martin, 1996; Solowij, 1998). Most studies in humans have observed changes consistent with a state of drowsiness, with increases in relative and absolute alpha power, particularly in frontal regions of cortex. In contrast, the CB_1 antagonist rimonabant was shown to induce EEG changes characteristic of arousal in rats, and increased the time spent in wakefulness as opposed to sleep (Santucci *et al.*, 1996). Mechoulam *et al.* (1997) have suggested that anandamide may play a role in the control of the sleep–waking cycle.

Studies of the effects of cannabis on perceptual abilities have yielded a variety of often conflicting results. While users often report a subjective enhancement of visual and auditory perception, sometimes with synaesthesia (sounds take on visual colourful qualities), laboratory studies have usually not shown marked changes in visual or auditory perception. One subjective effect that has been confirmed is the sensation that cannabis users experience time as passing more quickly relative to real time. In laboratory tests subjects overestimate the amount of elapsed time when asked to estimate, or produce shorter than required intervals when asked to signal a period of elapsed time (Hicks *et al.*, 1984; Mathew *et al.*, 1998). This curious effect can also be seen in animals. Han and Robinson (2001) trained rats to respond for food reward using a fixed-interval schedule. When treated with THC or WIN55 212-2, the animals shortened their response interval, whereas the antagonist rimonabant lengthened this interval.

There have been many studies of the acute and chronic effects of cannabis on human cognitive function (Jones, 1978; Solowij, 1998; Earleywine, 2002; and see Chapter 13). Performance on a variety of tests of cognitive function is impaired by the drug, but by comparison with alcohol, the effects of cannabis are subtle.

Effects of cannabinoids on hypothalamic control of appetite

Many subjective reports suggest that cannabis intoxication is associated with an increased appetite, particularly for sweet foods, even in subjects who were previously satiated. This effect can be confirmed under laboratory conditions (Hollister, 1971; Mattes *et al.*, 1994), although results from studies in human subjects have tended to be variable – perhaps because the increased appetite is focused on certain types of food. Nevertheless, controlled clinical trials showed that THC (dronabinol) had significant beneficial effects in counteracting the loss of appetite and reduction in body weight in patients suffering from the acquired immune deficiency syndrome (AIDS)-related wasting syndrome (Beal *et al.*, 1995) and this is one of the medical indications for which the drug has official approval in the USA.

THC also stimulates food intake in experimental animals, and again the effect is specific for high-fat or sweet high-fat diets and is not seen in animals offered standard rat chow (Koch, 2001). The endocannabinoid anandamide also stimulates food intake in rats, and the effect is blocked by rimonabant (Williams and Kirkham, 1999). Conversely, the CB_1 antagonist rimonabant, given on its own, suppressed food intake and led to reduced body weight in adult non-obese rats (Colombo *et al.*, 1998). Rimonabant (Ecopipam) is currently in clinical trials as a potential antiobesity agent. These results suggest that cannabinoids may play a role in the regulation of food intake and body weight (Mechoulam and Fride, 2001). At some stages during development these effects of endocannabinoids may be of critical importance. Fride *et al.* (2001) found that administration of the CB_1 antagonist rimonabant to newborn mouse pups had a devastating effect in decreasing milk ingestion and growth; continuing treatment with the antagonist led to death within 4–8 days. The effect of rimonabant could be almost fully reversed by coadministering THC.

Cannabis as an intoxicant and drug of dependence

Cannabis intoxication

There have been many subjective accounts of the cannabis 'high' (Iversen, 2000; Earlywine, 2002; and see Chapter 3). The experience is highly variable, depending on the dose of drug, the environment and the experience and expectations of the drug user. A typical 'high' is preceded initially by a transient stage of tingling sensations felt in the body and head, accompanied by a feeling of dizziness or lightheadedness. The 'high' is a complex experience, characterized by a quickening of mental associations and a sharpened sense of humour – sometimes described as a state of 'fatuous euphoria'. The user feels relaxed and calm, in a dreamlike state disconnected from the real world. The intoxicated subject often has difficulty in carrying on a coherent conversation, and may drift into daydreams and fantasies. Drowsiness and sleep may eventually ensue. The feelings of heightened perception, increased appetite and distortion of the sense of time have already been referred to. A survey of 1333 young British cannabis users (Atha and Blanchard, 1997) reported that the most common positive benefits reported were relaxation and relief from stress (25.6%), insight/personal development (8.7%) and euphoria (4.9%); more than half reported some positive benefits. But 21% also attributed some adverse effects to cannabis use – these included impaired memory (6.1%), paranoia (5.6%) and amotivation/laziness (4.8%).

As with other intoxicant drugs, little is known about the brain mechanisms that underlie the cannabis 'high'. The intoxicant effects are clearly mediated via CB_1 receptors. Huestis *et al.* (2001) carried out a well-controlled study in 63 healthy cannabis users, who received either rimonabant or placebo and smoked either a THC-containing or placebo marijuana cigarette. The CB_1 antagonist blocked the acute psychological effects of the active cigarettes. Interestingly, rimonabant itself, when given alone (with placebo cigarette), produced no significant psychological effects. The CB_1 receptor in brain also mediates the subjective effects of THC in animals. In rats trained to recognize oral THC as a discriminative cue ($ED_{50} =$ 0.64 mg/kg), the antagonist rimonabant blocked this behaviour, while a related compound SR140 098, which lacks brain penetration, was inactive (Perio *et al.*, 1996).

Mathew *et al.* (1997) used ^{15}O-water and positron emission tomography to measure changes in regional cerebral blood flow in a double-blind study in 32 volunteers comparing THC with placebo. Self-ratings of cannabis intoxication correlated most markedly with increased regional cerebral blood flow (rCBF) in the right frontal region. O'Leary *et al.* (2002), who also observed increased rCBF in insula, temporal poles and anterior cingulate – anterior paralimbic regions – reported similar findings. Decreased rCBF was seen in auditory regions of temporal lobe and in visual cortex, parietal cortex and thalamus. Studies of the effects of

THC on activity in rat brain, measured by the ^{14}C-deoxyglucose method, have also shown selective decreases in energy metabolism in structures related to sensory and limbic function and in hippocampus (Brett *et al.*, 2001; Freedland *et al.*, 2002).

Endocannabinoids and CB receptors are present in many regions of the limbic forebrain. For example, Katona *et al.* (2001) reported that CB receptors were expressed in high densities in lateral and basal nuclei in the rat amygdala. As in hippocampus, the CB receptors in these regions were located presynaptically on the terminals of cholecystokinin-containing GABAergic interneurones. Electrophysiological experiments showed that cannabinoids modulated GABAergic synaptic transmission. The authors suggested that such effects might underlie some of the actions of cannabinoids on emotional behaviour.

Other experiments have revealed that, in common with other euphoriant drugs, THC selectively activates dopaminergic neurons in the ventral tegmental area. In an electrophysiological study, French *et al.* (1997) reported that low doses of THC increased the firing of these cells. Tanda *et al.* (1997) used microdialysis probes to show that low doses of THC (0.15 mg/kg iv) caused an increased release of dopamine from the shell region of the nucleus accumbens, an effect that is also seen after administration of heroin, cocaine, *d*-amfetamine and nicotine. Tanda *et al.* (1997) found that the increased release of dopamine provoked by THC could be blocked by administration of the mu-opiate receptor antagonist naloxonazine, suggesting the involvement of an opioid mechanism. Electrophysiological studies showed that the cannabinoid WIN55 212-2 depressed the inhibitory GABAergic input to dopamine neurons in the ventral tegmental area in rat brain slice preparations in vitro, suggesting a mechanism that may underly their increased firing rate in vivo (Szabo *et al.*, 2002).

There is other evidence for an interaction between cannabinoid and opioid mechanisms. In tests of acute pain (Fuentes *et al.*, 1999) and chronic inflammatory pain (Welch and Stevens, 1992; Smith *et al.*, 1998) THC and morphine acted synergistically – one potentiated the antinociceptive actions of the other. This potentiation could be blocked by either SR 141 716 or naloxone, indicating that both CB_1 and opiate receptors were involved (Fuentes *et al.*, 1999). An electrophysiological analysis of the effects of cannabinoids on single-cell firing patterns in the rostral ventromedial medulla revealed that the effects of cannabinoids were similar to those elicited by morphine. The authors concluded that cannabinoids may produce analgesia through activation of a brainstem circuit that is also required for opiate analgesia, although the two mechanisms are pharmacologically distinct (Meng *et al.*, 1998).

One way of demonstrating the rewarding effects of drugs in animals is the conditioned place preference paradigm, in which an animal learns to approach an environment in which it had previously received a rewarding stimulus. Rats demonstrated a positive THC place preference after doses as low as 1 mg/kg (Lepore *et al.*, 1995). Studies of this behavioural effect of THC in mice lacking mu- or kappa-opioid receptors suggest that opioid mechanisms may play a key role in the reward-ing effects of THC. While the effects of THC on body temperature, pain sensitivity and reducing motor activity were unaffected in either opioid receptor knockout, the rewarding effects of THC, assessed by place preference, were abolished in the mu knockout mice, and enhanced in the kappa knockout animals (Ghozland *et al.*, 2002).

Tolerance and dependence

Many animal studies showed that tolerance develops to most of the behavioural and physiological effects of THC (for review, see Pertwee, 1991). The earlier clinical literature also suggested that tolerance also occurs after repeated administration of THC in humans – although many of these studies were poorly controlled (for reviews, see Jones, 1978; 1987; Hollister, 1986; 1998). But for many years cannabis was not considered to be a drug of addiction. Withdrawal of the drug did not lead to any obvious physical withdrawal symptoms either in people or in animals, and animals failed to self-administer the drug – a behaviour usually associated with drugs of addiction.

Attitudes have changed markedly in recent years. The *Diagnostic and Statistical Manual of Mental Disorders* (*DSM*-IV) (American Psychiatric Association, 1994) defines 'substance dependence' and 'substance abuse' rather than 'addiction'. When the *DSM*-IV criteria are applied to populations of regular cannabis users, surpris-ingly high proportions appear positive by these definitions (Anthony *et al.*, 1994; Swift *et al.*, 2001). More carefully controlled studies have also shown that a reliable and clinically significant withdrawal syndrome does occur in human cannabis users when the drug is withdrawn. The symptoms include craving for cannabis, decreased appetite, sleep difficulty and weight loss and may sometimes be accompanied by anger, aggression, increased irritability, restlessness and strange dreams (Budney *et al.*, 2001).

The existence of dependence on cannabinoids in animals is also much more clearly observable because of the availability of CB_1 receptor antagonist drugs that can be used to precipitate withdrawal. Thus, Aceto *et al.* (1996) described a behavioural withdrawal syndrome precipitated by rimonabant in rats treated for only 4 days with doses of THC as low as 0.5–4.0 mg/kg per day. The syndrome included scratching, face rubbing, licking, wet dog shakes, arched back and ptosis – many of the same signs are seen in rats undergoing opiate withdrawal. Similar withdrawal signs could be elicited by rimonabant in rats treated chronically with the synthetic cannabinoids CP-55 940 (Rubino *et al.*, 1998) or WIN55 212-2 (Aceto *et al.*, 2001). Rimonabant-induced withdrawal after 2 weeks of treatment of rats with the cannabinoid HU-120 was accompanied by marked elevations of release of the stress-related neuropeptide corticotrophin-releasing factor in the amygdala, a result also seen in animals undergoing heroin withdrawal (Rodríguez de Fonseca *et al.*, 1997). An electrophysiological study showed that precipitated withdrawal was also associated with reduced firing of dopamine neurons in the ventral tegmental area of rat brain (Diana *et al.*, 1998). These data clearly indicate that chronic administration of cannabinoids leads to adaptive changes in the brain, some of which are similar to those seen with other drugs of dependence. The ability of THC to cause a selective release of dopamine from the nucleus accumbens (Tanda *et al.*, 1997) also suggests some similarity between THC and other drugs in this category.

Furthermore, although many earlier attempts to obtain reliable self-administration behaviour with THC were unsuccessful (Pertwee, 1991), some success has been obtained recently. Squirrel monkeys were trained to self-administer low doses of THC (2 μg/kg per injection) – but only after the animals had first been trained to self-administer cocaine (Tanda *et al.*, 2000). THC is difficult to administer intravenously and these authors succeeded perhaps in part because they managed to deliver the drug intravenously in doses comparable to those to which human cannabis users are exposed. The potent synthetic cannabinoids are far more water-soluble than THC, which makes intravenous administration easier. Mice could be trained to self-administer intravenous WIN55 212-2 but CB_1 receptor knockout animals failed to exhibit this behaviour (Ledent *et al.*, 1999).

A number of studies have suggested that there may be links between the development of dependence to cannabinoids and to opiates. Some of the behavioural signs of rimonabant-induced withdrawal in THC treated rats can be mimicked by administration of the opiate antagonist naloxone (Kaymakçalan *et al.*, 1977). Conversely, the withdrawal syndrome precipitated by naloxone in morphine-dependent mice can be partly relieved by administration of THC (Hine *et al.*, 1975) or by endocannabinoids (Yamaguchi *et al.*, 2001). Rats treated chronically with the cannabinoid WIN55 212-2 became sensitized to the behavioural effects of heroin (Pontieri *et al.*, 2001). Such interactions can also be demonstrated acutely. A synergy between cannabinoids and opiate analgesics has already been described above. THC also facilitated the antinociceptive effects of RB 101, an inhibitor of enkephalin inactivation (Valverde *et al.*, 2001). These authors found that acute administration of THC caused an increased release of Met-enkephalin into microdialysis probes placed into the rat nucleus accumbens.

The availability of receptor knockout animals has also helped to illustrate cannabinoid–opioid interactions. CB_1 receptor knockout mice exhibited greatly reduced morphine self-administration behaviour and less severe naloxone-induced withdrawal signs than in wild-type animals, although the antinociceptive actions of morphine were unaffected in the knockout animals (Ledent *et al.*, 1999). The rimonabant-precipitated withdrawal syndrome in THC-treated mice was significantly attenuated in animals with knockout of the pro-enkephalin gene (Valverde *et al.*, 2000). Knockout of the μ-opioid receptor also reduced rimonabant-induced withdrawal signs in THC treated mice and there was an attenuated naloxone withdrawal syndrome in morphine-dependent CB$_1$ knockout mice (Lichtman *et al.*, 2001a, b).

Using other dosage regimes it is possible to observe behavioural sensitization to THC after repeated drug administration, and such animals also displayed heightened behavioural responses to morphine (Cadoni *et al.*, 2001).

These findings clearly point to interactions between the endogenous cannabinoid and opioid systems in the CNS, although the neural circuitry involved remains unknown. It is possible that the involvement of opioid mechanisms in mediating at least some of the effects of cannabinoids is relevant to understanding the euphoriant and addictive properties of these drugs.

Conclusions

Although we begin to understand some of the effects of cannabis on brain function, there is still much to be learned. Most of the CNS effects of the drug, including its intoxicant properties, appear to be due to its interactions with the CB$_1$ cannabinoid receptor, and the availability of CB$_1$ receptor knockout mice and CB$_1$ receptor antagonist drugs have provided powerful new tools for research on the central actions of cannabis. The interaction of the cannabinoid and opioid systems in the CNS may be relevant to understanding the dependence-liability associated with chronic cannabis use.

REFERENCES

Abel, E. L. (1971). Marihuana and memory: acquisition or retrieval? *Science*, **173**, 1038–1041.

Aceto, M. D., Scates, S. M., Lowe, J. A. and Martin, B. R (1996). Dependence on Δ^9-tetrahydrocannabinol: studies on precipitated and abrupt withdrawal. *J. Pharmacol. Exp. Ther.*, **278**, 1290–1295.

Aceto, M. D., Scates, S. M. and Martin, B. R. (2001). Spontaneous and precipitated withdrawal with a synthetic cannabinoid, WIN 55212-2. *Eur. J. Pharmacol.*, **416**, 75–81.

Adams, I. B. and Martin, B. R. (1996). Cannabis: pharmacology and toxicology in animals and humans. *Addiction*, **91**, 1585–1614.

Alger, B. E. and Pitler, T. A. (1995). Retrograde signaling at GABA$_A$-receptor synapses in the mammalian CNS. *Trends Neurosci.*, **18**, 333–340.

American Psychiatric Association (1994). *Diagnostic and Statistical Manual of Mental Disorders (DSM-IV)*, 4th edn. Washington, DC: American Psychiatric Association.

Anthony, J. C., Warner, L. A. and Kessler, R. C. (1994). Comparative epidemiology of dependence on tobacco, alcohol, controlled substances and inhalants. Basic findings from the National Comorbidity Survey. *Exp. Clin. Psychopharmacol.*, **2**, 244–268.

Atha, M. J. and Blanchard, S. (1997). *Self Reported Consumption Patterns and Attitudes Towards Drugs Among 1333 Regular Cannabis Users*. Wigan, UK: Independent Drug Monitoring Unit.

Beal, J. A., Olson, R., Laubenstein, L. *et al.* (1995). Dronabinol as a treatment for anorexia associated with weight loss in patients with AIDS. *J. Pain Symptom Manage.*, **10**, 89–97.

Bohme, G. A., Laville, M., Ledent, C., Paramentier, M. and Imperato, A. (2000). Enhanced long-term potentiation in mice lacking cannabinoid CB_1 receptors. *Neuroscience*, **95**, 5–7.

Breivogel, C. S. and Childers, S. R. (1998). The functional neuroanatomy of brain cannabinoid receptors. *Neurobiol. Dis.*, **5**, 417–431.

Brett, R., MacKenzie, F. and Pratt, J. (2001). Delta-9-tetrahydrocannabinol-induced alterations in limbic system glucose use in the rat. *Neuro-Report*, **12**, 3573–3577.

Budney, A. J., Hughes, J. R., Moore, B. A. and Novy, P. L. (2001). Marijuana abstinence effects in marijuana smokers maintained in their home environment. *Arch. Gen. Psychiatry*, **58**, 917–924.

Cadoni, C., Pisanu, A., Solinas, M., Acquas, E. and Di Chiara, G. (2001). Behavioural sensitization after repeated exposure to delta-9-tetrahydrocannabinol and cross-sensitization with morphine. *Psychopharmacology*, **158**, 259–266.

Colombo, G., Agabio, R., Diaz, G. *et al.* (1998). Appetite suppression and weight loss after the cannabinoid antagonist SR141716A. *Life Sci.*, **63**, PL113–PL117.

Compton, D. R., Aceto, M. D., Lowe, J. and Martin, B. R. (1996). In vivo characterization of a specific cannabinoid receptor antagonist (SR141716A) inhibition of Δ^9-tetrahydocannabinol-induced responses and apparent agonist activity. *J. Pharmacol. Exp. Ther.*, **277**, 586–594.

Deadwyler, S. A., Hampson, R. E. and Childers, S. R. (1995). Functional significance of cannabinoid receptors in brain. In *Cannabinoid Receptors*, ed. R. G. Pertwee, pp. 206–231. London: Academic Press.

DeSanty, K. P. and Dar, M. S. (2001). Cannabinoid-induced motor incoordination through the cerebellar CB_1 receptor in mice. *Pharmacol. Biochem. Behav.*, **69**, 251–259.

Diana, M., Melis, M., Muntoni, A. L. and Gessa, G. L. (1998). Mesolimbic dopaminergic decline after cannabinoid withdrawal. *Proc. Natl Acad. Sci. USA*, **95**, 10269–10273.

Dixon, W. E. (1899). The pharmacology of cannabis indica. *Br. Med. J.* **11**, 1354–1357.

D'Souza, D. C. and Kosten, T. R. (2001). Cannabinoid antagonists. *Arch. Gen. Psychiatry*, **58**, 330–331.

Earlywine, M. (2002). *Understanding Marijuana*. New York: Oxford University Press.

Egertová, M. and Elphick, M. R. (2000). Localisation of cannabinoid receptors in the rat brain using antibodies to the intracellular C-terminal tail of CB_1. *J. Comp. Neurol.*, **422**, 159–171.

Egertová, M., Giang, D. K., Cravatt, B. F. and Elphick, M. R. (1998). A new perspective on cannabinoid signaling: complementary localization of fatty acid amide hydrolase and the CB1 receptor in the rat brain. *Proc. R. Soc. Lond. B*, **265**, 2081–2085.

Elphick, M. R. and Egertová, M. (2001). The neurobiology and evolution of cannabinoid signaling. *Phil. Trans. R. Soc. Lond.*, **356**, 381–408.

Felder, C. C. and Glass, M. (1998). Cannabinoid receptors and their endogenous agonists. *Annu. Rev. Pharmacol. Toxicol.*, **38**, 179–200.

Freedland, C. S., Whitlow, C. T., Miller, M. D. and Porrino, L. J. (2002). Dose-dependent effects of delta-9-tetrahydrocannabinol on rates of local cerebral glucose utilization in rat. *Synapse*, **45**, 134–142.

French, E. D., Dillon, K. and Wu, X. (1997). Cannabinoids excite dopamine neurons in the ventral tegmentum and substantia nigra. *NeuroReport*, **8**, 649–652.

Fride, E., Ginzburg, Y., Breuer, A. *et al.* (2001). Critical role of the endogenous cannabinoid system in mouse pup suckling and growth. *Eur. J. Pharmacol.*, **419**, 207–214.

Fuentes, J. A., Ruiz-Gayo, M., Manzanares, J. *et al.* (1999). Cannabinoids as potential new analgesics. *Life Sci.*, **65**, 675–685.

Gerdeman, G. L.,Ronesi, J. and Lovinger, D. M. (2002). Postsynaptic endocannabinoid release is critical to long-term depression in the striatum. *Nature Neurosci.*, **5**, 446–451.

Ghozland, S., Matthes, H. W., Simonin, F. *et al.* (2002). Motivational effects of cannabinoids are mediated by mu-opioid and kappa-opioid receptors. *J. Neurosci.*, **22**, 1146–1154.

Gill, E. W., Paton, W. D. M. and Pertwee, R. G. (1970). Preliminary experiments on the chemistry and pharmacology of cannabis. *Nature*, **229**, 134–136.

Giuffrida, A. and Piomelli, D. (2000). The endocannabinoid system: a physiological perspective on its role in psychomotor control. *Chem. Physics Lipids*, **108**, 151–158.

Giuffrida, A., Parsons, L. H., Kerr, T. M. *et al.* (1999). Dopamine activation of endogenous cannabinoid signaling in dorsal striatum. *Nature Neurosci.*, **2**, 358–363.

Greenberg, H. S., Werness, S. A. S., Pugh, J. E. *et al.* (1994). Short-term effects of smoking marijuana on balance in patients with multiple sclerosis and normal volunteers. *Clin. Pharmacol. Ther.*, **55**, 324–328.

Hájos, N., Katona, I., Naiem, S. S. *et al.* (2000). Cannabinoids inhibit hippocampal GABAergic transmission and network oscillations. *Eur. J. Neurosci.*, **12**, 3239–3249.

Hampson, R. E. and Deadwyler, S. A. (1999). Cannabinoids, hippocampal function and memory. *Life Sci.*, **65**, 715–723.

Han, C. J. and Robinson, J. K. (2001). Cannabinoid modulation of time estimation in the rat. *Behav. Neurosci.*, **115**, 243–246.

Herkenham, M., Lynn, A. B., Johnson, M. R. *et al.* (1991). Characterization and localization of cannabinoid receptors in rat brain: a quantitative *in vitro* autoradiographic study. *J. Neurosci.*, **11**, 563–583.

Hicks, R. E., Gualtieri, C. T., Mayo, P. Jr and Perez-Reyes, M. (1984). Cannabis, atropine and temporal information processing. *Neuropsychobiology*, **12**, 229–237.

Hine, B., Friedman, E., Torrelio, M. and Gershon, S. (1975). Morphine-dependent rats: blockade of precipitated abstinence by tetrahydrocannabinol. *Science*, **187**, 443–445.

Hoffman, A. F. and Lupica, C. R. (2000). Mechanisms of cannabinoid inhibition of GABA$_A$ synaptic transmission in the hippocampus. *J. Neurosci.*, **20**, 2470–2479.

Hollister, L. E. (1971). Hunger and appetite after single doses of marihuana, alcohol and dextroamphetamine. *Clin. Pharmacol. Ther.*, **12**, 44–49.

   (1986). Health aspects of cannabis. *Pharmacol. Rev.*, **38**, 1–20.

   (1998). Health aspects of cannabis: revisited. *Int. J. Neuropsychopharmacol.*, **1**, 71–80.

Huestis, M. A., Gorelick, D. A., Heishman, S. J. *et al.* (2001). Blockade of effects of smoked marijuana by the CB$_1$-selective cannabinoid receptor antagonist SR141716. *Arch. Gen. Psychiatry*, **58**, 322–328.

Iversen, L. L. (2000). *The Science of Marijuana.* New York: Oxford University Press.

Jones, R. T. (1978). Marihuana: human effects. In *Handbook of Psychopharmacology*, vol. 12, ed. L. L. Iversen, S. D. Iversen and S. H. Snyder, pp. 373–412. New York: Plenum Press.

(1987). Drug of abuse profile: cannabis. *Clin. Chem.*, **33**, 72B–81B.

Katona, I., Sperlagh, B., Sik, A. *et al.* (1999). Presynaptically located CB$_1$ receptors regulate GABA release from axon terminals of specific hippocampal interneurons. *J. Neurosci.*, **19**, 4544–4558.

Katona, I., Sperlagh, B., Maglóczky, Z. *et al.* (2000). GABAergic interneurons are the targets of cannabinoid actions in the human hippocampus. *Neuroscience*, **100**, 797–804.

Katona, I., Rancz, E. A., Acsády, L. *et al.* (2001). Distribution of CB1 cannabinoid receptors in the amygdala and their role in the control of GABAergic transmission. *J. Neurosci.*, **21**, 9506–9518.

Kaymakçalan, S., Ayhan, I. H. and Tulunay, F. C. (1977). Naloxone-induced or postwithdrawal abstinence signs in Δ^9-tetrahydrocannabinol-tolerant rats. *Psychopharmacology*, **55**, 243–249.

Koch, J. E. (2001). Δ^9-THC stimulates food intake in Lewis rats. Effects on chow, high-fat and sweet high-fat diets. *Pharmacol. Biochem. Behav.*, **68**, 539–543.

Kreitzer, A. C. and Regehr, W. G. (2001a). Retrograde inhibition of presynaptic calcium influx by endogenous cannabinoids at excitatory synapses onto Purkinje cells. *Neuron*, **29**, 717–727.

(2001b). Cerebellar depolarization-induced suppression of inhibition is mediated by endogenous cannabinoids. *J. Neurosci.*, **21**, RC174–RC179.

Ledent, C., Valverde, O., Cossu, G. *et al.* (1999). Unresponsiveness to cannabinoids and reduced addictive effects of opiates in CB$_1$ receptor knockout mice. *Science*, **283**, 401–404.

Lenz, R. A., Wagner, J. J. and Alger, B. E. (1998). N- and L-type calcium channel involvement in depolarization-induced suppression of inhibition in rat hippocampal CA1 cells. *J. Physiol. (Lond.)*, **512**, 61–73.

Lepore, M., Vorel, S. R., Lowinson, J. and Gardner, E. L. (1995). Conditioned place preference induced by Δ^9-tetrahydrocannabinol: comparison with cocaine, morphine and food reward. *Life Sci.*, **56**, 2073–2080.

Lichtman, A. H. and Martin, B. R (1996). Δ^9-Tetrahydrocannabinol impairs spatial memory through a cannabinoid mechanism. *Psychopharmacology*, **126**, 125–131.

Lichtman, A. H., Fisher, J. and Martin, B. R. (2001a). Precipitated cannabinoid withdrawal is reversed by Δ^9-tetrahydrocannabinol or clonidine. *Pharmacol. Biochem. Behav.*, **69**, 181–188.

Lichtman, A. H., Sheikh, S. M., Loh, H. H. and Martin, B. R. (2001b). Opioid and cannabinoid modulation of precipitated withdrawal in Δ^9-tetrahydrocannabinol and morphine-dependent mice. *J. Pharmacol. Exp. Ther.*, **298**, 1007–1014.

Maejima, T., Hashimoto, K., Yoshida, T., Aiba, A. and Kano, M. (2001). Presynaptic inhibition caused by retrograde signal from metabotropic glutamate to cannabinoid receptors. *Neuron*, **31**, 463–475.

Mallet, P. E. and Beninger, R. J. (1998). The cannabinoid CB_1 receptor antagonist SR141716A attenuates the memory impairment produced by Δ^9-tetrahydrocannabinol or anandamide. *Psychopharmacology*, **140**, 11–19.

Manno, J. E., Glenn, M. S., Kiplinger, G. F. *et al.* (1970). Comparative effects of smoking marihuana or placebo on human motor and mental performance. *Clin. Pharmacol. Ther.*, **11**, 808–815.

Marsicano, G. and Lutz, B. (1999). Expression of the cannabinoid receptor CB_1 in distinct neuronal subpopulations in the adult mouse forebrain. *Eur. J. Neurosci.*, **11**, 4213–4225.

Marsicano, G., Wotjak, C. T., Azad, S. C. *et al.* (2002). The endogenous cannabinoid system controls extinction of aversive memories. *Nature*, **418**, 530–534.

Matsuda, L. A., Lolait, S. J., Brownstein, M. J., Young, A. C. and Bonner, T. I. (1990). Structure of a cannabinoid receptor and functional expression of the cloned cDNA. *Nature*, **346**, 561–564.

Mattes, R. D., Engelman, K., Shaw, L. M. and Elsohly, M. A. (1994). Cannabinoids and appetite stimulation. *Pharmacol. Biochem. Behav.*, **49**, 187–194.

Mathew, R. J., Wilson, W. H., Coleman, R. E., Turkington, T. G. and DeGrado, T. R. (1997). Marijuana intoxication and brain activation in marijuana smokers. *Life Sci.*, **60**, 2075–2089.

Mathew, R. J., Wilson, W. H., Turkington, T. G. and Coleman, R. E. (1998). Cerebellar activity and disturbed time sense after THC. *Brain Res.*, **797**, 183–189.

Mechoulam, R. and Fride, E. (2001). A hunger for cannabinoids. *Nature*, **410**, 763–765.

Mechoulam, R., Fride, E., Hanus, L. *et al.* (1997). Anandamide may mediate sleep induction. *Nature*, **389**, 25–26.

Mendelson, J. H., Babor, T. F., Kuehnle, J. C. *et al.* (1976). Behavioral and biological aspects of marijuana use. *Annal NY Acad. Sci.*, **282**, 186–210.

Meng, I. D., Manning, B. H., Martin, W. J. and Fields, H. L. (1998). An analgesia circuit activated by cannabinoids. *Nature*, **395**, 381–383.

Miller, L. L. and Branconnier, R. J. (1983). Cannabis: effects on memory and the cholinergic limbic system. *Psychol. Bull.*, **93**, 441–456.

Misner, D. L. and Sullivan, J. M. (1999). Mechanism of cannabinoid effects on long-term potentiation and depression in hippocampal CA1 neurons. *J. Neurosci.*, **19**, 6795–6805.

Munro, S., Thomas, K. L. and Abu-Shaar, M. (1993). Molecular characterization of a peripheral receptor for cannabinoids. *Nature*, **365**, 61–65.

Nakamura-Palacios, E. M., Winsauer, P. J. and Moerschbaecher, J. M. (2000). Effects of the cannabinoid ligand SR141716A alone or in combination with delta-9-tetrahydrocannabinol or scopolamine on learning in squirrel monkeys. *Behav. Pharmacol.*, **11**, 377–386.

Ohno-Shosaku, T., Maejima, T. and Kano M. (2001). Endogenous cannabinoids mediate retrograde signals from depolarized postsynaptic neurons to presynaptic terminals. *Neuron*, **29**, 729–738.

O'Leary, D. S., Block, R. I., Koeppel, J. A. *et al.* (2002). Effects of smoking marijuana on brain perfusion and cognition. *Neuropsychopharmacology*, **26**, 802–816.

Patel, S. and Hillard, C. J. (2001). Cannabinoid CB_1 receptor agonists produce cerebellar dysfunction in mice. *J. Pharmacol. Exp. Ther.*, **297**, 629–637.

Perio, A. A., Rinaldi-Carmona, M. M., Maruani, J. J. *et al.* (1996). Central mediation of the cannabinoid cue: activity of a selective CB1 antagonist SR 141716A. *Behav. Pharmacol.*, **7**, 65–71.

Pertwee, R. G. (1991). Tolerance to, and dependence on psychotropic cannabinoids. In *The Biological Basis of Drug Tolerance*, ed. J. Pratt, pp. 232–265. London: Academic Press.

(1999). Pharmacology of cannabinoid receptor ligands. *Curr. Med. Chem.*, **6**, 635–664.

Pettit, D. A. D., Harrison, M. P., Olson, J. M., Spencer, R. F. and Cabral, G. A. (1998). Immuno-histochemical localization of the neural cannabinoid receptor in rat brain. *J. Neurosci. Res.*, **51**, 391–402.

Pitler, T. A. and Alger, B. E. (1992). Postsynaptic spike firing reduces synaptic $GABA_A$ responses in hippocampal pyramidal cells. *J. Neurosci.*, **12**, 4122–4132.

(1994). Depolarization-induced suppression of GABAergic inhibition in rat hippocampal pyramidal cells: G protein involvement in a presynaptic mechanism. *Neuron*, **13**, 1447–1455.

Pontieri, F. E., Monnazzi, P., Scontrini, A., Buttarelli, F. R. and Patacchioli, F. R. (2001). Behavioral sensitization to heroin by cannabinoid pretreatment in the rat. *Eur. J. Pharmacol.*, **421**, R1–R3.

Reibaud, M., Obinu, M. C., Ledent, C. *et al.* (1999). Enhancement of memory in cannabinoid CB_1 receptor knock-out mice. *Eur. J. Pharmacol.*, **379**, 1–2.

Rinaldi-Carmona, M., Barth, F., Heaulme, M. *et al.* (1994). SR141716A, a potent and selective antagonist of the brain cannabinoid receptor. *FEBS Lett.*, **350**, 240–244.

Rodríguez de Fonseca, F., Rocio, M., Carrera, A. *et al.* (1997). Activation of corticotropin-releasing factor in the limbic system during cannabinoid withdrawal. *Science*, **276**, 2050–2054.

Rodríguez de Fonseca, F., Del Arco, I., Martín-Calderón, J. L., Gorriti, M. A. and Navarro, M. (1998). Role of the endogenous cannabinoid system in the regulation of motor activity. *Neurobiol. Dis.*, **5**, 483–501.

Roth, S. (1978). Stereoselective presynaptic inhibitory effect of delta-9-tetrahydrocannabinol on cholinergic transmission in the myenteric plexus of the guinea pig. *Can. J. Physiol. Pharmacol.*, **56**, 968–975.

Rubino, T., Patrini, G., Massi, P. *et al.* (1998). Cannabinoid-precipitated withdrawal: a time course study of the behavioral aspect and its correlation with cannabinoid receptors and G protein expression. *J. Pharmacol. Exp. Ther.*, **285**, 813–819.

Santucci, V., Storme, J. J., Soubrie, P. and Le Fur, G. (1996). Arousal-enhancing properties of the CB_1 cannabinoid receptor antagonist SR141716A in rats as assessed by electroencephalographic spectral and sleep-waking cycle analysis. *Life Sci.*, **58**, 103–110.

Sañudo-Peña, M. C., Tsou, K. and Walker, J. M. (2000). Motor actions of cannabinoids in the basal ganglia output nuclei. *Life Sci.*, **65**, 703–713.

Schlicker, E. and Kathmann, M. (2001). Modulation of transmitter release via presynaptic cannabinoid receptors. *Trends Pharmacol. Sci.*, **22**, 565–572.

Shen, M., Piser, T. M., Seybold, V. S. and Thayer, S. A. (1996). Cannabinoid receptor agonists inhibit glutamatergic synaptic transmission in rat hippocampal cultures. *J. Neurosci.*, **16**, 4322–4334.

Smith, F. L., Cichewicz, D., Martin, Z. L. and Welch, S. P. (1998). The enhancement of morphine antinociception in mice by delta-9-tetrahydrocannabinol. *Pharmacol. Biochem. Behav.*, **60**, 559–566.

Solowij, N. (1998). *Cannabis and Cognitive Functioning.* Cambridge: Cambridge University Press.

Stiglick, A. and Kalant, H. (1985). Residual effects of chronic cannabis treatment on behaviour in mature rats. *Psychopharmacology*, **85**, 436–439.

Swift, W., Hall, W. and Teesson, M. (2001). Cannabis use and dependence among Australian adults: results from the National Survey of Mental Health and Wellbeing. *Addiction*, **96**, 737–748.

Szabo, B., Siemes, S. and Wallmichrath, I. (2002). Inhibition of GABAergic neurotransmission in the ventral tegmental area by cannabinoids. *Eur. J. Neurosci.*, **15**, 2057–2061.

Tanda, G., Pontieri, F. E. and Di Chiara, G. (1997). Cannabinoid and heroin activation of meso-limbic dopamine transmission by a common μ_1 opioid receptor mechanism. *Science*, **276**, 2048–2050.

Tanda, G., Munzar, P. and Goldberg, S. R. (2000). Self-administration behavior is maintained by the psychoactive ingredient of marijuana in squirrel monkeys. *Nature Neurosci.*, **3**, 1073–1074.

Terranova, J. P., Michaud, J. C., Le Fur, G. *et al.* (1995). Inhibition of long-term potentiation in rat hippocampal slices by anandamide and WIN55 212-2; reversal by SR141 716-A, a selective antagonist of CB_1 cannabinoid receptors. *Naunyn Schmiedbergs Arch. Pharmacol.*, **352**, 576–579.

Terranova, J. P., Stomre, J. J., Lafon, N. *et al.* (1996). Improvement of memory in rodents by the selective CB_1 cannabinoid receptor antagonist SR141716A. *Psychopharmacology*, **126**, 165–172.

Valverde, O., Maldonado, R., Valjent, E., Zimmer, A. M. and Zimmer, A. (2000). Cannabinoid withdrawal syndrome is reduced in pre-proenkephalin knock-out mice. *J. Neurosci.*, **15**, 9284–9289.

Valverde, O., Noble, F. *et al.* (2001). Δ^9-Tetrahydrocannabinol releases and facilitates the effects of endogenous enkephalins: reduction in morphine withdrawal syndrome without change in rewarding effect. *Eur. J. Neurosci.*, **13**, 1816–1824.

Varma, N., Calrson, G. C., Ledent, C. and Alger, B. E. (2001). Metabotropic glutamate receptors drive the endocannabinoid system in hippocampus. *J. Neurosci.*, **21**, RC188–RC193.

Welch, S. P. and Stevens, D. L. (1992). Antinociceptive activity of intrathecally administered cannabinoids alone, and in combination with morphine, in mice. *J. Pharmacol. Exp. Ther.*, **262**, 10–18.

Williams, C. M. and Kirkham, T. C. (1999). Anandamide induces overeating: mediation by central cannabinoid (CB1) receptors. *Psychopharmacology*, **143**, 315–317.

Wilson, R. I. and Nicoll, R. A. (2001). Endogenous cannabinoids mediate retrograde signaling at hippocampal synapses. *Nature*, **410**, 588–592.

Yamaguchi, T., Hagiwara, Y., Tanaka, H. *et al.* (2001). Endogenous cannabinoid 2-arachidonylglycerol, attenuates naloxone-precipitated withdrawal signs in morphine-dependent mice. *Brain Res.*, **909**, 121–126.

Zimmer, A., Zimmer, A. M., Hohmann, A. G., Herkenham, M. and Bonner, T. I. (1999). Increased mortality, hypoactivity and hypoalgesia in cannabinoid CB1 receptor knockout mice. *Proc. Natl Acad. Sci. USA*, **96**, 5780–5785.

3

Acute and subacute psychomimetic effects of cannabis in humans

David J. Castle[1] and Nadia Solowij[2]

[1] University of Melbourne, Australia
[2] University of Wollongong, NSW, Australia

Cannabis sativa has been used for centuries for both its medicinal and psychomimetic effects. This chapter outlines the acute and subacute psychomimetic effects of cannabis in humans. Animal experiments with cannabis are not addressed here; the interested reader can find an account of such studies in Chapters 1 and 2 or refer to Adams and Martin (1996) or Chaperon and Thiebot (1999). Similarly, cannabis-associated psychotic disorders in humans are not dealt with here, as these are discussed in Chapters 5–7.

As we shall describe, the response of most people to cannabis is fairly stereotyped. Having said this, the experience of intoxication with any psychomimetic substance is influenced, *inter alia*, by dose; previous experience (and hence expectation of effect); the personal characteristics of the user (e.g. personality); and the context in which the drug is taken (O'Brien, 1996). Dose is particularly problematic with use of the plant *C. sativa*, as the proportional content of the major psychoactive compound (Δ^9-tetrahydrocannabinol, or THC) varies widely between different strains of the plant, as well as being dependent upon the conditions under which the plant was cultivated. Furthermore, the part of the plant or the type of plant product consumed also affects the amount of THC ingested: for example, cannabis resin has a THC content of up to 10 times that of the traditional cigarette (Ashton, 2001).

The route of administration also affects bioavailability. Thus, smoking is the most efficient form of administration as THC is delivered rapidly to the areas of the brain where it exerts its activity. Oral ingestion is inevitably slower in terms of onset of action, and there is significant first-pass hepatic metabolism, one of the end-products being 11-hydroxy-THC, itself psychoactive (Iversen, 2000).

Marijuana and Madness: Psychiatry and Neurobiology, ed. D. Castle and R. Murray. Published by Cambridge University Press. © Cambridge University Press 2004.

Table 3.1 Synopsis of effects of cannabis intoxication as recoded by Goode (*The Marijuana Smokers*, 1970) and Berke and Hernton (*The Cannabis Experience*, 1974)

- An initial 'buzz' with tingling and lightheadedness
- Euphoria and fatuous laughter
- An enhanced sensitivity of perception, for example, seeing colours very vividly
- An enhanced appreciation of art and music
- Synaesthesia: 'seeing' music, for example
- Visual and auditory hallucinations, which are usually transient and ill-formed
- Fantasies, which border on delusions, usually of a grandiose nature
- A feeling of 'double consciousness'

Data from Iversen (2000, pp. 79–87).

Historical accounts

Early reports of intoxication with cannabis are mostly individual accounts of experiences with the drug. One of the most extensive of these is that by Ludlow, who used cannabis regularly and in large doses and whose book, *The Hasheesh Eater* (1857), provides graphic descriptions of the effects of the drug. He states how he felt euphoric after imbibing cannabis such that 'I clapped my hands and shouted for joy . . . I glowed like a new-born soul'. He also experienced an alteration in sense of self, and an altered sense of the passage of time.

Marshall (1897) gave a vivid description of his experience with an extract of Indian charas (cannabis resin), emphasizing the euphoriant properties: 'I had the most irresistible desire to laugh. Everything seemed so ridiculously funny; even circumstances of a serious nature were productive of mirth . . . [I] . . . laughed incessantly . . . my cheeks ached'. He also described the characteristic prolongation of the sense of the passage of time, thinking that 'hours must have passed and only a few minutes had elapsed'. He alluded to grandiose beliefs whilst intoxicated, stating: 'My powers became superhuman; my knowledge covered the universe; my scope of sight was infinite'. He also described the 'horrors' after a very high dose of cannabis, during which he saw appalling visions, including demons.

The experiences of cannabis users in the USA during the 1960s have been recorded by Goode (1970) and, in the UK, by Berke and Hernton (1974). Iversen (2000) gives an excellent synopsis of these books (pp. 79–87), as outlined in Table 3.1.

Surveys of cannabis users

More recent studies have asked users generally about their experience whilst under the influence of cannabis. In a New Zealand study, Thomas (1996) surveyed 1000 people aged 18–25 years; 38% had used cannabis and reported various symptoms of intoxication, including panics (22%) and psychotic symptoms such as hearing voices or experiencing persecutory ideas (15%). An Australian study of 268 long-term cannabis users (median 19 years) by Reilly and colleagues (1998) found that they mostly used the drug to feel relaxed or relieve tension (61%), or for enjoyment and to feel good (27%); negative effects, including anxiety, paranoia and depression, were reported by 21% of the sample, and tiredness, lack of motivation and low energy by 21% also. In a large British study of 2794 cannabis users (Atha and Blanchard, 1997), nearly 60% reported positive effects, including relaxation and relief from stress (26%), insight and personal development (9%) and a positive effect on mood (5%) or sociability (2%). Again, adverse effects were common (21% overall) and included impairment of memory (6%), paranoia (6%), apathy/laziness (5%) and anxiety/panic (2%).

These reports of individuals' experiences with cannabis, whilst useful, do not give a comprehensive appraisal of the effects, nor do they allow comparison of effects across individuals receiving the same amount of drug under similar conditions. For these data, we need to turn to studies that have more rigorously assessed the effects of the drug under experimental conditions. We have selected representative studies spanning the last 50 years of such research.

Human experiments on psychomimetic effects of cannabis

In an early observational study, Ames (1958) gave 4–7 'grains' (sic) of oral cannabis to 12 medically trained volunteers, and recorded both their personal accounts of intoxication as well as the behaviours reported by non-intoxicated observers. Despite some personal differences in the experience of intoxication, all 12 volunteers reported a fairly stereotyped response, including the features detailed in Table 3.2.

Transient anxiety was also reported by some subjects, notably in the early stages of intoxication when there was an attempt to 'resist' the effects. Some subjects experienced visual hallucinations ('formed visual images, usually intricate') with eyes closed. Physical symptoms included tachycardia, postural hypotension, dry mouth, conjunctival suffusion, diuresis and paraesthesia of lips and extremities. Three subjects exposed twice to the same dose experienced the same symptoms on both exposures.

Isbell and colleagues (1967) were able to take advantage of the availability of synthetic THC to conduct studies on dose–response relationships. Subjects were former opiate addicts serving sentences for violation of US narcotic laws. They were administered various doses (120 and 480 μg/kg orally, and 50 and 200 μg/kg by smoking) of THC and the effects were measured both by questionnaire and by observation. Most subjects experienced a dose-related intensity of effects, including mood elevation, a sense of slowing of the passage of time and enhanced visual and auditory perception. At high doses, subjects reported 'marked distortion of

Table 3.2 Subjective reports of cannabis intoxication by 12 medical volunteers

• Disturbance of consciousness: this was described as a 'constriction of the field of awareness' with enhanced 'self observation'

• Disordered time perception, with a prolongation of the sense of the passage of time such that minutes 'seemed like an eternity' and subjects' estimate of time was later than actual time

• Impaired immediate recall, experienced as a 'fragmentation of thought' and apparent to observers as disjointed speech

• Mood disturbance, encompassing euphoria and often uncontrollable mirth, sometimes followed by short-lived depression

• A detachment from reality, probably best understood as depersonalization/derealization

Data from Ames (1958).

visual and auditory perception', depersonalization and derealization, and visual and auditory hallucinations. The effects were reproducible at the same doses in the same individuals upon re-exposure. Importantly, some people were vulnerable to a severe ('idiosyncratic') reaction to a relatively low dose of THC.

In a more recent observational study to explore the effects of the CB_1 receptor blocker SR141 716 on the experience of intoxication, Huestis *et al.* (2001) administered cannabis (2.64% THC) or placebo cigarettes to subjects who had received various doses of SR141 716. Peak experience of intoxication occurred within 60 min of smoking active cigarettes; 90 mg of SR141 716 reduced (by 38–43%) visual analogue scale ratings of 'how high do you feel now?'; 'how stoned on marijuana are you now?'; and 'how strong is the drug effect you feel now?' This study is the first to show in humans that the psychomimetic effects of cannabis are mediated by the CB_1 receptor.

In a study investigating the role of the dopamine system in cannabis intoxication, D'Souza *et al.* (2002) reported on the effect of pretreatment with the potent dopamine D2 receptor blocker haloperidol on the psychomimetic effects of THC in human volunteers. Ninety minutes following pretreatment with 0.05 mg/kg of haloperidol, subjects were given an intravenous dose of THC (0.035 mg/kg) or placebo. THC induced 'transient schizophrenia-like behavioural and cognitive symptoms', some of which were blocked by haloperidol, whilst others were enhanced. For further details, see Chapter 10.

Euphoria and laughter

As described above, one of the most characteristic effects of cannabis intoxication is euphoria, often associated with uncontrollable laughter. Ames and Castle (1996) point out how this infectious laughter is similar to that observed in young children. The neural mechanisms underlying this phenomenon are poorly understood. Paton and Pertwee (1973) suggested that cannabis causes 'a release of . . . the nerve networks subserving laughter' (p. 316), and they drew an analogy with the laughter associated with kuru, pseudobulbar palsy and gelastic epilepsy. In their study of patients with gelastic epilepsy, Arroya *et al.* (1993) found mirthful and mirthless forms, the mirthful one being associated with epileptic foci in the basal temporal area, whilst their patient with mirthless laughter had a focus in the left anterior cingulate. This raises the possibility that cannabis-induced mirthful laughter arises from an induced dysfunction in the basal temporal region of the brain (Ames and Castle, 1996).

An understanding of the euphoriant effect of THC has been attempted by a number of researchers. For example, Melges and colleagues (1971) gave three oral doses of THC (20, 40 and 60 mg) or placebo to eight male graduate students in random order on four separate days, each administration being separated by 1 week. Ratings of concentration (using the Present Concentration Inventory and Temporal Extension Inventory) were measured at 1.5, 3.5 and 5.5 h postingestion, and were positively correlated with mood elevation (as measured by the 'egotism', 'pleasantness', 'nonchalance' and 'social affection' subscales of the Mood Adjective Check Lists (Nowlis 1965)) in most subjects. This led these researchers to suggest that it is the 'concentration on the present' experienced by cannabis users that is, in general, associated with the drug's euphoriant effects. Of course, the small number of subjects and lack of consistent correlation between subjects limit this study.

The prominence of the euphoriant properties of cannabis begs the question of whether THC might be useful as an antidepressant. Iversen (2000) reports that one of the first medical uses of cannabis in the west was for the treatment of depression, and that such use continued until the discovery of the modern anti-depressant drugs in the 1950s. Grinspoon and Bakalar (1993) described 3 patients who found cannabis to be superior to conventional antidepressants in alleviating their depressed mood; one stated that after smoking marijuana he felt an almost immediate lightening of his mood, and subsequent regular use helped him to 'think clearly, to concentrate, and simply to enjoy the beauty of the world in a way I couldn't for years'. Other people find the anxiety and dysphoric effects outweigh the antidepressant effects, and no systematic trials of cannabis in depression provide supporting evidence for consistent antidepressant effects (Ames and Castle, 1996). Indeed, there is an association between cannabis consumption and depression, though causal pathways have not been elucidated (see Chapter 4).

Anxiety symptoms with cannabis intoxication

Cannabis is often used to relax and relieve anxiety (Reilly *et al.*, 1998; Ogborne *et al.*, 2000; Robson, 2001). Very-long-term users of cannabis report that they have continued to smoke into middle adulthood because they feel that cannabis relieves unpleasant feeling states such as anxiety and depression (Gruber *et al.*, 1997). Yet, as mentioned above, and perhaps paradoxically, anxiety and panic attacks are among the most common negative effects associated with cannabis use (Weil, 1970; Thomas, 1996; Hall and Solowij, 1998; Reilly *et al.*, 1998; Johns, 2001). These side-effects are greater in less experienced users and when large doses are consumed. There are suggestions that low doses may ameliorate anxiety, while higher doses may induce not only anxiety, but also paranoia and other positive psychotic symptoms (D'Souza *et al.*, 2002).

Cannabis use in the general population is associated with increased rates of anxiety and other mental health problems, but an association between cannabis use and overt anxiety disorder was not sustained in an epidemiological study after controlling for neuroticism, demographic and other substance use factors (Degenhardt *et al.*, 2001). Nevertheless, Troisi *et al.* (1998) found that the severity of symptoms of anxiety (and depression and alexythimia) increased as a function of the degree of involvement with cannabis, being greatest among cannabis-dependent persons. Stewart *et al.* (1997) found that cannabis use was associated with lower 'anxiety sensitivity', and Tucker and Westermeyer (1995) found fewer diagnostic criteria specific to cannabis dependence among comorbid substance use and anxiety disorder patients than in patients with substance use alone.

Clearly, smoked cannabis has the potential both to induce and to alleviate anxiety, but the factors that elicit these effects (e.g. biphasic, dose- and constituent-related), and determine individual susceptibilities to them, remain unclear. There are suggestions that anxiety and panic attacks as adverse reactions to (medicinal) cannabis are more common in the elderly, and less likely in children (Williams and Evans, 2000). There is also some suggestion that cannabidiol may reduce the anxiety induced by THC, and there is evidence that low doses of cannabidiol may operate as an antagonist at the cannabinoid (CB_1) receptor (Musty, 2002). There is speculation that CB_1 agonists (such as THC) may be anxiogenic (perhaps this is related to its propensity to induce tachycardia), while CB_1 antagonists may be anxiolytic (Musty, 2002). Huestis *et al.* (2001) reported no adverse effects from the administration of the antagonist SR141 716A to human volunteers, but they did not specifically assess anxiety. Animal research has found, on the contrary, that SR141 716A may increase anxiety-like behaviours in THC-naive rats (Navarro *et al.*, 1997). Further research is required to clarify these discrepancies.

Most recently, animal research has demonstrated involvement of the endogenous opioid system in the anxiolytic-like effects of THC (Berrendero and Maldonado, 2002), and that anxiety-like behaviours may be reduced by blockade of the enzymes involved in the breakdown of anandamide (Kathuria *et al.*, 2003); this paves the way for trialling these fatty-acid amide hydrolase (FAAH) inhibitors in human studies to treat anxiety.

Immediate effects on cognition and psychomotor functioning

Laboratory research generally supports the notion that cognition and psychomotor functioning are impaired in a dose-dependent fashion during acute intoxication after smoking or ingestion of cannabis (Solowij, 1998; Beardsley and Kelly, 1999; Heishman, 2002). Despite decades of research, however, precise data on the acute effects of cannabis remain obscure due to the variability inherent in human studies. Differences between studies may be due to differing methodologies and conditions of control in the laboratory, but inconsistencies may also arise as a function of individual variability in response to cannabis. Effects may differ in more or less experienced users, and the former may show reduced or enhanced effects due to tolerance or sensitization respectively (Beardsley and Kelly, 1999).

The evidence that cannabis slows reaction time on psychomotor tasks is mixed, and not necessarily in line with task difficulty, but it generally occurs in a dose-dependent manner. Pure sensory (e.g. critical flicker fusion) and motor functions (e.g. balance, hand steadiness, finger tapping) may be impaired or unaffected (Heishman, 2002). With an attentional component inherent in the task, choice reaction time is more consistently impaired (Heishman, 2002). Cannabis impairs focused, sustained selective and divided attention: speed and accuracy on the digit symbol substitution test have been shown to be impaired in some studies, but not others; vigilance is impaired in tasks of 30–60 min duration; at least one study showed detrimental performance on the Stroop; and speed or accuracy or both on divided attention tasks are often dose-dependently impaired under the influence of cannabis (Heishman, 2002). Impairments are seen most consistently in complex tasks requiring rapid shifts of attention; such tasks have been likened to the skills required when driving, and many studies of on-road and simulated or driving-related tasks have also demonstrated impaired performance under the influence of cannabis (Liguori et al., 1998; Kurzthaler et al., 1999). Cannabis impairs driving ability for at least an hour after smoking but there is also evidence that users are aware of their impairment and tend to compensate for it by driving more cautiously (Smiley, 1999).

As outlined above, cannabis has been shown to accelerate the 'internal clock', thereby increasing the subjective passage of time. This results in underestimation in time production tasks and overestimation in time judgement tasks. Recent animal research has confirmed the direct involvement of the endogenous cannabinoid system in the estimation of time, showing that CB_1 receptor agonists (including THC) shortened the estimation of the required response time interval, while the antagonist SR141716A lengthened the response time (Han and Robinson, 2001). Significant alterations in time sense during acute intoxication were found to be associated with decreased cerebellar blood flow (Mathew et al., 1998). It is unclear to what extent these temporal processing deficits are independent of memory dysfunction.

Memory is the function most consistently disrupted by acute cannabis intoxication. Free recall in immediate and delayed verbal learning tasks is impaired, with frequent intrusion of extraneous material (Solowij, 1998; Beardsley and Kelly, 1999; Heishman, 2002). Paired associate learning has been found to be affected in some studies but not others. Animal research has confirmed an impairing effect of cannabis on memory function through activation of cannabinoid receptors and resultant effects on other neuromodulator systems (Chaperon and Thiebot, 1999; Solowij, 2002).

Altered brain function and metabolism in humans have been demonstrated following acute and chronic use of marijuana by research utilizing cerebral blood flow (CBF), positron emission tomography (PET), and electroencephalographic (EEG) techniques (Solowij, 1998; 2002). Increased metabolism and CBF have been observed in prefrontal cortex during acute intoxication (Volkow *et al.*, 1996; Loeber and Yurgelun-Todd, 1999). In reviewing the combined literature on neuroimaging and animal receptor and neurochemical models, Loeber and Yurgelun-Todd (1999) concluded that the metabolism of component regions of the frontopontocerebellar network is altered by both acute and chronic exposure to cannabis through modulation of the cannabinoid and dopamine systems.

The impairing effects of cannabis on cognition are not severe, yet Beardsley and Kelly (1999) point out that such initially modest acute detriments in learning could 'cascade into a retarding developmental handicap in an adolescent user who progresses to chronic abuse' (p. 134). Residual effects after acute intoxication can be detected a day later (Heishman, 2002), and appear to linger for substantially longer following long-term chronic use of cannabis (see Chapter 13; Solowij, 2002).

The 'amotivational' syndrome

There is considerable debate about whether long-term cannabis abuse induces an 'amotivational syndrome'. The putative amotivational syndrome is a rather broader concept than merely cognitive impairment (the literature pertaining to cognition and schizophrenia in the long term is addressed in Chapter 13 and is not dealt with specifically here). As outlined by Schwartz (1987), the syndrome encompasses seven components, detailed in Table 3.3.

As Schwartz (1987) points out, studies from various parts of the world have reached different conclusions about the validity of this putative syndrome. Thus, some studies have presented data supporting a link between cannabis use and amotivation, whilst others have not. Mostly, such studies have been of unselected

Table 3.3 Components of the putative 'amotivational syndrome'

- Loss of interest in things in general, with associated apathy and passivity
- Loss of desire to work, and loss of concern with work performance, resulting in loss of productivity
- Loss of energy and easy fatigability
- Moodiness and irritability
- Impaired concentration
- Lack of concern for personal appearance and hygiene
- A lifestyle that prioritizes cannabis procurement and consumption

Data from Schwartz (1987).

groups of individuals, have not used rigorous diagnostic criteria and have not included a control group. In one of the few early controlled studies, Beaubrun and Knight (1973) examined 30 chronic cannabis users (at least 7 years of use) and 30 controls matched for age, sex, occupation, social class and income. There were no differences between subjects and controls in terms of mood disorder, thought disorder, mental illness and behavioural disturbance, and there was no evidence of decline in social or occupational functioning in either group.

The generalizability of the findings from this and other 'negative' studies have been questioned on the grounds that subjects were all from lower socioeconomic groups, including fishermen, farmers and unskilled and partly skilled workers. Some argue that the subtle impairments would only be seen in those engaged in more skilled work (Schwartz, 1987). However, in a study of college students, Pope *et al.* (1990) found that those who used illicit drugs (mostly cannabis) performed as well as non-users in terms of grades, athletic activities and other college activities. The users and non-users only differed on rates of attendance at a psychiatrist (18.8% versus 8.1% respectively) and having had sexual relations with at least one partner (85.8% versus 52.1% of non-users).

One of the problems with the Pope *et al.* (1990) study, however, is that amounts of cannabis consumption were not assessed, and arguably an 'amotivational syndrome' only occurs with prolonged heavy use. The study of Tennant and Groesbeck (1972) on the effects of cannabis use on US soldiers based in West Germany allowed an exploration of the effects of prolonged heavy use, as many soldiers were regular users of potent Middle-Eastern hashish (THC content of 5–10%). In 392 'occasional' users (around 10–12 g per month), essentially no long-term effects were noted. However, in 110 heavy users (dubbed 'hashoholics', using 50–600 g per month) a fairly consistent pattern emerged of apathy, listlessness, impairment of concentration and judgement and mild memory impairment. These individuals exhibited poor hygiene and slowed speech, lost interest in their personal appearance and showed a decline in job performance. Nine of these 110 soldiers were followed over several months after stopping cannabis use, and all but three showed a resolution of symptoms, with a restoration of memory function, alertness and concentration. The other three were also generally improved, but experienced occasional 'episodes of confusion'.

Thus, most of the evidence for the amotivational syndrome relies on naturalistic observational studies that inevitably have methodological limitations. In a laboratory study (Mendelson *et al.*, 1976), aimed at testing whether cannabis consumption impaired motivation to work, volunteers were assessed for productivity whilst smoking, and whilst not smoking, cannabis. In frequent users, smoking up to 12 cannabis cigarettes each day for 3 weeks had no negative impact on work output. This finding does not offer support for the amotivational syndrome, but again the dose and duration of cannabis might have been insufficient.

Another factor is that certain personality types might be predisposed to both cannabis consumption and to amotivation. For example, Dumas *et al.* (2002) assessed 232 healthy students aged 18–25 years, and found that past or occasional users, as well as heavy users, scored higher than non-users on scales measuring schizotypy; the effects were independent of anxiety and depression. Also, the literature on motivation for cannabis use (see Chapter 11) supports the notion that cannabis is used largely to alleviate negative affect (e.g. boredom, depression, lack of motivation), which might also be a factor in amotivation.

Thus, the issue of whether the amotivational syndrome is a true entity remains controversial. In reviewing this area, Castle and Ames (1996) concluded that it is probable that prolonged heavy use of cannabis can have 'amotivational' effects, but that these might reflect a subacute encephalopathy, consequent upon chronic intoxication with cannabis (being highly lipophilic, it is stored in fat cells for weeks) and reversible upon discontinuation. Hall and Solowij (1998) argued that there is therefore no need to invoke a syndrome – poor motivation may merely be symptomatic of chronic intoxication.

Conclusions

We have reviewed the acute and subacute psychomimetic properties of cannabis in humans. The effects on most users are fairly stereotyped and dose-dependent. Some of the features of intoxication have correlates with the intoxicating effects of other psychoactive compounds, and also with the so-called 'functional' psychoses. As such, the study of cannabis might enhance our understanding of the mood disorders, and of schizophrenia. The next chapter deals with the relationship between cannabis use and depression, and the following chapters focus more explicitly on the relationship with psychotic disorders.

REFERENCES

Adams, I. B. and Martin, B. R. (1996). Cannabis: pharmacology and toxicology in animals and humans. *Addiction*, **91**, 1585–1614.

Ames, F. R. (1958). A clinical and metabolic study of acute intoxication with *Cannabis sativa* and its role in the model psychoses. *J. Mental Sci.*, **104**, 972–999.

Ames, F. R. and Castle, D. J. (1996). Cannabis, mind, and mirth. *Eur. Psychiatry*, **11**, 329–334.

Arroya, S., Lesser, R. P., Gordob, B. *et al.* (1993). Mirth, laughter and gelastic seizures. *Brain*, **116**, 757–780.

Ashton, C. H. (2001). Pharmacology and effects of cannabis: a brief review. *Br. J. Psychiatry*, **178**, 101–106.

Atha, M. J. and Blanchard, S. (1997). *Regular Users. Self-Reported Consumption Patterns and Attitudes Towards Drugs Among 1333 Regular Cannabis Users.* London, UK: Independent Drug Monitoring Unit.

Beardsley, P. M. and Kelly, T. H. (1999). Acute effects of cannabis on human behavior and central nervous system functions. In *The Health Effects of Cannabis*, ed. H. Kalant, W. Corrigall, W. Hall and R. Smart, pp. 129–169. Toronto: Addiction Research Foundation, Centre for Addiction and Mental Health.

Beaubrun, M. H., and Knight, F. (1973). Psychiatric assessment of 30 chronic users of cannabis and 30 matched controls. *Am. J. Psychiatry*, **130**, 309–311.

Berke, J. and Hernton, C. (1974). *The Cannabis Experience.* London: Quartet Books.

Berrendero, F. and Maldonado, R. (2002). Involvement of the opioid system in the anxiolytic-like effects induced by delta (9)-tetrahydrocannabinol. *Psychopharmacology*, **163**, 111–117.

Castle, D. J. and Ames, F. R. (1996). Cannabis and the brain. *Aust. NZ J. Psychiatry*, **30**, 179–183.

Chaperon, F. and Thiebot, M. H. (1999). Behavioral effects of cannabinoid agents in animals. *Crit. Rev. Neurobiol.*, **13**, 243–281.

Degenhardt, L., Hall, W. and Lynskey, M. (2001). Alcohol, cannabis and tobacco use among Australians: a comparison of their associations with other drug use and use disorders, affective and anxiety disorders, and psychosis. *Addiction*, **96**, 1603–1614.

D'Souza, D. C., Wray, Y., MacDougall, L. *et al.* (2002). Cannabinoid–dopamine interactions and psychosis: effects of haloperidol in a cannabinoid 'model' psychosis. *Schizophrenia Res.*, **53**, 252–253.

Dumas, P., Saoud, M., Bouafia, S. *et al.* (2002). Cannabis use correlates with schizotypal personality traits in healthy students. *Psychiatry Res.*, **109**, 27–35.

Goode, E. (1970). *The Marijuana Smokers.* New York: Basic Books.

Grinspoon, L. and Bakalar, J. B. (1993). *Marihuana, the Forbidden Medicine.* New Haven, CT: Yale University Press.

Gruber, A. J., Pope, H. G. and Oliva, P. (1997). Very long-term users of marijuana in the United States: a pilot study. *Substance Use Misuse*, **32**, 249–264.

Hall, W. and Solowij, N. (1998). Adverse effects of cannabis. *Lancet*, **352**, 1611–1616.

Han, C. J. and Robinson, J. K. (2001). Cannabinoid modulation of time estimation in the rat. *Behavi. Neurosci.*, **115**, 243–246.

Heishman, S. J. (2002). Effects of marijuana on human performance and assessment of driving impairment. In *Biology of Marijuana: From Gene to Behaviour*, ed. E. S. Onaivi, pp. 308–332. New York: Taylor and Francis.

Huestis, M. A., Gorelick, D. A., Heishman, S. J. *et al.* (2001). Blockade of effects of smoked marijuana by the CB_1-selective cannabinoid receptor antagonist SR141716. *Arch. Gen. Psychiatry*, **58**, 322–328.

Isbell, H., Gorodetzsky, C. W., Jasinski, D. *et al.* (1967). Effects of delta-9-*trans*-tetrahydrocannabinol in man. *Psychopharmacologia*, **11**, 184–188.

Iversen, L. L. (2000). *The Science of Marijuana*. Oxford: Oxford University Press.

Johns, A. (2001). Psychiatric effects of cannabis. *Br. J. Psychiatry*, **178**, 116–122.

Kathuria, S., Gaetani, S., Fegley, D. *et al.* (2003). Modulation of anxiety through blockade of anandamide hydrolysis. *Nature Med.*, **9**, 76–81.

Kurzthaler, I., Hummer, M., Miller, C. *et al.* (1999). Effect of cannabis use on cognitive functions and driving ability. *J. Clin. Psychiatry*, **60**, 395–399.

Liguori, A., Gatto, C. P. and Robinson, J. H. (1998). Effects of marijuana on equilibrium, psychomotor performance and simulated driving. *Behav. Pharmacol.*, **9**, 599–609.

Loeber, R. T. and Yurgelun-Todd, D. A. (1999). Human neuroimaging of acute and chronic marijuana use: implications for frontocerebellar dysfunction. *Human Psychopharmacol. Clin. Exp.*, **14**, 291–301.

Ludlow, F. H. (1857). *The Hasheesh Eater: Being Passages from the Life of a Pythagorean*. New York: Harper.

Marshall, C. R. (1897). The active principle of Indian hemp: a preliminary communication. *Lancet*, **i**, 235–238.

Mathew, R. J., Wilson, W. H., Turkington, T. G. and Coleman, R. E. (1998). Cerebellar activity and disturbed time sense after THC. *Brain Res.*, **797**, 183–189.

Melges, F. T., Tinklenberg, J. R., Hollister, L. E. and Gillespie, H. K. (1971). Marijuana and the temporal span of awareness. *Arch. Gen. Psychiatry*, **24**, 564–567.

Mendelson, J. H., Kuehnle, J. C., Greenberg, I. and Mello, N. K. (1976). Operant acquisition of marihuana in man. *J. Pharmacol. Exp. Ther.*, **198**, 42–53.

Musty, R. E. (2002). Cannabinoid therapeutic potential in motivational processes, psychological disorders and central nervous system disorders. In *Biology of Marijuana: From Gene to Behavior*, ed. E. S. Onaivi, pp. 45–74. London: Taylor & Francis.

Navarro, M., Hernandez, E., Munoz, R. M. *et al.* (1997). Acute administration of the CB_1 cannabinoid receptor antagonist SR141716A induces anxiety-like responses in the rat. *Neuroreport*, **8**, 491–496.

Nowlis, V. (1965). Research with the mood adjective check list. In *Affect, Cognition, and Personality*, ed. S. Tomkins and C. Isard, pp. 352–389. New York: Springer.

O'Brien, C. P. (1996). Drug addiction and drug abuse. In *Goodman and Gilman's The Pharmacological Basis of Therapeutics* 9th edn, ed. J. G. Hardman, L. E. Limbird, P. B. Molinoff, R. W. Ruddon and A. G. Gilman, pp. 557–577. New York: McGraw-Hill.

Ogborne, A. C., Smart, R. G., Weber, T. and Birchmore-Timney, C. (2000). Who is using cannabis as a medicine and why: an exploratory study? *J. Psychoact. Drugs*, **32**, 435–443.

Paton, W. D. M. and Pertwee, R. G. (1973). The actions of cannabis in man. In *Marihuana*, ed. R. Mechoulam, pp. 287–333. New York: Academic Press.

Pope, H. G., Ionescu-Pioggia, M., Aizley, H. G. and Varma, D. K. (1990). Drug use and life style among college undergraduates in 1989: a comparison with 1969 and 1978. *Am. J. Psychiatry*, **147**, 998–1001.

Reilly, D., Didcott, P., Swift, W. and Hall, W. (1998). Long-term cannabis use: characteristics of users in an Australian rural area. *Addiction*, **93**, 837–846.

Robson, P. (2001). Therapeutic aspects of cannabis and cannabinoids. *Br. J. Psychiatry*, **178**, 107–115.

Schwartz, R. H. (1987). Marijuana: an overview. *Pediatr. Clin. North Am.*, **34**, 305–317.

Smiley, A. (1999). Marijuana: on-road and driving simulator studies. In *The Health Effects of Cannabis*, ed. H. Kalant, W. Corrigal, W. Hall and R. Smart, pp. 173–191. Toronto: Addiction Research Foundation, Centre for Addiction and Mental Health.

Solowij, N. (1998). *Cannabis and Cognitive Functioning*. Cambridge: Cambridge University Press.
  (2002). Cannabis and cognitive functioning. In *Biology of Marijuana: From Gene to Behaviour*, ed. E. S. Onaivi, pp. 308–332. New York: Taylor and Francis.

Stewart, S. H., Karp, J., Pihl, R. O. and Peterson, R. A. (1997). Anxiety sensitivity and self-reported reasons for drug use. *J. Substance Abuse*, **9**, 223–240.

Tennant, F. S. and Groesbeck, C. J. (1972). Psychiatric effects of hashish. *Arch. Gen. Psychiatry*, **27**, 133–136.

Thomas, H. (1996). A community survey of adverse effects of cannabis use. *Drug Alcohol Depend.*, **42**, 201–207.

Troisi, A., Pasini, A., Saracco, M. and Spalletta, G. (1998). Psychiatric symptoms in male cannabis users not using other illicit drugs. *Addiction*, **93**, 487–492.

Tucker, P. and Westermeyer, J. (1995). Substance-abuse in patients with comorbid anxiety disorder – a comparative study. *Am. J. Addict.*, **4**, 226–233.

Volkow, N. D., Gillespie, H., Mullani, N. *et al.* (1996). Brain glucose-metabolism in chronic marijuana users at baseline and during marijuana intoxication. *Psychiatry Res.: Neuroimaging*, **67**, 29–38.

Weil, A. (1970). Adverse reactions to marihuana. *N. Engl. J. Med.*, **282**, 997–1000.

Williams, E. M. and Evans, F. J. (2000). Cannabinoids in clinical practice. *Drugs*, **60**, 1303–1314.

The association between cannabis use and depression: a review of the evidence

Louisa Degenhardt[1], Wayne Hall[2], Michael Lynskey[3], Carolyn Coffey[4] and George Patton[4]

[1] University of New South Wales, Sydney, NSW, Australia
[2] University of Queensland, St Lucia, QLD, Australia
[3] Washington University School of Medicine, St Louis, MO, USA
[4] Murdoch Children's Research Institute, Parkville, VIC, Australia

Introduction

The association between cannabis and depression has not received as much attention as the links between cannabis use and psychosis. One of the reasons may be that the depressed are much less likely to come to the attention of treatment services than are those who are psychotic. Furthermore, some symptoms of cannabis dependence may mimic those of depression and so comorbid depression may go undiagnosed.

Rising rates of cannabis use (Donnelly and Hall, 1994; Hall et al., 1999; Degenhardt et al., 2000; Johns, 2001), depression (Andrews et al., 1998; Cicchetti and Toth, 1998) and suicide among young adults (Diekstra et al., 1995; Lynskey et al., 2000) have increased public concern about the role of substance abuse, including cannabis, in non-psychotic mental disorders. There has also been increasing advocacy for interventions to prevent and treat problematic cannabis use and depressed mood among young people. Given these parallel rises, recent speculation that the two may be linked is understandable.

Given the high prevalence of both cannabis use and depression there remains a question why any comorbid relationship has received little clinical attention? It may reflect a *lack* of association between the two. However, until recently, there was disagreement as to whether cannabis dependence (or problematic cannabis use) existed, with few treatments available. A lack of clinical attention may therefore have simply reflected a lack of services that might have detected an association. Lastly, due to its illegal status, cannabis use may remain unreported by clients presenting with depression.

Marijuana and Madness: Psychiatry and Neurobiology, ed. D. Castle and R. Murray. Published by Cambridge University Press. © Cambridge University Press 2004.

Some have suggested that cannabis use may be a contributory cause of depression and suicidal behaviours (Holden and Pakula, 2001; Johns, 2001). This hypothesis has some research support. A toxicological analysis of suicides in the USA detected cannabis in 16% of cases in California over a 2-year period, and 7% of cases in Alabama (Dhossche *et al.*, 2001) (although there were no analyses of the comparative rates of positive tests in the general population at any one point in time). A case-control study in New Zealand found higher rates of cannabis abuse/dependence among those who made serious suicide attempts (16%) than among controls (2%) (Beautrais *et al.*, 1999). The causal hypothesis would be consistent with the parallel increases in cannabis use among young adults (Degenhardt *et al.*, 2000) and in suicide rates among young males (Diekstra *et al.*, 1995; Lynskey *et al.*, 2000).

Given these concerns, this chapter evaluates the nature of the relationship between cannabis use and depression by addressing the following questions:

• Is there evidence of the association between cannabis use and depression?
• If there is, what are the potential explanations for the association?
• What evidence is needed to test these different explanations?
• What are the public health implications of the evidence to date?

Comorbidity between cannabis use and depression

Comorbidity has been defined by Feinstein as 'any distinct clinical entity that has co-existed or that may occur during the clinical course of a patient who has the index disease under study' (Feinstein, 1970, pp. 456–457). Within psychiatry, comorbidity is commonly used to refer to the overlap of two or more psychiatric disorders (Boyd *et al.*, 1984). However, as will become apparent in the following review, much of the research examining associations between cannabis use and depression have been studies which have examined relatively infrequent, low-level cannabis use. This distinction is one that will be further discussed later in the chapter.

Clinical samples

Case histories reporting associations between cannabis use and depressed mood have been reported in clinical literature for some decades (Pond, 1948; Ablon and Goodwin, 1974). The type of case reports has varied: some report persons developing *manic* symptoms after using cannabis (Stoll *et al.*, 1991; Bowers, 1998); some have reported cannabis being used as an antidepressant (Zelwer, 1994) while others have reported that persons with mania or bipolar disorder have used cannabis to *moderate* their manic symptoms (Grinspoon and Bakalar, 1998).

There is a very small literature on cannabis use in clinical populations with affective disorders. In one study of depressed outpatients, a history of substance use disorders was associated with a greater number of depressive episodes (Alpert *et al.*, 1994) but there was no difference in age of onset of depression, or in severity of depression at assessment (Alpert *et al.*, 1994). Studies of persons with bipolar disorder (Estroff *et al.*, 1985; Miller *et al.*, 1989; Brady *et al.*, 1991; Marken *et al.*, 1992; Mueser *et al.*, 1992; Sonne *et al.*, 1994) have found reported rates of cannabis abuse between 3% (Sonne *et al.*, 1994) and 19% (Marken *et al.*, 1992). Among a sample of heroin-dependent persons in methadone treatment, daily cannabis users reported the highest rates of depression (compared to occasional and non-users of cannabis; Bell *et al.*, 1995; Best *et al.*, 1999).

Convenience samples

Findings from convenience samples in the community have provided conflicting evidence on the association between cannabis use and depression. One study of a sample of persons from a primary care population found that *among females only*, lifetime use of cannabis more than five times doubled the risk of depression (Rowe *et al.*, 1995). One study of a sample of 88 high school seniors found that cannabis use was associated with greater suicidal ideation (Field *et al.*, 2001).

In contrast, a study of university students aged 19–21 years found no differences between light and heavy users in the number of depressive symptoms they reported (Musty and Kaback, 1995). Similarly, a study of high school students found that neither depression nor suicidal ideation was associated with the use of cannabis, tobacco or alcohol (Galaif *et al.*, 1998). One study used a sample of cannabis users attending college, with two groups: 45 'heavy users' (used cannabis daily for at least 2 years) and 44 'occasional users' (users who had never used cannabis more than 10 times per month; Kouri *et al.*, 1995); there were no significant differences between the groups for any psychiatric diagnoses.

A study of male army draftees using cannabis but no other illicit drugs found a relationship between increasing involvement with cannabis use (use, abuse and dependence) and increasing depression scores (Troisi *et al.*, 1998). However, the study did not compare these patterns to the rates of disorder among draftees who did not use cannabis or to draftees who used cannabis and other illicit drugs, who would presumably form a large proportion of cannabis users (Kandel *et al.*, 1997). In contrast, there was no association between the frequency of cannabis use and depression among a population sample of young adult males (Green and Ritter, 2000).

A study of young adults (aged 20 years) which grouped participants according to cannabis use (abstainers, experimenters and 'heavy' users) found that cannabis users had higher levels of depression (Milich *et al.*, 2000). However, these groups differed in more ways than their frequency of cannabis use. Heavy users were defined as those who had used cannabis at least 40 times *and at least one other illicit drug;*

experimenters had used cannabis less than 10 times and had not used more than one other illicit drug; and abstainers had not used cannabis or any other illicit drugs.

It is difficult for several reasons to project the findings of these studies to the general population. First, some of the samples were extremely small. Second, it is unclear how representative the samples were of the populations from which they came. Third, many of the groups sampled were specific populations such as college students (Kouri *et al.*, 1995), young adult males (Green and Ritter, 2000), army draftees (Troisi *et al.*, 1998) or commune members (Zablocki *et al.*, 1991). Fourth, some studies grouped participants so that they differed in drug use patterns other than cannabis use (Shedler and Block, 1990; Milich *et al.*, 2000), while other studies did not compare cannabis users with non-users (Zablocki *et al.*, 1991; Kouri *et al.*, 1995; Troisi *et al.*, 1998), or with those who used other drug types (Troisi *et al.*, 1998).

Representative samples of the general population

While such evidence suggests that there may be a 'greater than chance' association between cannabis use and depression, clinical samples are ill-suited to examining the question of whether comorbidity exists between the two. This is because it is not possible, using clinical samples, to distinguish between 'artefactual' comorbidity and 'true' comorbidity (Caron and Rutter, 1991). *Artefactual* comorbidity is comorbidity that arises because of the ways in which samples are selected or the behaviour is conceptualized, measured and classified. For example, artefactual comorbidity is made more likely if the criteria used to classify two disorders are the same or similar. *True* comorbidity refers to the actual co-occurrence of two separate conditions at a rate higher than expected by chance.

There are a number of reasons, related to sampling biases, which make artefactual comorbidity more likely in research in clinical populations. The first is Berkson's bias (Berkson, 1946). This refers to the fact that if a person has two disorders at a given point in time, then they are more likely to receive treatment simply because there are two separate disorders for which the person might seek help. Empirical work has demonstrated the existence of this bias (Roberts *et al.*, 1978).

The second reason is clinical bias (Galbaud Du Fort *et al.*, 1993). This refers to the fact that persons who have two disorders may be more likely to seek treatment *because* they have two disorders. Again, this source of bias has been demonstrated empirically (Galbaud Du Fort *et al.*, 1993).

Third, referral biases may exist, whereby some persons will be referred for treatment because of other background factors, such as having a family history of psychopathology. This may make it more likely that persons who are so referred will have a number of different mental health problems (Caron and Rutter, 1991).

In order to minimize the effects of sampling and selection biases, it is best to study the patterns of association between cannabis use and depression in representative samples of the general population (Berkson, 1946; Caron and Rutter, 1991; Galbaud Du Fort *et al.*, 1993). A number of large-scale surveys have examined associations between substance use disorders (including cannabis) and other mental disorders in the USA and other developed countries.

Recently, Chen and colleagues analysed the US National Comorbidity Survey data with a specific focus on cannabis use and major depressive episodes (Chen *et al.*, 2002). They found that a greater number of occasions of cannabis use were associated with a higher risk of having experienced a major depressive episode; and that lifetime cannabis dependence as defined by the American Psychiatric Association's classification system for mental disorders, the *Diagnostic and Statistical Manual of Mental Disorders* (*DSM*-III-R): American Psychiatric Association, was associated with a 3.4 times increased risk of major depression: 9.5% of those who had experienced a major depressive episode met criteria for cannabis dependence, compared to 4% of those who had never experienced such an episode (Chen *et al.*, 2002).

Grant (1995) found that persons meeting criteria for *DSM*-IV (American Psychiatric Association, 1994) cannabis abuse or dependence within the past year had 6.4 times the odds of meeting criteria for *DSM*-IV major depression than those without major depression (29% and 14%, compared to 3% overall).

Degenhardt and colleagues examined the relationship between different levels of cannabis use (no use, use, abuse or dependence) and depression in the Australian National Survey of Mental Health and Well-Being (NSMHWB). They found that those who were more heavily involved with cannabis use were more likely to meet criteria for *DSM*-IV mood disorders (Degenhardt *et al.*, 2001). Cannabis users were between two and three times more likely to meet criteria for a mood disorder than non-users and the prevalence of such disorders increased from 6% among non-users to 14% among those who met criteria for cannabis dependence.

The findings in adult samples have been mirrored by those in representative samples of adolescents and young adults. Research on drug use and mental disorders in a representative sample of Australians aged 13–17 years found that those who had *ever* used cannabis were three times more likely than those who had never used cannabis to meet criteria for depression (Rey *et al.*, 2002).

Fergusson and colleagues examined the association between cannabis use and major depression using data from a birth cohort of 1265 children born in mid-1977 in Christchurch, New Zealand (Fergusson *et al.*, unpublished manuscript; Fergusson and Horwood, 1997). They found that adolescents who had used cannabis 10 or more times by the age of 15–16 years were more likely also to meet criteria for a mood disorder at that age: 11% of those who had never used cannabis met such criteria, compared to 18% of those who had used cannabis 1–9 times, and 36% of those who had used it 10 or more times (Fergusson and Horwood, 1997). At age 20–21 years, 30% of those who were using cannabis at least weekly met criteria for depression, compared to 15% of those who did not use cannabis at that age (Fergusson et al., unpublished manuscript).

Similarly, the Zurich cohort study of young people (assembled when they were 20 years of age) found that, by age 30 years, those who met criteria for depression over the period of the study were 2.3 times more likely to report weekly cannabis use during this time (Angst, 1996).

A study by Patton and colleagues using a representative cohort of young adults (aged 20–21 years) in Victoria found that 68% of females who reported daily cannabis use in the past year were depressed – an odds of 8.6 compared to non-users (Patton et al., 2002). No other level of cannabis use was associated with an increased risk of depression and among males there was *no* association between cannabis use in the past year and depression (Patton et al., 2002).

In one cohort of American adolescents, those who had experimented with cannabis reported *better* social adjustment than those who had never used cannabis and those who were heavy cannabis users (Shedler and Block, 1990). This U-shaped curve needs to be considered within its social context: because this cohort had very high rates of cannabis use, the authors suggested that never having tried cannabis was an indicator of poor social adjustment, anxiety and emotional constriction, as was heavy cannabis use, while experimentation was an indicator of being socially well adjusted (Shedler and Block, 1990).

Two other US longitudinal studies have reported conflicting results. Brook and colleagues (Brook et al., 1998) found no relationship between cannabis use and *DSM*-III-R depressive disorders over 10 years of follow-up. In contrast, a study of students aged 12–14 years found that those reporting lifetime cannabis use had higher depression scores, and 42% met criteria for *DSM*-IV major depression at some point in their lives (Kelder et al., 2001).

Summary

There is increasing evidence that regular cannabis use and depression occur together more often than we might expect by chance. While not all studies have found a significant association, the weight of evidence indicates that there is an increased risk of depression among persons who report heavy cannabis use.

What explains the association between cannabis use and depression?

There are a number of reasons why cannabis use and depression might be associated (Caron and Rutter, 1991; Klein and Riso, 1994; Kessler, 1995; Neale and

Kendler, 1995): (1) cannabis use may be a contributory cause of depression (e.g. cannabis use precipitates depression); (2) depression may be a contributory cause of cannabis use (e.g. if depressed, individuals use cannabis to improve their mood); and (3) there is no direct relationship between the two and the association is explained by shared risk factors that increase the risk of both disorders.

Cannabis use causes depression

Heavy cannabis use could precipitate depression in at least two ways: (1) cannabis intoxication could produce depression indirectly by impairing psychological adjustment; or (2) large doses of the active ingredient of cannabis, Δ^9-tetrahydrocannabinol (Δ^9-THC), could affect serotonin and other neurotransmitters in a way that produces depressive symptoms.

Popular concerns about the effects of cannabis use on depression often implicitly assume the second of these hypotheses. There is as yet no animal model to support this contention but it is a hypothesis that cannot be excluded. None the less, this is not the only potential mechanism for a causal link between cannabis use and depression. Cannabis use may set in train a cascade of life events, such as leaving school early, early unplanned parenthood and reduced earning capacity, that in turn predispose to depression.

Evidence in support of either form of this hypothesis would include evidence from controlled studies: (1) that cannabis or Δ^9-THC worsens or does not improve mood; (2) that persons who use cannabis in adolescence are more likely to develop depression during early adulthood; (3) that persons who are depressed at baseline are *no* more likely to become cannabis users during a follow-up period; and (4) that associations between cannabis use and depression are not explained by potentially confounding variables.

Depression causes cannabis use

Most advocates of the notion that depression leads to cannabis use invoke the self-medication hypothesis, according to which persons who are depressed use cannabis to relieve their symptoms of depression (Mueser *et al.*, 1998). Research on self-reported reasons for substance use has provided some support for this idea (e.g. Warner *et al.* (1994); and see Chapter 11) but it can be argued that alleviating dysphoria is simply one among many factors – such as poor social skills, poor social functioning and peer group influences – that increase the likelihood of both substance use and mental disorders (Mueser *et al.*, 1998).

The self-medication hypothesis would be supported by evidence from controlled studies that: (1) cannabis or Δ^9-THC improves mood; (2) persons who are depressed at baseline are more likely to begin, continue or increase their cannabis use during follow-up; (3) persons who are cannabis users at baseline are no more likely to become depressed during follow-up; and (4) the associations in (2) are not explained by confounding variables.

Common factors increase the risk of both depression and cannabis use

The association between cannabis use and depression may arise because the same factors that predispose people to use cannabis also increase their risks of depression (Caron and Rutter, 1991; Kessler, 1995; Mueser *et al.*, 1998). These common factors might include biological, personality, social and environmental factors, or a combination of these factors.

This is a plausible hypothesis because there is a wealth of evidence that there are risk factors that are common to both mental and substance use disorders. For example, social disadvantage is more common among persons who are problematic substance users (Institute of Medicine, 1996) and who meet criteria for depressive disorders (Weissman *et al.*, 1991; Kessler *et al.*, 1994; Blazer, 1995). There are also higher rates of separation and divorce, and lower rates of being married or in a de facto relationship among persons with mental and substance use disorders (Jablensky *et al.* 1991; Weissman *et al.*, 1991; Kessler *et al.*, 1994; Blazer, 1995). Other factors that have been associated with both cannabis use disorders and depression include parental psychiatric illness and family dysfunction (Rutter, 1987; Velez *et al.*, 1989; Fergusson *et al.*, 1990; 1994).

If common risk factors explain the association between cannabis use and depression, then they would no longer be associated after these risk factors were taken into account. This explanation would be supported by evidence from controlled studies that: (1) the administration of cannabis or Δ^9-THC does not affect mood; (2) there is no temporal relationship between cannabis use and depressed mood (i.e. that cannabis use does not predict depression at a later point in time, and vice versa); and (3) the association between cannabis use and depression did not persist after statistical control for confounding or common risk factors.

A review of relevant evidence
Studies of the effects of cannabis use upon mood

Cannabis users often report increased well-being, euphoria and contentment after using cannabis (Hall *et al.*, 2001; and see Chapter 3) but controlled studies have not consistently shown that regular cannabis use affects mood for better or worse. One study found that cannabis had no effect upon mood in experienced cannabis users, while significantly worsening mood in inexperienced users (Mathew *et al.*, 1989). Controlled studies of persons with depression have found that THC significantly increases dysphoria (Pond, 1948; Ablon and Goodwin, 1974), while another found that Δ^9-THC given to a small sample of severely depressed inpatients did not improve depressed mood (Kotin *et al.*, 1973).

Cross-sectional surveys of the general population

Cross-sectional surveys may use multivariate statistical analysis to examine whether common factors explain any association observed between cannabis use and depression. In the Australian NSMHWB, for example, the observed relationship between cannabis use and depression among adults did not remain significant in multiple regression analyses that adjusted for potential confounders (Degenhardt *et al.*, 2001). Specifically, the relationship disappeared after controlling for alcohol, tobacco and other drug use and for neuroticism. This suggests that the association arose because cannabis users were more likely to meet criteria for an alcohol use disorder; to smoke tobacco regularly; to use other drug types; and to have higher neuroticism scores.

In the Australian child and adolescent survey, the increased risks of depression among lifetime cannabis users remained significant after statistical adjustment for confounders but the risk was reduced to 2 and the lower limit of the 95% confidence interval was close to 1 (Rey *et al.*, 2002). Among those who had used cannabis 10 or more times in the past month, this association was stronger, with a threefold increase in risk of depression (Rey *et al.*, 2001). A weak association observed between early initiation of cannabis use and depression among a sample of adult males was not significant after controlling for educational attainment, marital status, alcohol and tobacco use (Green and Ritter, 2000). Similarly, other research has found that, after accounting for demographics and other drug use, associations between cannabis use and depression no longer remain (Rowe *et al.*, 1995).

The use of longitudinal research to examine questions about causality

Longitudinal studies provide a more informative way to examine relationships between cannabis use and depression (Caron and Rutter, 1991; Merikangas and Angst, 1995). Evidence from such studies is reviewed in two sections: the first examines whether depression at one point in time predicts later cannabis use and the second examines whether cannabis use at one point in time predicts later depression. In each case, the 'common cause' hypothesis is examined by multivariate adjustment for confounders.

Does cannabis use predict later depression?

The results of longitudinal studies addressing this issue have not been wholly consistent, but the majority have found that *regular* early-onset cannabis use is associated with an increased risk of later depression.

Among the earliest work is that of Kandel and colleagues (1986) who followed up a cohort of adolescents in New York state. They found that cannabis use at age 15–16 years was *not* associated with depressive symptoms at age 24–25 years.

However, they did find that greater involvement with cannabis was associated with a lower degree of life satisfaction, and a higher chance of consulting a mental health professional or being hospitalized for a psychiatric disorder (Kandel, 1984). A study of a birth cohort from Dunedin, New Zealand, found that cannabis use by age 15 years was *not* associated with an increased risk of a mental disorder (depression, anxiety disorders, substance dependence or antisocial personality disorder) at age 18 years (McGee *et al.*, 2000).

The most comprehensive examination of the 'common cause' hypothesis has been conducted by Fergusson and colleagues using data on a wide range of possible confounding variables collected on a birth cohort followed from birth to young adulthood (Fergusson and Horwood, 2001). In an early report, the use of cannabis 10 or more times by age 15–16 years was *not* associated with either major depression or suicide attempts at age 16–18 years after controlling for the effects of confounding individual, familial, peer and sociodemographic variables (Fergusson and Horwood, 1997).

Fergusson and colleagues have more recently re-examined the association between cannabis use during adolescence and depression, suicidal ideation and suicide attempts at the age of 21 years (Fergusson *et al.*, unpublished manuscript). They examined the effects of heavier patterns of cannabis use than in their earlier study. They found that at age 20–21 years, 30% of those using cannabis weekly or more often met criteria for depression, compared to 15% of those who did not use cannabis at that age. They carried out fixed-effects regressions that adjusted for sociodemographic and individual factors, adverse life events, peer affiliation, school- and home-leaving age and alcohol dependence. The adjustments reduced the association substantially but a significant association remained between cannabis use during adolescence and depression, suicidal ideation and suicide attempts in the same year. After adjustment, at least weekly cannabis use in a given year was associated with a 1.7 times greater risk of reporting depression in the same year. For suicidal ideation and suicide attempts, there was an interaction between cannabis use and age: the association between weekly cannabis use in a given year and suicidal ideation/attempts in the same year was highest among those aged 14–15 years. This association declined as the cohort aged, so that by 20–21 years there was no significant association with weekly cannabis use.

Recently, similar analyses have been reported from an Australian cohort of adolescents who were followed up into young adulthood to examine the link between early-onset *regular* cannabis use and early adulthood depression (Patton *et al.*, 2002). It found that among *females only*, weekly cannabis use in adolescence predicted a twofold increase in rates of depression at 20–21 years, while daily use predicted a fourfold increased risk. These relationships were adjusted for confounding factors including sociodemographic variables, alcohol use, gender and antisocial behaviour.

The only prospective study examining the relationship between cannabis use and depression in *adulthood* was recently reported by Bovasso. This study used data from a follow-up of the Baltimore site of the Epidemiological Catchment Area study in which a subsample of 1920 people from the original 1980 study were reassessed 14–16 years later (Bovasso, 2001). Those who reported cannabis use and at least one symptom of cannabis abuse/dependence at baseline were 4.5 times more likely to report depressive symptoms and 4.6 times more likely to report suicidal ideation in the follow-up period than those who were 'non-abusers'. This relationship remained after adjusting for baseline depressive symptoms and demographic variables (Bovasso, 2001). Approximately 4% of those who reported depressive symptoms during the follow-up period had met criteria for cannabis abuse at baseline, compared to 1% of those who did not report depressive symptoms.

Does depression predict later cannabis use?

A number of longitudinal studies of representative samples of children and adolescents, or birth cohorts, have examined the association between depression and later cannabis use. In general, these studies have failed to find a significant association.

Paton and colleagues found no significant relationship between depressive mood and cannabis use either cross-sectionally or prospectively (over 6 months of follow-up) in a cohort of adolescents (16–17 years) from New York state (Paton *et al.*, 1977). However, they did find that depressed mood was related to the *onset* of cannabis use among those who had not used it previously (Paton *et al.*, 1977). In a later analysis, Kandel and Davies (1986) found that depression at age 16–17 years was not associated with higher rates of cannabis use at age 24–25 years. Indeed, males with depression at the first assessment were *less* likely to have used cannabis than those without a history of depression. Later analyses of this cohort revealed that, at age 34–35 years, depression at age 15–16 years was *not* associated with either early onset or current heavy cannabis use (Kandel and Chen, 2000).

A study of a cohort of African-American students followed from grade 6 to grade 10 found that depression in sixth grade was not associated with subsequent cannabis use (Miller-Johnson *et al.*, 1998). Similarly, a study of a cohort of Dutch children found that depression did not predict later substance dependence (including cannabis) (Hofstra *et al.*, 2002). The Dunedin, New Zealand, birth cohort study analysed the relationships between depression at age 15 years and alcohol or cannabis dependence at age 21 years in females (Bardone *et al.*, 1998). There was no significant association between the early-onset depression and later cannabis dependence, with or without statistically controlling for covariates.

A longitudinal study of children with prepubertal major depression found that there was no significant association with drug abuse or dependence by the time they were in their mid to late 20s (Weissman *et al.*, 1999). The same results were found by Brook and colleagues when they analysed the association between adolescent depression and later cannabis use (ranging from 'light' to 'heavy'), after controlling for age and gender (Brook *et al.*, 1998). Most recently, Patton and colleagues analysed the strength of association between depression between ages 14 and 18 and use of cannabis either weekly or daily at age 20–21 years (Patton *et al.*, 2002). There was no significant relationship between adolescent depression and weekly or daily cannabis use in young adulthood, after adjusting for sociodemographic variables, alcohol use, gender, adolescent cannabis use and antisocial behaviour. The Bovasso study cited above also found that, among those who did not meet criteria for cannabis abuse at baseline, depressive symptoms at baseline did not significantly predict an increased risk of cannabis abuse during follow-up (Bovasso, 2001).

Summary

Cross-sectional and longitudinal studies have provided mixed evidence on the nature of the association between cannabis use and depression. Cross-sectional studies have suggested that the relationship can be explained by other factors, such as the use of other drugs. Longitudinal studies have suggested that the 'self-medication' hypothesis does not fit the pattern of cannabis use over time *among cohorts of adolescents and young adults.* There is some evidence that heavy cannabis use increases the risk of depression during follow-up, and that this relationship is partly, but not *completely,* explained by confounding variables.

The Bovasso study (Bovasso, 2001) allows some estimation of the population attributable risk for this association. Approximately 67% of those with cannabis abuse but no depressive symptoms at baseline developed depression *during 14–16 years of follow-up*, compared to 31% of those without cannabis abuse (it is not clear why Bovasso only examined cannabis abuse, and not dependence). The number of persons who met criteria for cannabis abuse at baseline without also reporting depressive symptoms was extremely small (only 15 out of 849 who did not report depressive symptoms at baseline).

As a result, 0.6% of the sample developed depressive symptoms over 14–16 years, *possibly* as a consequence of their cannabis use. These figures are likely to be overestimates of the effect of problematic cannabis use as they assume a strong causal relationship when a variety of potentially confounding factors were not assessed in the study. Given current rates of cannabis use, assuming that the link is causal, then 1.9% of the depressive symptoms that developed over 15 years could be attributed to cannabis abuse. Thus, in a population in which problematic cannabis use is uncommon (as is still the case in most developed countries), then heavy cannabis use may explain only a small proportion of depression in the population. These estimates of attributable risk need to be improved upon in future longitudinal studies.

Implications for future research

Our review of the literature has identified a number of limitations in the available research on cannabis use and depression. In the following section, we outline these limitations, and make suggestions for ways in which future research might overcome them.

Measurement of cannabis use

Limitations with the measurement of cannabis use in previous research include the following. First, some epidemiological studies have grouped cannabis with other drugs (Anthony and Helzer, 1991; Kessler *et al.*, 1996), so it is not clear what contribution has been made by cannabis use. Second, some studies have grouped cannabis abuse and dependence into 'use disorders' (Anthony and Helzer, 1991), although some epidemiological research has examined cannabis abuse and dependence separately for comorbidity with major depression (Grant, 1995; Degenhardt *et al.*, 2001). Third, some studies have examined only cannabis *use* without distinguishing between increasing levels of involvement (Abel, 1971; Gale and Guenther, 1971; Shedler and Block, 1990; Zablocki *et al.*, 1991; Gruber *et al.*, 1997; Milich *et al.*, 2000).

It is also important to consider the *level* of cannabis use. It has been most typical to examine patterns of comorbidity between the problematic or regular use of drugs, and other mental health problems, most probably because it is at higher levels of use that we might expect to see associations with other problems, and the clinical concept of comorbidity itself imports the co-occurrence of two *disorders*.

In support of this distinction between low level or lifetime use and regular/problematic use, studies reporting relatively low levels of cannabis use have usually failed to find a significant relationship with depression, so it is a reasonable hypothesis that: (1) low-level cannabis use is *not* associated with a *significant* increase in the risk of depression; and (2) it is only when persons are using cannabis heavily (perhaps weekly or more often) that the risk of depression is increased. Future work needs to test these hypotheses directly.

Measurement of depression

One issue that has complicated our review of the evidence has been the variety of different ways in which depression has been assessed. Some studies have assessed major depression as defined by *DSM* (Fergusson and Horwood, 1997; Degenhardt *et al.*, 2001; Fergusson *et al.*, unpublished manuscript). However, others have used measures of 'depressive symptoms' (Kandel and Davies, 1986; Kandel *et al.*, 1986; Bovasso, 2001), continuous measures of depression (Troisi *et al.*, 1998; Milich *et al.*, 2000), and cut-off scores on continuous depression scales (Patton *et al.*, 2002). It is possible that some of the discrepant findings have reflected these differences in measurement.

Study designs

Convenience samples are not appropriate for examining associations between cannabis use and depression. Well-designed surveys of the general population have indicated that heavy cannabis use and depression occur at a level greater than chance, but these studies are less well-suited to testing causal hypotheses. Two study methods that are more appropriate for this task are longitudinal studies (Fergusson and Horwood, 2001) and analyses of data from genetically informative research designs (Neale and Kendler, 1995; Rutter *et al.*, 2001).

Longitudinal studies

To date most longitudinal studies have used adolescent or young adult samples. From a public health perspective, this group is important because of the high rates of incident cannabis use and depression in this age group. In this age group there is clearly emerging evidence that frequent cannabis use predicts depression. This relationship may change with time. It is likely that many frequent users will reduce or cease using when detrimental consequences such as depression become evident. Whether their high risk for depression resolves with cessation of use is an important and as yet unanswered question. The one available study in adults was limited in terms of the number of participants in some groups (only 15 participants were 'cannabis abusers' without depressive symptoms at baseline) and the lack of precision about the measurement of depression during a long follow-up (a 14–16-year interval between baseline and follow-up; Bovasso, 2001).

The use of genetically informative designs to examine causality

There is mounting evidence for a substantial genetic component in many behaviours and behavioural disorders (Kendler, 2001; Rutter *et al.*, 2001). Standard genetic modelling of twin data has indicated a moderate to high heritability of both cannabis use/dependence and liability to depression. Specifically, estimates of the heritability of cannabis dependence have ranged from 45% to 62% (Kendler and Prescott, 1998; Kendler *et al.*, 2000; Lynskey *et al.*, 2002) and a recent meta-analysis of twin studies of major depression has suggested that 37% of the liability to major depression is due to heritable factors (Sullivan *et al.*, 2000). A recent study suggests that the association between major depression and cannabis dependence may be partially explained by a high degree of overlap in the genetic factors predisposing to cannabis use and depressive disorders (Fu *et al.*, 2002).

Given these findings, further genetically informative research designs may make substantial contributions to our understanding of the relationship between cannabis use and depression. The potential research designs include the study of twins, either reared together or apart, adoption studies and studies of the children of twins and other extended family designs. These study designs (recently summarized by Rutter and colleagues (2001)) have not, as yet, been applied to the study of the relationship between cannabis use and depression. The need for such research is reinforced by recent findings that much of the association between depression and both tobacco (Kendler *et al.*, 1993a) and alcohol (Kendler *et al.*, 1993b) dependence can be explained by common genetic factors.

Conclusions

Surveys of representative samples of the general population have established that rates of depression are elevated in those who use cannabis frequently or who are cannabis-dependent. The extent of this comorbidity exceeds levels we would expect to see by chance. There does not appear to be an increased risk of depression associated with infrequent cannabis use.

The reasons for this comorbidity are uncertain. Research does not provide support for the self-medication hypothesis. It may be too early to rule out shared risk factors since not all cross-sectional studies have adequately controlled for confounding variables, and the results of cohort studies to date have been mixed.

There appears to be a modest association between early-onset regular or problematic cannabis use and later depression. There are at least two broad classes of explanation: the first of these is biological, in which cannabis use causes changes in neurotransmitter systems that make depressed mood more likely. There is little research evidence to support this possibility. Greater evidence exists to support the other form of this causal hypothesis, in which the effects of regular or problematic cannabis use are socially mediated. There is increasing evidence to suggest that regular and early-onset cannabis use are associated with reduced educational attainment (Lynskey and Hall, 2000), unemployment and crime (Fergusson and Horwood, 1997; Lynskey and Hall, 2000), all factors that may lead to increased risks of later mental health problems. However, the evidence on this issue is limited, and future research needs to examine both possibilities.

There is a need for longitudinal and twin studies that better assess the relationship between cannabis use, depression and confounding factors. Furthermore, there is a need to examine relationships among *adult* samples, since nearly every cohort study has not extended into middle or late adulthood, and associations have only been reported for adolescents or young adults.

If we assume that cannabis use and depression are causally related, the proportion of depression that is attributable to cannabis use is very modest. On the basis of the current literature, and on current patterns of cannabis use in the general population (in which few people use cannabis heavily), regular cannabis use explains only a small proportion of depression in the population.

REFERENCES

Abel, E. (1971). Changes in anxiety feelings following marihuana smoking. *Br. J. Addict.*, **66**, 185–187.

Ablon, S. L. and Goodwin, F. K. (1974). High frequency of dysphoric reactions to tetrahydro-cannabinol among depressed patients. *Am. J. Psychiatry*, **131**, 448–453.

Alpert, J., Maddocks, A., Rosenbaum, J. and Fava, M. (1994). Childhood psychopathology retrospectively assessed among adults with early onset depression. *J. Affect. Disord.*, **31**, 165–171.

American Psychiatric Association (1987). *Diagnostic and Statistical Manual of Mental Disorders*, 3rd edn revised (DSM-III-R). Washington, DC: American Psychiatric Association.

American Psychiatric Association (1994). *Diagnostic and Statistical Manual of Mental Disorders*, 4th edn. Washington, DC: American Psychiatric Association.

Andrews, G., Mathers, C. and Sanderson, K. (1998). The burden of disease. *Med. J. Aust.*, **169**, 156–158.

Angst, J. (1996). Comorbidity of mood disorders: a longitudinal prospective study. *Br. J. Psychiatry*, **168** (suppl. 30) 31–37.

Anthony, J. C. and Helzer, J. (1991). Syndromes of drug abuse and dependence. In *Psychiatric Disorders in America*, ed. L. N. Robins and D. A. Regier, pp. 116–154. New York: The Free Press.

Bardone, A. Moffitt, T., Caspi, A. *et al.* (1998). Adult physical health outcomes of adolescent girls with conduct disorder, depression, and anxiety. *J. Am. Acad. Child Adolescent Psychiatry*, **37**, 594–601.

Beautrais, A. L., Joyce, P. R. and Mulder, R. T. (1999). Cannabis abuse and serious suicide attempts. *Addiction*, **94**, 1155–1164.

Bell, J., Ward, J., Mattick, R. P. *et al.* (1995) *An Evaluation of Private Methadone Clinics*. Canberra: Australian Government Publishing Service.

Berkson, J. (1946). Limitations of the application of fourfold table analysis to hospital data. *Biometrics Bull.*, **2**, 47–53.

Best, D., Gossop, M., Greenood, J. *et al.* (1999). Cannabis use in relation to illicit drug use and health problems among opiate users in treatment. *Drug Alcohol Rev.*, **18**, 31–38.

Blazer, D. (1995). Mood disorders: epidemiology. In *Comprehensive Textbook of Psychiatry*, VIth edn., vol. 1, ed. H. Kaplan and B. Sadock, pp. 1079–1089. Baltimore, MD: Williams and Wilkins.

Bovasso, G. (2001). Cannabis abuse as risk factor for depressive symptoms. *Am. J. Psychiatry*, **158**, 2033–2037.

Bowers, M. (1998). Family history and early psychotogenic response to marijuana. *J. Clin. Psychiatry*, **59**, 198–199.

Boyd, J. H., Burke, J. D., Gruenberg, E. *et al.* (1984). Exclusion criteria of DSM-III: a study of co-occurrence of hierarchy-free syndromes. *Arch. Gen. Psychiatry*, **41**, 983–989.

Brady, K. T., Casto, S., Lydiard, R. B. *et al.* (1991). Substance abuse in an inpatient psychiatric sample. *Am. J. Drug Alcohol Abuse*, **17**, 389–397.

Brook, J. S., Cohen, P. and Brook, D. W. (1998). Longitudinal study of co-occurring psychiatric disorders and substance use. *J. Am. Acad. Child Adolescent Psychiatry*, **37**, 322–330.

Caron, C. and Rutter, M. (1991). Comorbidity in child psychopathology: concepts, issues and research strategies. *J. Child Psychol. Psychiatry*, **32**, 1063–1080.

Chen, C.-Y., Wagner, F. and Anthony, J. (2002). Marijuana use and the risk of major depressive episode: epidemiological evidence from the United States National Comorbidity Survey. *Social Psychiatry Psychiatric Epidemiol.*, **37**, 199–206.

Cicchetti, D. and Toth, S. (1998). The development of depression in children and adolescents. *Am. Psychol.*, **53**, 221–241.

Degenhardt, L., Lynskey, M. and Hall, W. (2000). Cohort trends in the age of initiation of drug use in Australia. *Aust. NZ J. Public Health*, **24**, 421–426.

Degenhardt, L., Hall, W. and Lynskey, M. (2001). The relationship between cannabis use, depression and anxiety among Australian adults: findings from the National Survey of Mental Health Well-Being. *Social Psychiatry Psychiatric Epidemiol.*, **36**, 219–227.

Dhossche, D., Rich, C. and Isacsson, G. (2001). Psychoactive substances in suicides: comparison of toxicologic findings in two samples. *Am. J. Forensic Med. Pathol.*, **22**, 239–243.

Diekstra, R., Kienhorst, C. and de Wilde, E. (1995). Suicide and suicidal behaviour among adolescents. In *Psychosocial Disorders Among Young People: Time Trends and their Causes*, ed. M. Rutter and D. J. Smith, pp. 686–761. Chichester: John Wiley.

Donnelly, N. and Hall, W. (1994). *Patterns of Cannabis Use in Australia. NCADA Monograph Series no. 27*. Canberra: Australian Government Publishing Service.

Estroff, T., Dackis, C., Gold, M. and Pottash, A. (1985). Drug abuse and bipolar disorders. *Int. J. Psychiatry Med.*, **15**, 37–40.

Feinstein, A. R. (1970). The pre-therapeutic classification of comorbidity in chronic disease. *J. Chronic Dis.*, **23**, 455–468.

Fergusson, D. M. and Horwood, L. J. (1997). Early onset cannabis use and psychosocial adjustment in young adults. *Addiction*, **92**, 279–296.

Fergusson, D. M. and Horwood, L. J. (2001). The Christchurch Health and Development Study: review of findings on child and adolescent mental health. *Aust. NZ J. Psychiatry*, **35**, 287–296.

Fergusson, D., Horwood, J. and Lawton, M. (1990). Vulnerability to childhood problems and family social background. *J. Child Psychol. Psychiatry*, **31**, 1145–1160.

Fergusson, D., Horwood, L. and Lynskey, M. (1994). Parental separation, adolescent psychopathology and problem behaviours. *J. Am. Acad. Child Adolescent Psychiatry*, **33**, 1122–1131.

Fergusson, D. M., Horwood, J. and Swain-Campbell, N. (2002). Cannabis use and psychosocial adjustment in adolescence and young adulthood. *Addiction*, **97**, 1123–1135.

Field, T., Diego, M. and Sanders, C. (2001). Adolescent suicidal ideation. *Adolescence*, **36**, 241–248.

Fu, Q., Heath, A. C., Bucholz, K. K. *et al.* (2002). Shared genetic risk of major depression, alcohol dependence and marijuana dependence: the contribution from antisocial personality disorder in men. *Arch. Gen. Psychiatry*, **59**, 1125–1132.

Galaif, E., Chou, C.-P., Sussman, S. and Dent, C. (1998). Depression, suicidal ideation, and substance use among continuation high school students. *J. Youth Adolescence*, **27**, 275–299.

Galbaud Du Fort, G., Newman, S. and Bland, R. (1993). Psychiatric comorbidity and treatment seeking: sources of selection bias in the study of clinical populations. *J. Nerv. Ment. Dis.*, **181**, 464–474.

Gale, E. N. and Guenther, G. (1971). Motivational factors associated with the use of cannabis (marihuana). *Br. J. Addict.*, **66**, 188–194.

Grant, B. F. (1995). Comorbidity between *DSM*-IV drug use disorders and major depression: results of a national survey of adults. *J. Substance Abuse*, **7**, 481–497.

Green, B. E. and Ritter, C. (2000). Marijuana use and depression. *J. Health Social Behav.*, **41**, 40–49.

Grinspoon, L. and Bakalar, J. B. (1998). The use of cannabis as a mood stabilizer in bipolar disorder: anecdotal evidence and the need for clinical research. *J. Psychoactive Drugs*, **30**, 171–177.

Gruber, A. J., Pope, H. G. and Oliva, P. (1997). Very long-term users of marijuana in the United States: a pilot study. *Substance Use Misuse*, **32**, 249–264.

Hall, W., Johnston, L. and Donnelly, N. (1999). Epidemiology of cannabis use and its consequences. In *The Health Effects of Cannabis*, ed. H. Kalant, W. Corrigall, W. Hall and R. Smart, pp. 71–125. Toronto, Canada: Centre for Addiction and Mental Health.

Hall, W., Degenhardt, L. and Lynskey, M. (2001). *The Health and Psychological Consequences of Cannabis Use*. NCADA Monongraph no. 44. Canberra: Australian Publishing Service.

Hofstra, M., van der Ende, J. and Verhultz, F. (2002). Child and adolescent problems predict *DSM*-IV disorders in adulthood: a 14-year follow-up of a Dutch epidemiological sample. *J. Am. Acad. Child Adolescent Psychiatry*, **41**, 182–189.

Holden, R. and Pakula, I. (2001). Marijuana, stress and suicide: a neuroimmunological explanation. *Aust. NZ J. Psychiatry*, **36**, 465–466.

Institute of Medicine (1996). *Pathways of Addiction*. Washington, DC: National Academy Press.

Jablensky, A. Sartorius, N. and Ernberg, G. (1991). Schizophrenia: manifestations, incidence and course in different cultures. A World Health Organization ten-country study. *Psychol. Med.* (suppl. 20).

Johns, A. (2001). Psychiatric effects of cannabis. *Br. J. Psychiatry*, **178**, 116–122.

Kandel, D. B. (1984). Marijuana users in young adulthood. *Arch. Gen. Psychiatry*, **41**, 200–209.

Kandel, D. and Chen, K. (2000). Types of marijuana users by longitudinal course. *J. Studies Alcohol*, **61**, 367–378.

Kandel, D. and Davies, M. (1986). Adult sequelae of adolescent depressive symptoms. *Arch. Gen. Psychiatry*, **43**, 255–262.

Kandel, D. B., Davies, M., Karus, D. and Yamaguchi, K. (1986). The consequences in young adulthood of adolescent drug involvement. *Arch. Gen. Psychiatry*, **43**, 746–754.

Kandel, D., Chen, K., Warner, L. A., Kessler, R. C. and Grant, B. (1997). Prevalence and demographic correlates of symptoms of last year dependence on alcohol, nicotine, marijuana and cocaine in the U.S. population. *Drug Alcohol Dependence*, **44**, 11–29.

Kelder, S., Murray, N., Orpinas, P. *et al.* (2001). Depression and substance use among minority middle-school students. *Am. J. Public Health*, **91**, 761–766.

Kendler, K. S. (2001). Twin studies of psychiatric illness: an update. *Arch. Gen. Psychiatry*, **58**, 1005–1014.

Kendler, K. S. and Prescott, C. A. (1998). Cannabis use, abuse, and dependence in a population-based sample of female twins. *Am. J. Psychiatry*, **155**, 1016–1022.

Kendler, K., Neale, M., MacLean, C. *et al.* (1993a). Smoking and major depression: a causal analysis. *Arch. Gen. Psychiatry*, **50**, 36–43.

Kendler, K. S., Heath, A. C., Neale, M. C., Kessler, R. C. and Eaves, L. J. (1993b). Alcoholism and major depression in women. A twin study of the causes of comorbidity. *Arch. Gen. Psychiatry*, **50**, 690–698.

Kendler, K., Karkowski, L., Neale, M. and Prescott, C. (2000). Illicit psychoactive substance use, heavy use, abuse and dependence in a US population-based sample of male twins. *Arch. Gen. Psychiatry*, **57**, 261–269.

Kessler, R. C. (1995). Epidemiology of psychiatric comorbidity. In *Textbook in Psychiatric Epidemiology*, ed. M. T. Tsuang, M. Tohen and G. E. P. Zahner, pp. 179–197. New York: Wiley.

Kessler, R. C., McGonagle, K. A., Zhao, S. *et al.* (1994). Lifetime and 12-month prevalence of DSM-III-R psychiatric disorders in the United States. Results from the National Comorbidity Survey. *Arch. Gen. Psychiatry*, **51**, 8–19.

Kessler, R. C., Nelson, C. B., McGonagle, K. A., *et al.* (1996). The epidemiology of co-occurring addictive and mental disorders: implications for prevention and service utilization. *Am. J. Orthopsychiatry*, **66**, 17–31.

Klein, D. and Riso, L. (1994). Psychiatric disorders: problems of boundaries and comorbidity. In *Basic Issues in Psychopathology*, ed. G. Costello, pp. 19–66. New York: Guilford.

Kotin, J., Post, R. and Goodwin, F. (1973). Δ9-Tetrahydrocannabinol in depressed outpatients. *Arch. Gen. Psychiatry*, **28**, 345–348.

Kouri, E., Pope, H., Yurgelun-Todd, D. and Gruber, S. (1995). Attributes of heavy vs. occasional marjiuana smokers in a college population. *Biol. Psychiatry*, **38**, 475–481.

Lynskey, M. and Hall, W. (2000). The effects of adolescent cannabis use on educational attainment: a review. *Addiction*, **95**, 1621–1630.

Lynskey, M., Degenhardt, L. and Hall, W. (2000). Cohort trends in youth suicide in Australia 1964 to 1997. *Aust. NZ J. Psychiatry*, **34**, 408–412.

Lynskey, M. T., Heath, A. C., Nelson, E. C. *et al.* (2002). Genetic and environmental contributions to cannabis dependence in a national young adult twin sample. *Psychol. Med.*, **32**, 195–207.

Marken, P., Stanislav, S. *et al.* (1992). Profile of a sample of subjects admitted to an acute care psychiatric facility with manic symptoms. *Psychopharmacol. Bull.*, **28**, 201–205.

Mathew, R., Wilson, W. and Tant, S. (1989). Acute changes in cerebral blood flow associated with marijuana smoking. *Acta Psychiatr. Scand.*, **79**, 118–128.

McGee, R., Williams, S., Poulton, R. and Moffitt, T. (2000). A longitudinal study of cannabis use and mental health from adolescence to early adulthood. *Addiction*, **95**, 491–503.

Merikangas, K. and Angst, J. (1995). The challenge of depressive disorders in adolescence. In *Psychosocial Disturbances in Young People*, ed. M. Rutter, Cambridge: Cambridge University Press.

Milich, R., Lynam, D. Zimmerman, R. *et al.* (2000). Differences in young adult psychopathology among drug abstainers, experimenters, and frequent users. *J. Substance Abuse*, **11**, 69–88.

Miller, F., Busch, F. and Tanenbaum, J. (1989). Drug abuse in schizophrenia and bipolar disorder. *Am. J. Drug Alcohol Abuse*, **15**, 291–295.

Miller-Johnson, S., Lochman, J., Coie, J., Terry, R. and Hyman, C. (1998). Comorbidity of conduct and depressive problems at sixth grade: substance use outcomes across adolescence. *J. Abnormal Child Psychol.*, **26**, 221–232.

Mueser, K., Yarnold, P. and Bellack, A. (1992). Diagnostic and demographic correlates of substance abuse in schizophrenia and major affective disorder. *Acta Psychiatr. Scand.*, **85**, 48–55.

Mueser, K. T., Drake, R. E. and Wallach, M. A. (1998). Dual diagnosis: a review of etiological theories. *Addict. Behav.*, **23**, 717–734.

Musty, R. E. and Kaback, L. (1995). Relationships between motivation and depression in chronic marijuana users. *Life Sci.*, **56**, 2151–2158.

Neale, M. C. and Kendler, K. S. (1995). Models of comorbidity for multifactorial disorders. *Am. J. Hum. Genet.*, **57**, 935–953.

Paton, S., Kessler, R. and Kandel, D. (1977). Depressive mood and adolescent illicit drug use: a longitudinal analysis. *J. Genet. Psychol.*, **131**, 267–289.

Patton, G., Coffey, C., Carlin, J. *et al.* (2002). Cannabis use and mental health in young people: cohort study. *Br. Med. J.*, **325**, 1195–1198.

Pond, D. (1948). Psychological effects in depressive patients of the marijuana homologue, synhexyl. *J. Neurol., Neurosurg. Psychiatry*, **11**, 271–279.

Rey, J., Sawyer, M., Clark, J. and Baghurst, P. (2001). Depression among Australian adolescents. *Med. J. Aust.*, **175**, 19–23.

Rey, J., Sawyer, M., Raphael, B., Patton, G. and Lynskey, M. (2002). Mental health of teenagers who use cannabis: results of an Australian survey. *Br. J. Psychiatry*, **180**, 216–221.

Roberts, R. S., Spitzer, W. O., Delmore, T. and Sackett, D. L. (1978). An empirical demonstration of Berkson's bias. *J. Chron. Dis.*, **31**, 119–128.

Rowe, M., Fleming, M., Barry, K., Manwell, L. and Kropp, S. (1995). Correlates of depression in primary care. *J. Fam. Pract.*, **41**, 551–558.

Rutter, M. (1987). Parental mental disorder as a psychiatric risk factor. In *Psychiatric Update: American Psychiatric Association: Annual Review*, vol. 6, ed. R. Hales and A. Frances, pp. 647–663. Washington, DC: American Psychiatric Press.

Rutter, M., Pickles, A., Murray, R. and Eaves, L. (2001). Testing hypotheses on specific environmental causal effects on behavior. *Psychol. Bull.*, **127**, 291–324.

Shedler, J. and Block, J. (1990). Adolescent drug use and psychological health: a longitudinal inquiry. *Am. Psychol.*, **45**, 612–630.

Sonne, S., Brady, K. and Morton, W. (1994). Substance abuse and bipolar affective disorder. *J. Nerv. Ment. Dis.*, **182**, 349–352.

Stoll, A., Cole, J. and Lukas, S. (1991). A case of mania as a result of fluoxetine–marijuana interaction. *J. Clin. Psychiatry*, **52**, 280–281.

Sullivan, P. F., Neale, M. C. and Kendler, K. S. (2000). Genetic epidemiology of major depression: review and meta-analysis. *Am. J. Psychiatry*, **157**, 1552–1562.

Troisi, A., Pasini, A., Saracco, M. and Spalletta, G. (1998). Psychiatric symptoms in male cannabis users not using other illicit drugs. *Addiction*, **93**, 487–492.

Velez, C., Johnson, J. and Cohen, P. (1989). A longitudinal analysis of selected risk factors for childhood psychopathology. *J. Am. Acad. Child Adolescent Psychiatry*, **28**, 861–864.

Warner, R., Taylor, D. and Wright, J. (1994). Substance use among the mentally ill: prevalence, reasons for use and effects on illness. *Am. J. Orthopsychiatry*, **74**, 30–39.

Weissman, M. Livingston Bruce, M., Leaf, P. Florio, L. and Holzer, C. (1991). Affective disorders. In *Psychiatric Disorders in America*, ed. L. Robins and D. Regier, pp. 53–80. New York: MacMillan.

Weissman, M. M., Wolk, S., Wickramaratne, P. *et al.* (1999). Children with prepubertal-onset major depressive disorder and anxiety grown up. *Arch. Gen. Psychiatry*, **56**, 794–801.

Zablocki, B., Aidala, A., Hansell, S. and White, H. (1991). Marijuana use, introspectiveness, and mental health. *J. Health Social Behav.*, **32**, 65–79.

Zelwer, A. (1994). Depression and marijuana. *Aust. and NZ J. Psychiatry*, **28**, 528.

5

Cannabis and psychosis proneness

Hélène Verdoux

University Victor Segalen, Bordeaux, France

In many countries, a large proportion of the general population is now exposed to cannabis, as a result of its widespread recreational use (Webb *et al.*, 1996; Smart and Ogborne, 2000). From a public health point of view, a careful assessment of the impact of cannabis on mental health in general-population subjects is thus warranted, in order to decide whether prevention strategies aimed at reducing exposure to this drug are justified. Investigation of the mental health characteristics of cannabis users in the general population is especially important for identification of a potential aetiological risk factor for severe mental illness. Converging findings obtained by prospective population-based cohort studies suggest that cannabis use may be an independent risk factor for the onset of psychosis (Andreasson *et al.*, 1987; Arseneault *et al.*, 2002; van Os *et al.*, 2002; Weiser *et al.*, 2002).

However, the nature of the link between cannabis use and psychosis is far from being elucidated. Findings drawn from clinical samples of subjects identified as cases of psychosis have limited value in shedding light on the mechanisms underlying this association, as the potential confounding factors linked to the clinical status of the subjects are difficult to control in such samples. Thus, studies exploring factors modulating the expression of psychosis in non-clinical populations may better identify causal risk factors for psychosis than studies carried out in clinical samples (Verdoux *et al.*, 1998b, van Os *et al.*, 2000; 2001; Verdoux and van Os, 2002). This review will focus on the studies that have investigated the relationships between cannabis use and occurrence of psychotic experiences in non-clinical populations.

Psychosis proneness in cannabis users

As no consensual definition of psychosis proneness exists (Claridge, 1997), a broad definition of this term will be used to describe psychotic experiences occurring in

Marijuana and Madness: Psychiatry and Neurobiology, ed. D. Castle and R. Murray. Published by Cambridge University Press. © Cambridge University Press 2004.

subjects without a clinical diagnosis of psychosis. Hence, this definition includes so-called schizotypal signs (Venables *et al.*, 1990), as well as full-blown or attenuated psychotic symptoms that are experienced at least once by a relatively large proportion (ranging from 15 to 20%) of subjects without clinical psychosis (Eaton *et al.*, 1991; Tien, 1991; Verdoux *et al.*, 1998a; Poulton *et al.*, 2000; van Os *et al.*, 2000).

Is there a cross-sectional association between cannabis use and psychosis proneness?

The links between psychosis proneness and cannabis use in non-clinical populations have been explored by a limited number of cross-sectional studies. The first studies focused on the associations between cannabis and 'positive' psychosis proneness. For example, Williams *et al.* (1996) explored the associations between cannabis use and schizotypal scores measured using the Schizotypy-A (STA) scale (Claridge and Beech, 1995) in 211 subjects from the general population recruited through advertisement. The STA explores 'positive' schizotypal signs such as perceptual anomalies and magical or paranoid ideation. Higher total scores were found in subjects who ever used cannabis as compared to never-users, and this association remained significant after exclusion of subjects who ever used other drugs. Kwapil (1996) performed a 10-year follow-up of students who had been assessed at baseline by the scales developed by Chapman and collaborators (Chapman *et al.*, 1994) measuring the positive schizotypal dimension ('perceptual aberration' and 'magical ideation' scales/Per-Mag) and the negative schizotypal dimension ('physical anhedonia' and 'social anhedonia' scales). Subjects with deviant Per-Mag scores (at least 1.96 above the mean, $n = 34$) presented with a higher frequency of substance use over the ensuing 10 years compared to subjects with lower Per-Mag scores ($n = 139$). However, the reverse association did not hold true; that is, substance use at baseline did not predict subsequent psychosis over the follow-up period.

Recent studies investigating the associations between cannabis use and psychosis proneness have focused on the links between cannabis use and dimensions of psychosis proneness. A study by Skosnik *et al.* (2001) measured dimensions of psychosis using the nine subscales of the Schizotypal Personality Questionnaire (SPQ) (Raine, 1991) in 15 current cannabis users (at least one use per week), 10 past cannabis users (no use in the 45 days prior to assessment) and 15 drug-free subjects recruited through advertisements. Subjects with current cannabis use had higher SPQ total scores than past or non-users. Significant differences were found between the three groups regarding 'positive' schizotypal scores (magical thought, perceptual distortion, ideas of reference) as well as on the subscales scores 'odd behaviour' and 'odd speech' (this last score was lower in current cannabis users). No association was found between cannabis use status and 'negative' schizotypal scores (suspiciousness, anxiety, constricted affect, lack of close friends).

Nunn *et al.* (2001) performed a study on the link between dimensions of psychosis proneness and substance use in a sample of 196 students. The subjects were categorized into cannabis and alcohol users (at least two uses of each substance per week); cannabis users; alcohol users; and subjects with neither cannabis nor alcohol use. Subjects who had used other drugs on more than one occasion were excluded. The Oxford–Liverpool Inventory of Feelings and Experiences (O-LIFE psychosis proneness) (Mason *et al.*, 1995) was used to assess four schizotypal dimensions: unusual experiences (positive dimension), introverted anhedonia (negative dimension), cognitive disorganization and impulsivity–non-conformity. Also, the Peters *et al.* Delusion Inventory (PDI) was employed as a measure of delusional ideation (Verdoux *et al.*, 1998b; Peters *et al.*, 1999). Subjects using only cannabis had higher scores on scales assessing positive symptoms (unusual experiences and PDI scores). Such an association was not found in subjects using only alcohol. Subjects using both cannabis and alcohol scored lower than non-users on the introverted anhedonia scale.

Dumas *et al.* (2002) interviewed students ($n = 232$) who were categorized according to level of cannabis use (never, past or occasional users, and regular users – at least two uses per week). Psychosis proneness was assessed using the SPQ (Raine, 1991) and by the scales developed by Chapman *et al.* (1994). Subjects who never used cannabis scored significantly lower than the two other groups on most scales assessing the positive dimension, and on two scales assessing the negative dimension (SPQ constricted affect and physical anhedonia). These two latter associations were no longer significant after adjustment for self-reported anxiety and/or depression.

Our own study (Verdoux *et al.*, 2003b) explored the pattern of associations between cannabis use and dimensions of psychosis in a sample of 571 female undergraduate students. A standardized self-report questionnaire was used to collect information on use of alcohol and of illicit substances, including cannabis. The subjects were asked to specify the frequency of use of each substance over the last month, ranging from one (never in the past 30 days) to seven (several times a day). Dimensions of psychosis were measured by the Community Assessment of Psychic Experiences (CAPE) (Stefanis *et al.*, 2002), a 42-item self-report questionnaire derived from the PDI-21 (Peters *et al.*, 1999). In view of our previous studies using the PDI-21 in non-clinical populations (Verdoux *et al.*, 1998a; 1999; van Os *et al.*, 1999), we excluded or reworded ambiguous PDI-21 items and added others exploring hallucinations. The CAPE includes a total of 20 items of positive psychotic experiences, to which were added 14 items exploring negative experiences derived from the Subjective Experience of Negative Symptoms (SENS) (Selten *et al.*, 1998) and eight items exploring cognitive depressive experiences discriminating between depressive and negative symptoms (Kibel *et al.*, 1993). Each item explores the frequency of the experience on a four-point scale of never, sometimes,

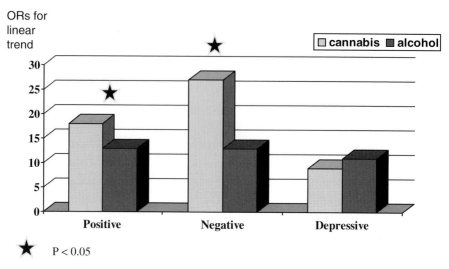

ORs for
linear
trend

□ cannabis ■ alcohol

★ P < 0.05

Figure 5.1   Cannabis use and dimensions of psychosis in a non-clinical population.

often and nearly always. Principal components factor analysis of the CAPE gives a three-factor model of separate depressive, positive and negative factors (Stefanis *et al.*, 2002). Cannabis use was categorized according to the frequency of use as 'no use over the last month', 'once a month to once a week', and 'more than once a week'. For each psychosis dimension (positive, negative, depressive), we tested the hypothesis that there would be a linear trend in the association between cannabis use and psychosis dimension score, i.e. the more frequent the use of cannabis, the higher the score on that dimension. To assess the specificity of any association between cannabis use and psychosis dimensions, we also used the same method to explore the associations between psychosis dimensions and alcohol use.

Significant associations were found between cannabis use and positive and negative dimension scores, such that increased levels of cannabis use were associated with higher positive and negative dimension scores (Fig. 5.1). There was no association between cannabis use and depressive dimension score. To take into account the correlations between the dimensions, we tested whether there were independent effects of cannabis use on the three dimensions of psychosis by estimating the effect of cannabis on each dimension while adjusting for the two other dimensions. The associations between frequency of cannabis use and higher positive and higher negative dimension scores were still significant, indicating that positive and negative dimensions were independently associated with cannabis use. Consonant with the results reported by Nunn *et al.* (2001), the specificity of the findings for cannabis use was suggested by the lack of association between alcohol use and dimensions of psychosis.

Methodological considerations

Studies exploring cross-sectional associations between cannabis use and psychosis proneness in non-clinical populations provide strikingly consistent findings regarding the positive dimension of psychosis proneness. Irrespective of differences in sampling procedure and in the scales used to measure schizotypy, all the reviewed studies found that subjects with cannabis use have higher positive psychosis proneness scores than non-users. More discrepant findings have been obtained regarding the negative dimension. Thus, Skosnik *et al.* (2001) found no association between cannabis use and negative psychosis proneness, but that study was limited by the use of a large number of univariate statistical tests (thus not taking into account potential confounders) on a small sample of subjects (see above) and only a limited number of items were explored to measure the negative dimension. Nunn *et al.* (2001) found that subjects with both cannabis and alcohol use had lower anhedonia scores than non-users. In contrast, Dumas *et al.* (2002) and Verdoux *et al.* (2003b) both reported that cannabis users had higher scores at scales assessing the negative dimension of psychosis proneness; however, these associations were no longer significant after adjusting for anxiety/depression in the study by Dumas *et al.* (2002).

Such discrepant findings may reflect the fact that negative signs may be less easily captured than positive ones by self-rating scales, and that their measurement may be more highly dependent on the method of assessment. The main drawback in the measurement of the negative dimension in clinical as well as in non-clinical samples is linked to the ability of the scale to discriminate between negative and depressive symptoms. No association was found between depressive symptoms and cannabis use in the studies investigating this association (Nunn *et al.*, 2001; Dumas *et al.*, 2002; Verdoux *et al.*, 2003b). Thus, assessments of the negative dimension mixing up negative and depressive symptoms may attenuate the strength of association between negative symptoms and cannabis use. To address this problem, the CAPE was designed by selecting items discriminating between depressive and negative symptoms; items loading on the CAPE negative dimension were 'being untalkative', 'lack of spontaneity', 'lack of emotion', 'blunted feelings', 'having no interest in others', 'lack of motivation', 'lack of activity', 'lack of hygiene', 'being unable to terminate things' and 'lacking hobbies' (Verdoux *et al.*, 2003b). Another potential explanation for the discrepancies between our findings and those obtained by the other studies is that the negative dimension measured using these items was based on a quasi-dimensional model of psychosis proneness taking the abnormal state as the reference point (Claridge and Beech, 1995). In other words, the negative items were based on a measure of attenuated negative psychotic symptoms rather than on a measure based upon a fully dimensional model taking 'normality' as the reference point, as used in the other schizotypal scales. A final point is that we cannot exclude the possibility of the association between negative symptoms and cannabis use in our sample being due to the sample being exclusively female; however, none of the other studies reported that the associations between cannabis use and dimensions of psychosis were modified by gender, making this unlikely.

Implications

A persisting 'amotivational syndrome' (Tennant and Groesbeck, 1972), character-ized by loss of motivation and interests, and impaired occupational achievement, has been described in heavy cannabis users, probably induced by the subacute encephalopathy linked to chronic cannabis intoxication (Castle and Ames, 1996; Hall and Solowij, 1997; Johns, 2001; and see Chapter 3). This so-called 'amoti-vational syndrome' has a striking phenomenological similarity with the negative dimension of psychosis and the dose–response relationship between the frequency of cannabis use and the intensity of the negative symptoms found in our sample of students may indirectly confirm the existence of such a phenomenon.

Several studies have reported that subjects with psychosis using cannabis are more likely to present with prominent positive symptoms and fewer negative symptoms than non-users (Mathers and Ghodse, 1992; Peralta and Cuesta, 1992; Allebeck et al., 1993; Kirkpatrick et al., 1996; Salyers and Mueser, 2001). It has been suggested on the basis of these findings that subjects with psychosis may use cannabis to self-medicate negative symptoms (Peralta and Cuesta, 1992; Skosnik et al., 2001). However, the association seen in clinical settings may be explained by other factors independently associated with cannabis use and negative symptoms. Subjects with a dual diagnosis are also characterized by a better premorbid adjustment and a less severe form of illness (Mueser et al., 1990; Dixon et al., 1991; Arndt et al., 1992; Salyers and Mueser, 2001). Thus, the lower frequency of cannabis use in subjects with prominent negative symptoms might be a consequence of negative symptoms and poor premorbid adjustment. A certain level of social competence is required to obtain illicit drugs, and subjects with prominent negative symptoms may have a limited access to these drugs due to impairments in this domain of functioning.

Does cannabis induce the occurrence of psychotic experiences in non-clinical subjects?

The main limitation of cross-sectional studies reporting that non-clinical subjects with cannabis use are more likely to present with psychotic experiences is that the direction of causality, if any, cannot be definitely established. Heavy cannabis use may be a consequence, rather than a cause, of more frequent positive and/or negative psychotic experiences. Alternatively, a propensity to use cannabis and to present with psychotic experiences may be independently associated with similar risk factors such as personality characteristics (Liraud and Verdoux, 2000).

To find answers to these unsolved questions, it is necessary to investigate the effects of cannabis on the occurrence of psychotic experiences in non-clinical populations, prospectively. Anecdotal experimental evidence suggests that the administration of tetrahydrocannabinol or cannabis to volunteers may induce positive psychotic symptoms in a limited number of subjects (Thornicroft, 1990). A systematic review of randomized controlled trials comparing the antiemetic effects of cannabis with placebo or other antiemetics showed that 6% of patients receiving cannabis presented with hallucinations and 5% with 'paranoia', while no patient treated with control drugs presented with such side-effects (Tramèr et al., 2001).

In order to characterize better the temporal relationship between cannabis use and psychotic symptoms, we have explored the impact of cannabis use on the onset of psychotic experiences using the Experience Sampling Method (ESM: Verdoux et al., 2003a). ESM is a structured diary technique that was developed to investigate subjective experience over time in the stream of daily life and across naturally occurring situations (Csikszentmihalyi and Larson, 1987; Delespaul, 1995; Swendsen and Norman, 1998; Swendsen et al., 2000). In an ESM study, subjects are asked to self-report variables such as environment, activity and feelings several times a day over consecutive days. The validity of ESM in collating information on psychotic experiences in daily life has now been demonstrated by several studies (Delespaul, 1995; Myin-Germeys et al., 2001a, b).

Among the baseline sample of 649 students previously described, we selected a stratified random sample of 79 subjects, depending on 'low' (no use over the past month) versus 'high' (use at least 2–3 times a week) cannabis consumption, and on level of psychosis proneness, assessed using the CAPE. Responding to randomly programmed 'bips' from a wristwatch, subjects were asked to describe their present substance use and psychotic experiences five times a day over 7 consecutive days (Fig. 5.2). Substance use was explored by the question: 'Over the last period, did you use some substances?' (yes/no), followed by an open question ('if, yes, which substance(s) did you use?'). Psychotic experiences were explored by four questions rated on seven-point Likert scales: (1) 'How would you describe the social ambience and the persons you met?' (1 = very friendly/7 = very hostile); (2) 'Did you have the impression that something strange happened to you or around you that you could not explain?' (1 = nothing strange/7 = very strange); (3) 'Did you have unusual sensorial or perceptual experiences?' (1 = not at all/7 = very often); (4) 'Did you have the impression that your thoughts or emotions could be read or influenced?' (1 = not at all/7 = very often).

Regardless of the level of psychosis proneness, the likelihood of reporting unusual perceptions within a given 3-h ESM period was increased if cannabis was used

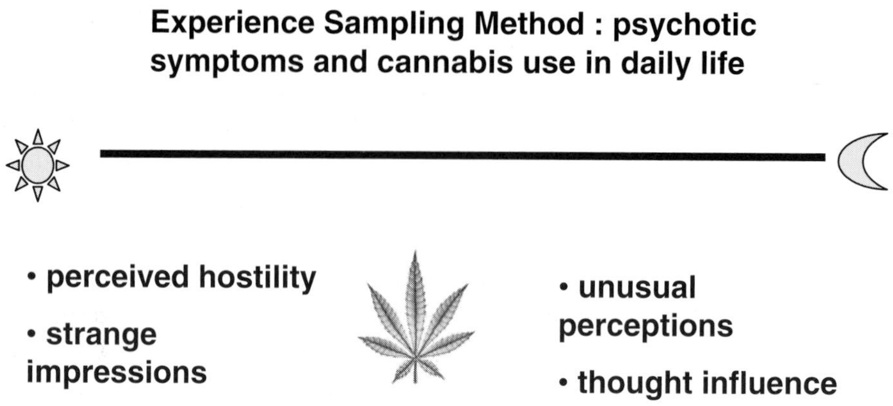

Experience Sampling Method : psychotic symptoms and cannabis use in daily life

 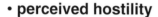

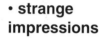
• perceived hostility

• strange impressions

• unusual perceptions

• thought influence

Figure 5.2 Experience Sampling Method: psychotic symptoms and cannabis use in daily life.

within the same ESM assessment period. Subjects were also significantly less likely to report perceived hostility; that is, they were more likely to find the atmosphere and the people friendly in the periods marked by cannabis use, than in those without cannabis use. In order to characterize better the temporal association between cannabis use and occurrence of psychotic experiences, we further explored this association across sequential assessment periods within the same day. There was no increased risk of psychotic experiences for a given ESM assessment if cannabis was consumed during the previous assessment period, and there was no evidence that cannabis use was increased in the periods following the occurrence of any of the psychotic experiences. Our findings demonstrate that cannabis use is a risk factor for the acute occurrence of abnormal perceptions in daily life, and that this effect is consistent with the estimated duration of the pharmacological effects of cannabis (Ashton, 2001). Moreover, these findings do not support the self-medication model, hypothesizing that cannabis is a consequence rather than a cause of psychotic symptoms. However, the present study only explored the acute effects of cannabis in the induction of psychotic experiences, and we can only speculate as to whether there is a continuum between the short-term and the long-term effects of cannabis with regard to increased risk of psychosis.

Is the risk of acute psychotic experiences induced by cannabis increased in subjects with a pre-existing psychosis vulnerability?

Although there is good evidence that cannabis is a risk factor for psychosis, an unresolved question regarding the link between cannabis use and psychosis is whether the impact of cannabis on subsequent psychosis is stronger in subjects with a pre-existing vulnerability for psychosis (McGuire *et al.*, 1995).

Is there an interaction between cannabis use and psychosis vulnerability in their effects on psychotic experiences in daily life?

We used the ESM sample previously described to examine the interaction between cannabis use and psychosis vulnerability (Verdoux *et al.*, 2003a). The 79 subjects included in this study were interviewed using the Mini International Neuropsychiatric Interview (MINI, 4.4 version). Psychosis vulnerability was defined by the MINI criteria for identifying a possible psychotic condition among subjects from the general population (Amorin *et al.*, 1998): (1) at least one bizarre psychotic symptom over the previous month; or (2) at least two non-bizarre psychotic symptoms over the previous month. We found that the acute effects of cannabis were modified by the level of psychosis vulnerability. Subjects with high psychosis vulnerability were more likely to experience unusual perceptions or thought influence during periods of cannabis use, but such effects were not found in subjects with low psychosis vulnerability.

Is there an interaction between cannabis use and psychosis vulnerability in their effects on increased incidence of psychotic disorder?

The previous ESM study explored only the short-term effects of cannabis on occurrence of psychotic experiences in vulnerable subjects. In order to characterize better the long-term effects of cannabis exposure in the interaction with psychosis vulnerability on psychosis outcome, we investigated this interaction in a longitudinal study of a population-based sample from the Dutch general population (Netherlands Mental Health Survey and Incidence Study, NEMESIS: van Os *et al.*, 2002). The subjects were interviewed at baseline (T_1) by lay interviewers using the Composite International Diagnostic Interview (CIDI). Clinical re-interviews were conducted by telephone by an experienced clinician for a subsample of individuals who had evidence of CIDI psychotic symptoms. Of the 4848 subjects who were followed up over 3 years, 59 presented with *Diagnostic and Statistical Manual of Mental Disorders* (*DSM*-III-R: American Psychiatric Association, 1987) diagnoses of any affective or non-affective psychotic disorder at baseline. This group included individuals who were clinical cases of psychosis but also individuals with subclinical psychotic experiences (no assessment of need for treatment was made at baseline). Thus, we considered these subjects as individuals with established vulnerability for psychosis. Cases of psychosis at the end of the follow-up (T_2) were identified using the Brief Psychiatric Rating Scale (BPRS) items 'unusual thought content', 'hallucinations' and 'conceptual disorganization', categorized according to the intensities of symptoms as 'BPRS any psychosis' or 'BPRS pathology-level psychosis'. The *DSM*-III-R diagnosis of psychosis was also established at the end of the follow-up using the same diagnostic interview procedure (CIDI and clinical re-interview);

assessment of need for mental health care in the context of psychotic symptoms was defined by the Camberwell Assessment of Need (Slade *et al.*, 1996). Substance use at baseline was assessed using the CIDI L section.

The effect of baseline cannabis on the psychosis outcomes at T_2 was estimated in 59 subjects with baseline *DSM*-III-R lifetime diagnosis psychotic disorder, and then compared with the effect of cannabis in individuals with no psychosis vulnerability at baseline ($n = 4045$). The biological synergism between cannabis use and psychosis vulnerability at baseline on psychosis outcome was estimated by calculating the additive statistical interaction between these two factors, taking into account the degree of parallelism (i.e. the degree to which cannabis use and psychosis vulnerability 'compete' for psychosis outcome). We found that the impact of cannabis on psychosis outcome was especially marked in subjects with established vulnerability for psychosis. The difference in risk of follow-up psychosis between those who did and did not use cannabis was much stronger in those with a baseline vulnerability for psychosis (BPRS any psychosis 46.7%, BPRS pathology-level psychosis 54.7%; needs-based diagnosis of psychotic disorder 23.3%) than in those without a baseline experience of psychosis (BPRS any psychosis 1.8%; BPRS pathology-level psychosis 2.2%; needs-based diagnosis of psychotic disorder 1.3%). Around 80% of the psychosis outcome in individuals exposed to both cannabis and established psychosis vulnerability was attributable to the synergistic action of these two factors. In other words, this prospective study showed that subjects with established vulnerability for psychotic disorder are particularly sensitive to the effects of cannabis, resulting in an increased risk of presenting with clinical psychosis.

Implications

These studies provide evidence supporting the hypothesis that exposure to cannabis may precipitate the onset of psychosis in vulnerable subjects. Investigations of the short- and long-term effects of cannabis exposure demonstrate that cannabis interacts with psychosis vulnerability not only in the acute induction of psychotic experiences, but also in the onset of clinical psychosis. These findings suggest that a continuum may exist between the short-term and the long-term effects of cannabis in subjects with psychosis vulnerability. Cumulative exposure to cannabis may induce persistent psychotic symptoms in vulnerable subjects, and the subsequent course of these symptoms may become at least in part independent of the exposure to cannabis.

Conclusions

Studies conducted in non-clinical samples show that cannabis users are more likely to present with attenuated psychotic symptoms than non-users, suggesting that a continuum may exist between the increased prevalence of cannabis use in subjects with clinical psychosis, and the cross-sectional association between cannabis use and psychosis proneness in subjects without clinical psychosis. Furthermore, the direction of the link between cannabis and psychosis is clarified by these studies, which support the hypothesis that cannabis use may be an independent risk factor for psychosis, at least in subjects with a pre-existing vulnerability for such a disorder. The mechanisms underlying the interaction between vulnerability for psychosis and cannabis use in the onset of psychosis need to be further explored. For example, it would be of interest to investigate whether high-risk subjects with a familial vulnerability for psychosis are more prone to experience psychotic symptoms when using cannabis than subjects with a low familial morbid risk. Further research on cannabis and psychosis proneness should also focus on the interaction between development and cannabis use, as the risk of psychosis in cannabis users may be at least in part age-related, dependent on the stage of brain maturation. This issue is of public health importance, as there is widespread use of cannabis in adolescents and young adults, coinciding with the peak period for the onset of psychosis.

REFERENCES

Allebeck, P., Adamsson, C., Engstrom, A. and Rydberg, U. (1993). Cannabis and schizophrenia: a longitudinal study of cases treated in Stockholm County. *Acta Psychiatr. Scand.*, **88**, 21–24.

American Psychiatric Association (1987). *Diagnostic and Statistical Manual of Mental Disorders*, 3rd edn. Washington, DC: American Psychiatric Association.

Amorin, P., Lecrubier, Y., Weiller, E., Hergueta, T. and Sheehan, D. (1998). DSM-III-R psychotic disorders: procedural validity of the MINI International Neuropsychiatric Interview (MINI). Concordance and causes for discordance with the CIDI. *Eur. Psychiatry*, **13**, 26–34.

Andreasson, S., Allebeck, P., Engstrom, A. and Rydberg, U. (1987). Cannabis and schizophrenia. A longitudinal study of Swedish conscripts. *Lancet*, **2**, 1483–1486.

Arndt, S., Tyrrell, G., Flaum, M. and Andreasen, N. C. (1992). Comorbidity of substance abuse and schizophrenia: the role of pre-morbid adjustment. *Psychol. Med.*, **22**, 379–388.

Arseneault, L., Cannon, M., Poulton, R. *et al.* (2002). Cannabis use in adolescence and risk for adult psychosis: longitudinal prospective study. *Br. Med. J.*, **325**, 1212–1213.

Ashton, C. (2001). Pharmacology and effects of cannabis: a brief review. *Br. J. Psychiatry*, **178**, 101–106.

Castle, D. J. and Ames, F. R. (1996). Cannabis and the brain. *Aust. NZ J. Psychiatry*, **30**, 179–183.

Chapman, L., Chapman, J., Kwapil, T., Eckblad, M. and Zinser, M. (1994). Putatively psychosis-prone subjects 10 years later. *J. Abnormal Psychol.*, **103**, 171–183.

Claridge, G. (1997) Theoretical background and issues. In: *Schizotypy. Implications for Illness and Health*, ed. G. Claridge, pp. 3–18. Oxford: Oxford University Press.

Claridge, G. and Beech, T. (1995) Fully and quasi-dimensional constructions of schizotypy. In *Schizotypal Personality*, ed. A. Raine, T. Lencz and S. A. Mednick, pp. 192–216. Cambridge: Cambridge University Press.

Csikszentmihalyi, M. and Larson, R. (1987). Validity and reliability of the Experience-Sampling Method. *J. Nerv. Ment. Dis.*, **175**, 526–536.

Delespaul, P. (1995) *Assessing Schizophrenia in Daily Life*. Maastricht: Universitaire Press.

Dixon, L., Haas, G., Weiden, P. J., Sweeney, J. and Frances, A. J. (1991). Drug abuse in schizophrenic patients: clinical correlates and reasons for use. *Am. J. Psychiatry*, **148**, 224–230.

Dumas, P., Saoud, M., Bouafia, S. *et al.* (2002). Cannabis use correlates with schizotypal personality traits in healthy students. *Psychiatry Res.*, **109**, 27–35.

Eaton, W., Romanoski, A., Anthony, J. C. and Nestadt, G. (1991). Screening for psychosis in the general population with a self-report interview. *J. Nerv. Ment. Dis.*, **179**, 689–693.

Hall, W. and Solowij, N. (1997). Long-term cannabis use and mental health. *Br. J. Psychiatry*, **171**, 107–108.

Johns, A. (2001). Psychiatric effects of cannabis. *Br. J. Psychiatry*, **178**, 116–122.

Kibel, D. A., Laffont, I. and Liddle, P. F. (1993). The composition of the negative syndrome of chronic schizophrenia. *Br. J. Psychiatry*, **162**, 744–750.

Kirkpatrick, B., Amador, X. F., Flaum, M. *et al.* (1996). The deficit syndrome in the DSM-IV field trial: I. Alcohol and other drug abuse. *Schizophr. Res.*, **20**, 69–77.

Kwapil, T. R. (1996). A longitudinal study of drug and alcohol use by psychosis-prone and impulsive-nonconforming individuals. *J. Abnormal Psychol.*, **105**, 114–123.

Liraud, F., and Verdoux, H. (2000). Which temperamental characteristics are associated with substance use in subjects with psychotic and mood disorders? *Psychiatry Res.*, **93**, 63–72.

Mason, G., Claridge, G. and Jackson, M. (1995). New scales for the assessment of schizotypy. *Personal. Individ. Differ.*, **18**, 7–13.

Mathers, D. C. and Ghodse, A. H. (1992). Cannabis and psychotic illness. *Br. J. Psychiatry*, **161**, 648–653.

McGuire, P. K., Jones, P., Harvey, I. *et al.* (1995). Morbid risk of schizophrenia for relatives of patients with cannabis-associated psychosis. *Schizophr. Res.*, **15**, 277–281.

Mueser, K. T., Yarnold, P. R., Levinson, D. F. *et al.* (1990). Prevalence of substance abuse in schizophrenia: demographic and clinical correlates. *Schizophr. Bull.*, **16**, 31–56.

Myin-Germeys, I., Delespaul, P. and de Vries, M. (2001a). The context of delusional experiences in the daily life of patients with schizophrenia. *Psychol. Med.*, **31**, 489–498.

Myin-Germeys, I., van Os, J., Schwartz, J., Stone, A. and Delespaul, P. (2001b). Emotional reactivity to daily life stress in psychosis. *Arch. Gen. Psychiatry*, **58**, 1137–1144.

Nunn, J., Rizza, F. and Peters, E. R. (2001). The incidence of schizotypy among cannabis and alcohol users. *J. Nerv. Ment. Dis.*, **189**, 741–748.

Peralta, V. and Cuesta, M. J. (1992). Influence of cannabis abuse on schizophrenic psychopathology. *Acta Psychiatr. Scand.*, **85**, 127–130.

Peters, E. R., Joseph, S. A. and Garety, P. A. (1999). Measurement of delusional ideation in the normal population: introducing the PDI (Peters *et al.* Delusions Inventory). *Schizophr. Bull.*, **25**, 553–576.

Poulton, R., Caspi, A., Moffitt, T. *et al.* (2000). Children's self-reported psychotic symptoms and adult schizophreniform disorder. *Arch. Gen. Psychiatry*, **57**, 1053–1058.

Raine, A. (1991). The SPQ: a scale for the assessment of schizotypal personality based on DSM-III-R criteria. *Schizophr. Bull.*, **17**, 556–563.

Salyers, M. and Mueser, K. (2001). Social functioning, psychopathology, and medication side effects in relation to substance use and abuse in schizophrenia. *Schizophr. Res.*, **48**, 109–123.

Selten, J. P., Gernaat, H. B., Nolen, W. A., Wiersma, D. and van den Bosch, R. J. (1998). Experience of negative symptoms: comparison of schizophrenic patients to patients with a depressive disorder and to normal subjects. *Am. J. Psychiatry*, **155**, 350–354.

Skosnik, P. D., Spatz-Glenn, L. and Park, S. (2001). Cannabis use is associated with schizotypy and attentional disinhibition. *Schizophr. Res.*, **48**, 83–92.

Slade, M., Phelan, M., Thornicroft, G. and Parkman, S. (1996). The Camberwell Assessment of Need (CAN): comparison of assessments by staff and patients of the needs of the severely mentally ill. *Soc. Psychiatry Psychiatric Epidemiol.*, **31**, 109–113.

Smart, R. and Ogborne, A. (2000). Drug use and drinking among students in 36 countries. *Addict. Behav.*, **25**, 455–460.

Stefanis, N., Hanssen, M., Smyonis, N. *et al.* (2002). Evidence that three dimensions of psychosis have a distribution in the general population. *Psychol. Med.*, **32**, 347–358.

Swendsen, J. D. and Norman, S. (1998). Preparing for community violence: mood and behavioral correlates of the second Rodney King verdicts. *J. Traumatic Stress*, **11**, 57–70.

Swendsen, J. D., Tennen, H., Carney, M. A. *et al.* (2000). Mood and alcohol consumption: an experience sampling test of the self-medication hypothesis. *J. Abnormal Psychol.*, **109**, 198–204.

Tennant, F. S. Jr and Groesbeck, C. J. (1972). Psychiatric effects of hashish. *Arch. Gen. Psychiatry*, **27**, 133–136.

Thornicroft, G. (1990). Cannabis and psychosis. Is there epidemiological evidence for an association? *Br. J. Psychiatry*, **157**, 25–33.

Tien, A. (1991). Distributions of hallucinations in the population. *Soc. Psychiatry Psychiatric Epidemiol.*, **26**, 287–292.

Tramèr, M., Carroll, D., Campbell, F. *et al.* (2001). Cannabinoids for control of chemotherapy induced nausea and vomiting: quantitative systematic review. *Br. Med. J.*, **323**, 16.

van Os, J., Verdoux, H., Maurice-Tison, S. *et al.* (1999). Self-reported psychosis-like symptoms and the continuum of psychosis. *Soc. Psychiatry Psychiatric Epidemiol.*, **34**, 459–463.

van Os, J., Hanssen, M., Bijl, R. and Ravelli, A. (2000). Strauss (1969) revisited: a psychosis continuum in the general population? *Schizophr. Res.*, **45**, 11–20.

van Os, J., Hanssen, M., Bijl, R. and Vollebergh, W. (2001). Prevalence of psychotic disorder and community level of psychotic symptoms. *Arch. Gen. Psychiatry*, **58**, 663–668.

van Os, J., Bak, M., Hanssen, M. *et al.* (2002). Cannabis and psychosis: a longitudinal population-based study. *Am. J. Epidemiol.*, **156**, 319–327.

Venables, P., Wilkins, S., Mitchell, D., Raine, A. and Bailes, K. (1990). A scale for the measurement of schizotypy. *Personality Individ. Differ.*, **11**, 481–495.

Verdoux, H. and van Os, J. (2002). Psychotic symptoms in non-clinical populations and the continuum of psychosis. *Schizophr. Res.*, **54**, 59–65.

Verdoux, H., Maurice-Tison, S., Gay, B. *et al.* (1998a). A survey of delusional ideation in primary care patients. *Psychol. Med.*, **28**, 127–134.

Verdoux, H., van Os, J., Maurice-Tison, S. *et al.* (1998b). Is early adulthood a critical developmental stage for psychosis proneness? A survey of delusional ideation in normal subjects. *Schizophr. Res.*, **29**, 247–254.

Verdoux, H., van Os, J., Maurice-Tison, S. *et al.* (1999). Increased occurrence of depression in psychosis-prone subjects. A follow-up study in primary care settings. *Comp. Psychiatry*, **40**, 462–468.

Verdoux, H., Gindre, C., Sorbara, F., Tournier, M. and Swendsen, J. (2003a). Cannabis use and the expression of psychosis vulnerability in daily life. *Psychol. Med.*, **33**, 23–32.

Verdoux, H., Sorbara, F., Gindre, C., Swendsen, D. and van Os, J. (2003b). Cannabis and dimensions of psychosis in a non-clinical population of female subjects. *Schizophr. Res.*, **59**, 77–84.

Webb, E., Ashton, C., Kelly, P. and Kamali, F. (1996). Alcohol and drug use in UK university students. *Lancet*, **348**, 922–925.

Weiser, M., Reichenberg, A., Rabinowitz, J. *et al.* (2002). Self-reported drug abuse in male adolescents with behavioural disturbances, and follow-up for future schizophrenia. *Schizophr. Res.*, **53** (suppl.), 227.

Williams, J. H., Wellman, N. A. and Rawlins, J. N. (1996). Cannabis use correlates with schizotypy in healthy people. *Addiction*, **91**, 869–877.

6

Is there a specific 'cannabis psychosis'?

Wayne Hall[1] and Louisa Degenhardt[2]

[1] University of Queensland, St Lucia, QLD, Australia
[2] University of New South Wales, Sydney, NSW, Australia

There are good reasons to be concerned about the possibility that cannabis use may be a cause of psychotic disorders. Psychoses are serious and disabling disorders (Bromet *et al.*, 1995). Cannabis is widely used during late adolescence in many developed societies (Hall *et al.*, 1999), and high doses of tetrahydrocannabinol (THC) – the psychoactive substance in cannabis – have been reported to produce psychotic symptoms such as visual and auditory hallucinations, delusional ideas and thought disorder in normal volunteers (Hall *et al.*, 2001; and see Chapter 5).

There are a number of hypotheses about the relationship between cannabis use and psychosis that need to be distinguished (Thornicroft, 1990). The strongest hypothesis in causal terms is that heavy cannabis use causes a specific 'cannabis psychosis'. It assumes that these psychoses would not occur in the absence of cannabis use, and that the causal role of cannabis can be inferred from the symptoms and their relationship to cannabis use; that is, they are preceded by heavy cannabis use and remit after abstinence. It also assumes that cannabis psychoses are qualitatively different from other psychotic disorders. This hypothesis is the subject of this chapter. The potential role of cannabis as a causal agent for schizophrenia *per se* is the subject of Chapter 7.

Making causal inferences

In order to infer that cannabis use is a cause of a specific psychotic disorder, we need evidence: that there is an association between cannabis use and psychosis; that chance is an unlikely explanation of the association; that cannabis use preceded the psychosis; and that plausible alternative explanations of the association can be excluded (Hall, 1987).

Marijuana and Madness: Psychiatry and Neurobiology, ed. D. Castle and R. Murray. Published by Cambridge University Press. © Cambridge University Press 2004.

Evidence that cannabis use and psychosis are associated and that chance is an unlikely explanation of the association is readily available. There are a small number of prospective studies that show that cannabis use precedes psychoses. The most difficult task is to exclude the hypothesis that the relationship between cannabis use and psychosis is due to other factors (e.g. other drug use, or a genetic predisposition to develop schizophrenia and use cannabis).

The discovery of an 'amfetamine psychosis' provides an instructive example of how such a strong relationship between drug use and psychosis was tested between the 1950s and the early 1970s. The first case report of a psychosis following amfetamine use was as long ago as 1938 (Young and Scovell, 1938) but it was not until Connell's series of 42 cases in 1958 that the association became more widely known (Connell, 1958). Connell reported cases of psychosis following very heavy oral use of amfetamine or methamfetamine (average dose of 325 mg daily) sold over the counter. The symptoms of psychosis (most commonly including ideas of reference, delusions of persecution, auditory and visual hallucinations) remitted quickly following abstinence after admission (usually after 2 weeks; Connell, 1958).

Sceptical US investigators argued that Connell's series did not exclude the alternative hypothesis that persons at risk of psychosis were more likely to use amfetamines. This alternative hypothesis became harder to sustain after provocation studies (that would nowadays be regarded as unethical) were done in Australia and the USA. Bell (1973) showed (initially inadvertently and later deliberately) that he could reproduce the psychosis in amfetamine users by injecting large amounts of methamfetamine. Studies by Angrist and colleagues in normal volunteers showed that large doses of amfetamine given by injection produced characteristic psychotic symptoms (Angrist and Gershon, 1970; Angrist et al., 1974). The case for the hypothesis was strengthened by evidence of its biological plausibility: excess dopamine levels (which were produced by chronic amfetamine administration in animals) have been implicated in schizophrenia (Julien, 2001).

It is difficult to extend such studies to resolve the 'cannabis psychosis' controversy in the same way. Ethical constraints preclude experimental studies in humans using large doses of THC to see if its use produces psychotic symptoms. Observational studies of the effects of cannabis use on psychotic symptoms in psychosis-prone individuals (see Chapter 5) are the nearest ethically acceptable alternative. The next best alternative has been experimental studies in which small doses of THC are given to healthy controls and persons with schizophrenia whose performance is compared on certain psychological tasks (Emrich et al., 1997). At present, there are no suitable animal models to reproduce the phenomena, although research is increasingly examining this issue (see section on biological plausibility, below).

It is necessary to examine the relationship between cannabis use and psychosis using statistical research methods to rule out common causal hypotheses. This chapter reviews the best epidemiological and clinical studies on 'cannabis psychosis'. We begin by reviewing case reports of 'cannabis psychosis'. We then review controlled clinical studies and finally epidemiological studies of the association between cannabis use and psychotic symptoms and disorders. The epidemiological studies estimate the relationship between cannabis use and the risk of psychosis after adjusting for confounding variables such as personal characteristics prior to using cannabis, family history of psychotic illness and other drug use. We conclude the chapter with a brief discussion of the biological plausibility of an association between cannabis use and psychosis. The reader is also referred to Chapters 5 and 8.

Studies of 'cannabis psychosis'

Case reports

There are numerous case reports of a putative 'cannabis psychosis' (Talbott and Teague, 1969; Kolansky and Moore, 1971; Bernardson and Gunne, 1972; Tennant and Groesbeck, 1972; Chopra and Smith, 1974; Carney *et al.*, 1984; Tunving, 1985; Drummond, 1986; Onyango, 1986; Cohen and Johnson, 1988; Solomons *et al.*, 1990; Eva, 1992; Wylie *et al.*, 1995). These describe individuals who develop psychotic symptoms or disorders after using cannabis.

Chopra and Smith (1974), for example, described 200 patients who were admitted to a psychiatric hospital in Calcutta between 1963 and 1968 with psychotic symptoms following the use of cannabis (Chopra and Smith, 1974). The most common symptoms 'were sudden onset of confusion, generally associated with delusions, hallucinations (usually visual) and emotional lability . . . amnesia, disorientation, depersonalisation and paranoid symptoms' (p. 24). Most psychoses were preceded by the ingestion of a large dose of cannabis and there was amnesia for the period between ingestion and hospitalization. The authors argued that it was unlikely that excessive cannabis use was a sign of pre-existing psychopathology because a third of their cases had no prior psychiatric history, the symptoms were remarkably uniform regardless of prior psychiatric history and those who used the most potent cannabis preparations experienced psychotic reactions after the shortest period of use.

The findings of Chopra and Smith (1974) have received some support from other case series that suggest that large doses of potent cannabis products can be followed by a 'toxic' psychotic disorder with 'organic' features of amnesia and confusion. These disorders have been reported from a variety of different places, including the Caribbean (Spencer, 1971; Harding and Knight, 1973), India (Chopra and Smith, 1974), New Zealand (Eva, 1992), Scotland (Wylie *et al.*, 1995), South Africa (Solomons *et al.*, 1990), Sweden (Bernardson and Gunne, 1972; Palsson *et al.*, 1982;

Tunving, 1985; 1987), the UK (Carney *et al.*, 1984; Drummond, 1986; Onyango, 1986) and the USA (Talbott and Teague, 1969; Tennant and Groesbeck, 1972).

These disorders have been attributed to cannabis use for combinations of the following reasons: the onset of the symptoms followed closely upon ingestion of large quantities of cannabis; the affected individuals often exhibited 'organic' symptoms such as confusion, disorientation and amnesia; some had no reported personal or family history of psychosis prior to using cannabis; their symptoms remitted rapidly (usually within several days to several weeks) after a period of enforced abstinence from cannabis use; recovery was usually complete with the person having no residual psychotic symptoms of the type often seen in persons with schizophrenia; and if the disorder recurred, it was after the individual used cannabis again.

Some commentators have been critical of this evidence (Lewis, 1968; Thornicroft, 1990; Gruber and Pope, 1994; Schuckit, 1994; Poole and Brabbins, 1996). They criticize the poor quality of information on cannabis use and its relationship to the onset of psychosis, and the person's premorbid adjustment and family history of psychosis. They also emphasize the wide variety of clinical pictures of 'cannabis psychosis' reported by different observers. These weaknesses impair the evidential value of these case series.

Controlled clinical studies

A small number of controlled studies have been conducted over the past 20 years to test the 'cannabis psychosis' hypothesis. Some case-control studies have either compared persons with 'cannabis psychosis' with persons who have schizophrenia, or compared psychoses occurring in persons who do and do not have biochemical evidence of cannabis use prior to presenting for treatment. Their results have been mixed.

Controlled studies of 'cannabis psychosis'

Thacore and Shukla (1976) reported a case-control study of 25 cases who had a 'cannabis psychosis' with 25 controls who were diagnosed as having paranoid schizophrenia with no history of cannabis use. The cases had a paranoid psychosis resembling schizophrenia in which there was a clear temporal relationship between the prolonged use of cannabis and the development of psychosis on more than two occasions. Patients with 'cannabis psychosis' displayed more odd and bizarre behaviour, violence and panic, but exhibited less formal thought disorder and had better insight than those with schizophrenia. They also responded swiftly to neuroleptic drugs and recovered completely.

In contrast to these positive findings, a number of controlled studies have not found such a clear association. Imade and Ebie (1991), for example, compared the symptoms of 70 patients with cannabis-associated functional psychoses, 163 patients with schizophrenia and 39 patients with mania. They reported that there were no symptoms that were unique to cannabis psychosis, and none that enabled them to distinguish a 'cannabis psychosis' from schizophrenia.

Controlled studies of psychosis in users and non-users of cannabis

Rottanburg et al. (1982) compared the symptoms of 20 psychotic patients with cannabinoids in their urine with those of 20 psychotic patients who did not have cannabinoids in their urine. Subjects with cannabinoids in their urine had more symptoms of hypomania and agitation, and less auditory hallucinations, flattening of affect, incoherent speech and hysteria than controls. They also showed marked improvements in symptoms by the end of a week, whereas there was no change in symptomatology in the patients whose urine did not contain cannabinoids.

Chaudry et al. (1991) compared 15 psychotic bhang (cannabis tea) users with 10 bhang users without psychosis. They found that their cases were more likely to have a history of chronic cannabis use and past psychotic episodes. They were also more likely to be uncooperative and to have symptoms of excitement, hostility, grandiosity, hallucinations, disorientation and unusual thought content. All cases remitted within 5 days and had no residual psychotic symptoms.

Mathers et al. (1991) reported a study of patients presenting to two London hospitals and whose urine was analysed for the presence of cannabinoids. They found a relationship between the presence of cannabinoids in urine and having a psychotic diagnosis. Rolfe et al. (1993) reported a similar association between urinary cannabinoids and psychosis in 234 patients admitted to a Gambian psychiatric unit.

Thornicroft (1992) compared 45 cases who had a psychotic episode and urine positive for cannabinoids with 45 controls who had psychotic symptoms but either had urine negative for cannabinoids or reported no cannabis use. They found very few demographic or clinical differences between the groups.

A comparison of 52 persons with schizophrenia and current substance abuse/dependence with 78 persons without any history of abuse or dependence found that those with a comorbid diagnosis were more likely to have higher scores on the Symptom Checklist 90 – revised (SCL-90-R) scales of paranoid ideation and psychoticism (Fowler et al., 1998). In contrast, a sample of consecutively admitted psychotic patients grouped according to presence of cannabinoids in urine ($n = 11$ positive, $n = 29$ negative) found that those with positive urine tests were less likely to be thought-disordered, suspicious or deluded, as assessed by the Brief Psychiatric Rating Scale (Sembhi and Lee, 1999).

A study of persons identified in a census survey of Westminister, UK, with schizophrenia similarly found that those with 'non-alcohol substance misuse' (the most commonly misused substance was cannabis) were not significantly different from those without such a history to have positive or negative symptoms of schizophrenia or symptoms of disorganization (Duke et al., 2001).

Recently, Soyka and colleagues (2001) compared a sample of 447 persons with schizophrenia grouped according to the presence of a substance use disorder (around one-third of comorbid cases involved problematic cannabis use). The two groups were compared for the presence of over 100 symptoms at both admission and discharge from inpatient treatment. Subjects with a comorbid substance use disorder were significantly more likely (at $P < 0.05$ level) than those without such a disorder to have the following symptoms at admission: sudden delusional ideas, visual hallucinations, thought withdrawal, thought insertion, irritability and increased drive. They were significantly *less* likely to have the following symptoms at admission: delusions of guilt, anxiety, parathymia, inhibition of drive, mannerisms and mutism (Soyka *et al.*, 2001). At discharge from treatment, those with a comorbid substance use disorder were still more likely to have visual hallucinations, thought withdrawal and thought insertion, and irritability and less likely to have delusions of guilt and parathymia. However, *none* of the differences were significant at the level of $P < 0.001$, the level that the authors chose as the criterion of clear statistical difference due to the very large number of comparisons. The findings of this study therefore do not give any clear evidence of symptom differences according to comorbid substance use disorders.

McGuire *et al.* (1995) compared 23 cases of psychoses occurring in persons whose urines were positive for cannabinoids with 46 psychotic patients whose urines were negative for cannabinoids or who reported no cannabis use. The two groups did not differ in their psychiatric histories or symptoms profile, as assessed by 'blind' ratings of clinical files using the Present State Examination (PSE). The cases (7.1%), however, were more likely than controls (0.7%) to have a family history of schizophrenia.

Contrasting findings were obtained in a recent study by Miller and colleagues (2001) examining a cohort of young people recruited according to risk of schizophrenia, with 'high risk' defined as at least two relatives with a history of schizophrenia, compared to an age-, gender- and socioeconomically matched sample of controls. Recent frequent cannabis use was associated with an overall increase in the likelihood of reporting psychotic symptoms. However, current cannabis use was reported by similar proportions of the groups and there was no increase in the likelihood of the high-risk group experiencing psychotic symptoms if they were current users (Miller *et al.*, 2001).

Two studies have reported no difference in the prevalence of psychotic disorders in chronic cannabis users and controls. Beaubruhn and Knight (1973) compared the rate of psychosis in 30 chronic daily Jamaican cannabis users with that in 30 non-cannabis-using controls. Stefanis *et al.* (1976, 1977) reported a study of 47 chronic cannabis users in Greece and 40 controls. The small number of cases and the low prevalence of psychosis in the population make these negative findings unconvincing.

Epidemiological studies

A small number of studies have examined the relationship between cannabis use and psychotic symptoms in samples from the general population. One limitation of these studies is that they examined whether cannabis users were more likely to report psychotic symptoms without examining whether cannabis users' symptoms were qualitatively different from non-users' patterns.

Tien and Anthony (1990) used data from the US Epidemiologic Catchment Area study to compare the drug use of individuals who reported 'psychotic experiences' during a 12-month period. These psychotic experiences comprised four types of hallucinations and seven types of delusional belief. They compared 477 cases who reported one or more psychotic symptoms in the 1-year follow-up with 1818 controls who did not. Cases and controls were matched for age and social and demographic characteristics. Daily cannabis use was found to double the risk of reporting psychotic symptoms (after statistical adjustment for alcohol use and psychiatric diagnoses at baseline).

Thomas (1996) reported the prevalence of psychotic symptoms among cannabis users in a random sample of people drawn from the electoral roll of a large city in the North Island of New Zealand. One in seven (14%) cannabis users reported 'strange, unpleasant experiences such as hearing voices or becoming convinced that someone is trying to harm you or that you are being persecuted' after using cannabis. Unfortunately, only cannabis users in the sample were asked these questions so it was not possible to compare rates of psychotic symptoms among persons who had and had not used cannabis.

Degenhardt and Hall (2001) found, in an Australian adult population, that persons who used cannabis were more likely to screen positively for psychosis, as determined by a screening questionnaire. Around one in 143 persons who were non-users screened positively, with the prevalence increasing as involvement with cannabis increased, such that one in 15 persons who met criteria for cannabis dependence also screened positively for psychosis. After controlling for demographics, neuroticism and other drug use, this relationship was still significant. Dependent cannabis users reported twice the rate of psychotic symptoms of non-cannabis users.

Time trends in the incidence and prevalence of schizophrenia

If cannabis use causes psychosis *de novo*, then the incidence and prevalence of schizophrenia and other psychoses should increase as the prevalence of cannabis increases in the age group at risk. Because there has been a dramatic increase in the prevalence of cannabis use in successive birth cohorts in Australia since the early 1970s (Degenhardt *et al.*, 2000), this hypothesis predicts an increased incidence and prevalence of psychosis among younger Australians. Degenhardt and colleagues

(2001) evaluated this hypothesis by modelling trends in the number of persons with psychosis in Australia since the prevalence of regular cannabis use began to increase. There was no significant increase in the incidence of schizophrenia and other psychoses over the past 30 years in Australia, suggesting that cannabis use was *not* causally related to the incidence of any significant number of psychosis 'cases' (i.e. there is a low population attributable fraction).

Biological plausibility of the association between cannabis use and psychosis

The principal psychoactive ingredient of cannabis is Δ^9-tetrahydrocannabinol, which acts upon a specific cannabinoid receptor (CB_1) in the brain (Hall *et al.*, 2001; and see Chapters 1 and 2). While historically the dopaminergic system of the brain has been considered to play an important role in psychotic disorders (Julien, 2001), there is increasing evidence that the cannabinoid system may be involved in schizophrenia and related psychotic disorders (Fritzsche, 2001; Glass, 2001; Skosnik *et al.*, 2001). Animal research has shown that CB_1 receptor knockout mice have behaviours consistent with some of the symptoms of schizophrenia, such as reduced goal-directed activity and impaired memory for temporal representations (Fritzsche, 2001).

Elevated levels of anandamide, an endogenous cannabinoid agonist, have been found in the cerebrospinal fluid of persons with schizophrenia (Leweke *et al.*, 1999) and a recent case-control study found that persons with schizophrenia had a greater density of CB_1 receptors in the prefrontal cortex than controls (Dean *et al.*, 2001).

Finally, a recent laboratory study of the effects of cannabis use on a previously drug-free person with schizophrenia (as ascertained via urinalysis) found that several hours after smoking cannabis (without the knowledge of the researchers), this person developed positive psychotic symptoms (Voruganti *et al.*, 2001). Examination of brain scans before and after cannabis use showed a significant increase in dopaminergic transmission, suggesting that cannabis may be linked to positive psychotic symptoms via increased dopaminergic transmission in the brain (Voruganti *et al.*, 2001).

Conclusions

The existence of a discrete 'cannabis psychosis' is still a matter for debate. In its favour are case series of 'cannabis psychosis', and a small number of controlled studies that compare the characteristics of 'cannabis psychosis' with those of psychoses in individuals who were not using cannabis at the time of manifestation of psychotic symptoms (Boutros and Bowers, 1996). Critics of the hypothesis emphasize the fallibility of clinical judgements about aetiology, the poorly specified criteria used in diagnosing these psychoses, the dearth of controlled studies and the striking variations in the clinical features of 'cannabis psychosis' (Poole and Brabbins, 1996).

It is a plausible hypothesis that high doses of cannabis can produce psychotic symptoms (see Chapters 3 and 5). There is no compelling evidence, however, that there is a specific clinical syndrome that is identifiable as a 'cannabis psychosis'. The clinical symptoms reported by different observers have been mixed. These symptoms seem to remit rapidly, with full recovery after abstinence from cannabis.

If cannabis-induced psychoses exist, they are rare or they only rarely receive medical intervention in western societies (American Psychiatric Association, 1994; Lishman, 1987). The total number of cases of putative 'cannabis psychosis' in the 12 case series reviewed by Hall *et al.* (2001) was 397, and 200 of these came from a single series collected over 6 years from a large geographic area in which heavy cannabis use was endemic (Chopra and Smith, 1974).

There are a number of likely reasons for the rarity of 'cannabis psychosis' in western societies. One is that they occur after the use of large doses of THC, or long periods of sustained heavy use. Although lifetime use of cannabis has increased in western societies, the pattern of heavy cannabis use remains rare (Donnelly and Hall, 1994). A second possibility is that cannabis psychosis only occurs in persons who have a pre-existing vulnerability to psychotic disorder. A third possibility is that heavy sustained use and vulnerability are both required.

REFERENCES

American Psychiatric Association (1994). *Diagnostic and Statistical Manual of Mental Disorders*, 4th ed. Washington, DC: American Psychiatric Association.

Angrist, B. M. and Gershon, S. (1970). The phenomenology of experimentally induced amphetamine psychosis – preliminary observation. *Biol. Psychiatry*, **2**, 95–107.

Angrist, B., Sathanthen, G., Wilks, S. and Gerson, S. (1974). Amphetamine psychosis: behavioral and biochemical aspects. *J. Psychiatric Res.*, **11**, 13–23.

Beaubruhn, M. and Knight, F. (1973). Psychiatric assessment of 30 chronic users of cannabis and 30 matched controls. *Am. J. Psychiatry*, **130**, 309–311.

Bell, D. (1973). The experimental reproduction of amphetamine psychosis. *Arch. Gen. Psychiatry*, **29**, 35–40.

Bernardson, G. and Gunne, L. M. (1972). Forty-six cases of psychosis in cannabis abusers. *Int. J. Addict.*, **7**, 9–16.

Boutros, N. N. and Bowers, M. B. (1996). Chronic substance-induced psychotic disorders: state of the literature. *J. Neuropsychiatry Clin. Neurosci.*, **8**, 262–269.

Bromet, E., Dew, A. and Eaton, W. (1995). Epidemiology of psychosis with special reference to schizophrenia. In *Textbook in Psychiatric Epidemiology*, ed. M. Tsuang, M. Tohen and G. Zahner, pp. 283–300. New York: Wiley.

Carney, M. W. P., Bacelle, L. and Robinson, B. (1984). Psychosis after cannabis use. *Br. Med. J.*, **288**, 1047.

Chaudry, H. R., Moss, H. B., Bashir, A. and Suliman, T. (1991). Cannabis psychosis following bhang ingestion. *Br. J. Addict.*, **86**, 1075–1081.

Chopra, G. S. and Smith, J. W. (1974). Psychotic reactions following cannabis use in East Indians. *Arch. Gen. Psychiatry*, **30**, 24–27.

Cohen, S. and Johnson, K. (1988). Psychosis from alcohol or drug abuse. *Br. Med. J.*, **297**, 1270–1271.

Connell, P. H. (1958). *Amphetamine Psychosis*. Maudsley Monograph number 5. London: Chapman & Hall.

Dean, B., Sundram, S., Bradbury, R., Scarr, E. and Copolov, D. (2001). Studies on [3H]CP-55940 binding in the human central nervous system: regional specific changes in density of cannabinoid-1 receptors associated with schizophrenia and cannabis use. *Neuroscience*, **103**, 9–15.

Degenhardt, L. and Hall, W. (2001). The association between psychosis and problematical drug use among Australian adults: findings from the National Survey of Mental Health and Well-Being. *Psychol. Med.*, **31**, 659–668.

Degenhardt, L., Lynskey, M. and Hall, W. (2000). Cohort trends in the age of initiation of drug use in Australia. *Aust. NZ J. Public Health*, **24**, 421–426.

Degenhardt, L., Hall, W. and Lynskey, M. (2001). *Modelling some Possible Relationships between Cannabis Use and Psychosis*. NDARC technical report no. 121. Sydney: National Drug and Alcohol Research Centre, University of NSW.

Donnelly, N. and Hall, W. (1994). *Patterns of Cannabis Use in Australia*. NCADA monograph series no. 27. Canberra: Australian Government Publishing Service.

Drummond, L. (1986). Cannabis psychosis: a case report. *Br. J. Addict.*, **81**, 139–140.

Duke, P., Pantelis, C., McPhillips, M. and Barnes, T. (2001). Comorbid non-alcohol substance misuse among people with schizophrenia: epidemiological study in central London. *Br. J. of Psychiatry*, **179**, 509–513.

Emrich, H., Leweke, F. and Schneider, U. (1997). Towards a cannabinoid hypothesis of schizophrenia: cognitive impairments due to dysregulation of the endogenous cannabinoid system. *Pharmacol., Biochem. Behav.*, **56**, 803–807.

Eva, J. (1992). Cannabis psychosis. *Psychiatric Bull.*, **16**, 310–311.

Fowler, I., Carr, V., Carter, N. and Lewin, T. (1998). Patterns of current and lifetime substance use in schizophrenia. *Schizophr. Bull.*, **24**, 443–455.

Fritzsche, M. (2001). Are cannabinoid receptor knockout mice animal models for schizophrenia? *Med. Hypotheses*, **56**, 638–643.

Glass, M. (2001). The role of cannabinoids in neurodegenerative diseases. *Progr. Neuro-Psychopharmacol. Biol. Psychiatry*, **25**, 743–765.

Gruber, A. J. and Pope, H. G. (1994). Cannabis psychotic disorder: does it exist? *Am. J. Addict.*, **3**, 72–83.

Hall, W. (1987). A simplified logic of causal inference. *Aust. NZ J. Psychiatry*, **21**, 507–513.

Hall, W., Johnston, L. and Donnelly, N. (1999). Epidemiology of cannabis use and its conse-quences. In *The Health Effects of Cannabis*, ed. H. Kalant, W. Corrigall, W. Hall and R. Smart, pp. 71–125. Toronto, Canada: Centre for Addiction and Mental Health.

Hall, W., Degenhardt, L. and Lynskey, M. (2001). *The Health and Psychological Consequences of Cannabis Use.* National Drug Strategy monograph number 44. Canberra: Australian Publishing Service.

Harding, T. and Knight, F. (1973). Marijuana-modified mania. *Arch. Gen. Psychiatry*, **29**, 635–637.

Imade, A. G. T. and Ebie, J. C. (1991). A retrospective study of symptom patterns of cannabis-induced psychosis. *Acta Psychiatr. Scand.*, **83**, 134–136.

Julien, R. (2001). *A Primer of Drug Action*, 9th edn. New York: Worth.

Kolansky, H. and Moore, W. (1971). Effects of marihuana on adolescents and young adults. *J.A.M.A.*, **216**, 486–492.

Leweke, F. M., Giuffrida, A., Wurster, U., Emrich, H. M. and Piomelli, D. (1999). Elevated endogenous cannabinoids in schizophrenia. *Neuroreport*, **10**, 1665–1669.

Lewis, A. (1968). A review of the international clinical literature. In *Cannabis: Report by the Advisory Committee on Drug Dependence*. London: Her Majesty's Stationery Office.

Lishman, W. A. (1987). *Organic Psychiatry: The Psychological Consequences of Cerebral Disorder*, 2nd ed. Oxford: Blackwell Scientific Publications.

Mathers, D., Ghodse, A., Caan, A. and Scott, S. (1991). Cannabis use in a large sample of acute psychiatric admissions. *Br. J. Addict.*, **86**, 779–784.

McGuire, P., Jones, R., Harvey, I. *et al.* (1995). Morbid risk of schizophrenia for relatives of patients with cannabis associated psychosis. *Schizophr. Res.*, **15**, 277–281.

Miller, P., Lawrie, S. M., Hodges, A. *et al.* (2001). Genetic liability, illicit drug use, life stress and psychotic symptoms: preliminary findings from the Edinburgh study of people at high risk for schizophrenia. *Soc. Psychiatry Psychiatric Epidemiol.*, **36**, 338–342.

Onyango, R. S. (1986). Cannabis psychosis in young psychiatric inpatients. *Br. J. Addic.*, **81**, 419–423.

Palsson, A., Thulin, S. O. and Tunving, K. (1982). Cannabis psychoses in South Sweden. *Acta Psychiatr. Scand.*, **66**, 311–321.

Poole, R. and Brabbins, C. (1996). Drug induced psychosis. *Br. J. Psychiatry*, **168**, 135–138.

Rolfe, M., Tang, M., Sabally, S. *et al.* (1993). Psychosis and cannabis abuse in the Gambia: a case-control study. *Br. J. Psychiatry*, **163**, 798–801.

Rottanburg, D., Robins, A. H., Ben-Arie, O., Teggin, A. and Elk, R. (1982). Cannabis-associated psychosis with hypomanic features. *Lancet*, **2**, 1364–1366.

Schuckit, M. A. (1994). Can marijuana cause a long-lasting psychosis? *Drug Abuse Alcoholism Newslett.*, **23**, 1–4.

Sembhi, S. and Lee, J. W. Y. (1999). Cannabis use in psychotic patients. *Aust. NZ J. Psychiatry*, **33**, 529–532.

Skosnik, P. D., Spatz-Glenn, L. and Park, S. (2001). Cannabis use is associated with schizotypy and attentional dysinhibition. *Schizophr. Res.*, **48**, 83–92.

Solomons, K., Neppe, V. M. and Kuyl, J. M. (1990). Toxic cannabis psychosis is a valid entity. *South Afr. Med. J.*, **78**, 476–481.

Soyka, M., Albus, M., Immler, B., Kathmann, N. and Hippius, H. (2001). Psychopathology in dual diagnosis and non-addicted schizophrenics – are there differences? *Eur. Arch. Psychiatriy Clin. Neurosci.*, **251**, 232–238.

Spencer, D. J. (1971). Cannabis-induced psychosis. *Int. J. Addict.*, **6**, 323–326.

Stefanis, C., Boulougouris, J. and Liakos, A. (1976). Clinical and psychophysiological effects of cannabis in long term users. In *Pharmacology of Marihuana*, ed. M. Braude and S. Szara, pp. 659–665. New York: Raven Press.

Stefanis, C., Dornbush, R. and Fink, M. (1977). *Hashish: Studies of Long-Term Use.* New York: Raven Press.

Talbott, J. A. and Teague, J. W. (1969). Marihuana psychosis: acute toxic psychosis associated with the use of cannabis derivatives. *J.A.M.A.*, **210**, 299–302.

Tennant, F. S. and Groesbeck, C. J. (1972). Psychiatric effects of hashish. *Arch. Gen. Psychiatry*, **27**, 133–136.

Thacore, V. R. and Shukla, S. R. P. (1976). Cannabis psychosis and paranoid schizophrenia. *Arch. Gen. Psychiatry*, **33**, 383–386.

Thomas, H. (1996). A community survey of adverse effects of cannabis use. *Drug Alcohol Depend.*, **42**, 201–207.

Thornicroft, G. (1990). Cannabis and psychosis: is there epidemiological evidence for an association? *Br. J. Psychiatry*, **157**, 25–33.

Thornicroft, G. (1992). Is "cannabis psychosis" a distinct category? *Eur. Psychiatry*, **7**, 277–282.

Tien, A. Y. and Anthony, J. C. (1990). Epidemiological analysis of alcohol and drug use as risk factors for psychotic experiences. *J. Nerv. Ment. Dis.*, **178**, 473–480.

Tunving, K. (1985). Psychiatric effects of cannabis use. *Acta Psychiatr. Scand.*, **72**, 209–217.

Tunving, K. (1987). Psychiatric aspects of cannabis use in adolescents and young adults. *Pediatrician*, **14**, 83–91.

Voruganti, L. N. P., Slomka, P., Zabel, P., Mattar, A. and Awad, A. G. (2001). Cannabis induced dopamine release: an in-vivo SPECT study. *Psychiatry Res. Neuroimaging*, **107**, 173–177.

Wylie, A. S., Scott, R. T. A. and Burnett, S. J. (1995). Psychosis due to 'skunk'. *Br. Med. J.*, **311**, 125.

Young, D. and Scovell, W. (1938). Paranoid psychosis in narcolepsy and possible danger of benzadrine treatment. *Med. Clin. North Am.*, **22**, 637–646.

7

Cannabis as a potential causal factor in schizophrenia

Louise Arseneault, Mary Cannon, John Witton and Robin Murray

Institute of Psychiatry, King's College London, UK

For many decades, the debate about whether cannabis use can cause schizophrenia has remained unresolved. Fifteen years after the publication of the first evidence that cannabis may be a causal risk factor for later schizophrenia, three further epidemiological studies have recently provided supportive evidence. This chapter reviews the evidence that cannabis use can cause schizophrenia, within the framework of established criteria for determining causality.

What is a cause?

The precise definition of what constitutes a cause and the elaboration of criteria for determining causality have a long and contentious history. Epidemiologists have often skirted the controversial topic by referring to 'risk factors' or 'exposures' rather than 'causes'. Nevertheless, we do indeed want to find causes.

Rothman and Greenland (1998), in their influential textbook of epidemiology, offered a clear definition of causation:

We can define a cause of a specific disease event as an antecedent event, condition, or characteristic that was necessary for the occurrence of the disease at the moment it occurred, given that other conditions are fixed. In other words, a cause for a disease occurrence is an event, condition or characteristic that preceded that disease occurrence, and without which the disease would either not have occurred at all, or would not have occurred until some later time.

Rothman and Greenland (1998) used pictures of 'causal pies' as a device to explain the concept of necessary and sufficient causes (Fig. 7.1). Each pie can be thought of as a constellation of causes that inevitably leads to disease occurrence, each constellation being sufficient for causation. Each slice in the pie represents a component cause. Each component is necessary for the disease to occur from that particular causal constellation. A disease may have many different sufficient causes.

Marijuana and Madness: Psychiatry and Neurobiology, ed. D. Castle and R. Murray. Published by Cambridge University Press. © Cambridge University Press 2004.

Schizophrenia

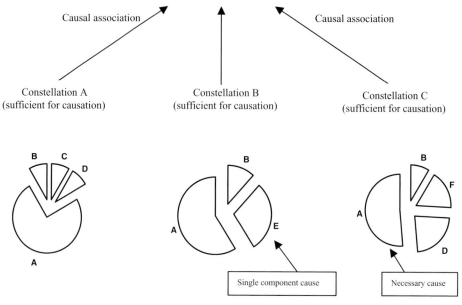

Figure 7.1   Causal pie model. Adapted with permission from Rothman and Greenland (1998).

A particular component cause may also be part of several different sufficient causes and therefore lead to a disease in conjunction with different component causes. Any component cause that is an active agent in all the sufficient causes for a disease outcome is deemed a necessary cause. The disease will not occur without it.

Meehl (1977) employed the following example to illustrate the concept of necessary and sufficient causes. A team of experts, investigating the cause of a warehouse fire, concludes that the cause of the fire was a short circuit in a fuse box. Clearly a short in a fuse box was not a necessary cause as there are many other ways in which a fire can start (including arson). This cause is also not sufficient for the warehouse to burn down because, under many conditions, a short would not cause a fire at all – for example, if there were no flammable materials in the vicinity of the fuse box, or if a sprinkler system was automatically activated. The short in the fuse box was a cause in that it was part of the complex series of events leading to the fire in the warehouse. At that time, the fire would not have occurred without the short in the fuse box, but the short in the fuse box was not sufficient for the fire to occur. It was only the totality of the conditions in the warehouse at that time – flammable materials near the box, no sprinkler system, wooden walls – that was sufficient for the fire to occur. The short circuit in the fuse was therefore a necessary component of a complex constellation that was sufficient for the fire to occur.

In this chapter we will seek to determine from the best evidence that is currently available whether cannabis is a cause of schizophrenia, and if so, whether it is a sufficient, necessary or component cause.

What are the defining criteria of a cause?

Causal criteria that deal with the exposure–disease relationship are often used as general guidelines for ascertaining causes. Hill (1965) listed the following criteria: strength, consistency, specificity, biological gradient, temporality, coherence and plausibility. Support for each criterion strengthens the case for a causal association, but, as Rothman and Greenland (1998) point out, only one criterion, temporality, is a sine qua non for causality. Susser (1991) subsequently used the Hill criteria to distil three properties that may serve to define causes: association, temporal priority and direction.

Association is the requirement that a cause and a disease appear together. When the putative cause is present, the disease rate is higher than when the putative cause is absent. There is no requirement for the putative cause to be present in every case of the disease, just that the rate of disease is higher in those with it than without it.

Temporal priority is the property that the putative cause be present before the disease. Associations between the putative cause and the disease can occur not only because the cause leads to the disease, but also because the disease leads to the cause – i.e. schizophrenia could lead to cannabis use. To rule out this possibility, the fundamental property of a cause is that it is present prior to the outcome under study.

Direction is the property referring to the fact that changes in the putative cause will actually lead to change in the outcome. In other words, the association of the putative cause with the disease derives from this putative cause and not from a third factor associated with both. Epidemiologists refer to the latter phenomenon as 'confounding'.

We shall examine the empirical evidence supporting the assumption that cannabis is a causal factor in schizophrenia under these three headings.

Evidence for association

There is little dispute that cannabis intoxication can trigger brief episodes of psychotic symptoms and that it can produce short-term exacerbation or recurrences of pre-existing psychotic symptoms (Negrete *et al.*, 1986; Thornicroft, 1990; Mathers and Ghodse, 1992; and see Chapter 6). However, there remains controversy over the existence of chronic psychotic states persisting beyond cessation of cannabis use and resembling schizophrenia (Johns, 2001).

More than 10 years ago, in a review article, Thornicroft (1990) reported some evidence supporting an association between cannabis and psychosis from clinical and epidemiological studies. He concluded by stressing the importance of longitudinal population cohort studies with prospective design to help elucidate the potential causal influences of cannabis on psychosis. Since then, four major national surveys (from the USA, the UK, Australia and the Netherlands) provided evidence that rates of cannabis use are higher among people with schizophrenia than the general population.

The US National Epidemiological Catchment Area study (Robins and Regier, 1991), conducted in the first half of the 1980s, collected data on 20 000 community and institutional residents. This study indicated that 50% of those identified with schizophrenia also had a diagnosis of substance use disorder (abuse or dependence), compared to 17% of the general population (Regier *et al.*,1990). Using the same sample, another study showed that people who reported at least one psychotic symptom had a higher rate of daily cannabis use (10.1%), compared to those who did not have any psychotic symptoms (4.8%) (Tien and Anthony, 1990). The authors reported that people who used cannabis on a daily basis were 2.4 times more likely to report psychotic experiences than non-daily cannabis users. This result held even after controlling for a variety of confounding variables such as sociodemographic factors, social role and psychiatric conditions.

The UK National Psychiatric Morbidity Survey collected data from three different groups of individuals: a group representative of the UK general population (household survey), a group of homeless people and a group of long-term residents of psychiatric institutions. The survey showed that 5% of patients with schizophrenia or delusional disorders and 5% of homeless people with psychosis reported using cannabis during the year prior to interview. Similarly, 5% of the general population also reported using cannabis (Farrell *et al.*, 1998). Low rates of cannabis use reported in this study might be explained by the exclusive use of self-reports to assess cannabis use among the two high-risk groups. This strategy may create a problem of underreported cannabis use, especially in clinical settings and with homeless people.

The more representative Australian National Survey of Mental Health and Well-Being found that 12% of those diagnosed with schizophrenia also had met *International Classification of Disease* (*ICD*-10) criteria (World Health Organization, 1992) for cannabis use disorder (Hall and Degenhardt, 2000). Furthermore, after statistically adjusting for other disorders and sociodemographic factors, individuals who met the *ICD*-10 criteria for cannabis dependence were nearly three times as likely to report that they had been diagnosed with schizophrenia than those without cannabis dependence disorder. Finally, a longitudinal population-based study conducted in the Netherlands also provided rates of cannabis use among individuals representative of the Dutch general population (Van Os *et al.*, 2002). Cannabis use was more prevalent among those subjects with a vulnerability to psychosis at the initial assessment (15.3%) than those without (7.7%).

Similarly, local surveys have found high rates of cannabis use in psychiatric patients under treatment. For example, of those in a study of patients with psychotic illnesses in contact with mental health services in South London, 40.4% reported trying cannabis at least once in their life (Menezes *et al.*, 1996). Fifty-one per cent of a patient sample detained under the 1983 Mental Health Act reported lifetime use of cannabis (Wheatley, 1998). A recent study in Scotland compared rates of substance misuse in patients with schizophrenia with rates in the general population drawn from rural, suburban and urban settings (McCreadie, 2002). Findings indicated that 7% of patients reported problematic use of drugs (4% related specifically to cannabis use) compared to 2% of controls. High rates of cannabis use, along with other non-alcohol substances, were found in a cohort study of 352 people suffering from schizophrenia and other related psychoses in a central London area (Duke *et al.*, 2001). This group included individuals living in the community as well as hospitalized patients and took place in areas with notable deprivation. Nearly 20% of the group reported lifetime cannabis use. Unfortunately, the absence of controls prevents us from comparing this rate with that for the general population. Finally, a study examining psychotic patients from London and Malta showed that 38.8% of patients and 21.9% of controls were using cannabis (Grech *et al.*, 1998).

Elevated rates of cannabis use among people with schizophrenia raises important questions about the reason for this association – is the cannabis use a consequence or a cause of the condition? Studies examining temporal priority between these two events will help to answer this question.

Evidence for temporal priority and direction

Retrospective studies

Two studies of clinical samples have examined retrospective reports of drug use in individuals who developed schizophrenia. First, Hambrecht and Hafner (1996) reported on a retrospective study of 232 patients with schizophrenia. Data showed that one-third of the sample used drugs at least 1 year before the onset of the illness, another third used drugs and subsequently developed the illness within 1 year, and another third started using cannabis after the occurrence of schizophrenia symptoms. In a second study, Cantwell *et al.* (1999) investigated a group of 168 schizophrenic first-episode patients and found that 37% showed evidence of substance use and alcohol use before their presentation to services.

However, studies based on retrospective self-reports are prone to recall bias and, in order to establish temporal priority, we need to have prospective reports of cannabis use, collected before the onset of schizophrenia and, hence, unbiased by later outcome. Ideally we should also use population-based samples.

Prospective studies

At present, there are three population-based samples in which use of cannabis was assessed in adolescence, before diagnosis of schizophrenia outcomes: two cohort studies and one longitudinal population-based survey. These samples are described below and summarized in Table 7.1. We will use the evidence from these samples to establish temporal priority and direction for the association between cannabis use and schizophrenia.

The Swedish conscript cohort

For many years the only evidence that cannabis use might predispose to later psychosis came from a cohort study of 50 087 Swedish conscripts who were followed up using record-linkage techniques based on inpatient admissions for psychiatric care (Andréasson *et al.*, 1987). A dose–response relationship was observed between cannabis use at conscription (age of 18) and schizophrenia diagnosis 15 years later. Self-reported 'heavy cannabis users' (i.e. those who had used cannabis more than 50 times) were six times more likely than non-users to have been diagnosed with schizophrenia 15 years later. However, more than half of these heavy users had a psychiatric diagnosis other than psychosis at conscription and, when this confound was controlled for, the relative risk decreased to 2.3 (but none the less remained statistically significant). Of note, very few heavy cannabis users (3%) went on to develop schizophrenia, indicating that cannabis use may serve to increase the risk for schizophrenia only among individuals already vulnerable to developing psychosis. The authors concluded that 'Cannabis should be viewed as an additional clue to the still elusive aetiology of schizophrenia'. However, it took more than 15 years for further evidence to emerge in support of a causal association. This probably reflects the difficulty of obtaining such prospective data on cannabis use as well as an initial lack of interest on the part of the research community in this issue.

A follow-up study of the same Swedish Conscript Cohort has recently been carried out (Zammit *et al.*, 2002). Consistent with previous findings, this report showed that by the age of 18 years 'heavy cannabis users' were 6.7 times more likely than non-users to be diagnosed with schizophrenia 27 years later. This risk held when the analysis was repeated on a subsample of men who used cannabis only, as opposed to using other drugs as well. The risk was reduced but remained significant after controlling for other potential confounding factors such as disturbed behaviour,

Table 7.1 Epidemiological studies on cannabis use and schizophrenia

	Authors	Study design, year of enrolment (n)	Sex	Number of participants	Follow-up (years)	Age of cannabis users	Outcome	n (%) of outcome	Diagnostic criteria
Swedish conscript cohort (Sweden)	Andréasson et al. (1987)	Conscript cohort 69–70 (~50 000)	Males	45 570	15	18	1. Inpatient admission for schizophrenia	246 (0.5)	ICD-8
	Zammit et al. (2002)	Conscript cohort 69–70 (~50 000)	Males	50 053	27	18	1. Hospital admission for schizophrenia	362 (0.7)	ICD-8/9
NEMESIS (the Netherlands)	Van Os et al. (2002)	Population-based study 96 (7076)	Males and females	4104	3	Between 18 and 64	1. Any level of psychotic symptoms	38 (0.9)	Brief Psychiatric Rating Scale
							2. Pathology level of psychotic symptoms	10 (0.3)	
							3. Need for care	7 (0.2)	
Dunedin Study (New Zealand)	Arseneault et al. (2002)	Birth cohort 72–73 (1037)	Males and females	759	11	15	Schizophreniform disorder 1. Symptoms 2. Diagnosis	25 (3.3)	DSM-IV

NEMESIS, Netherlands Mental Health Interview Survey and Incidence Study; ICD, International Classification of Disease; DSM-IV, Diagnostic and Statistical Manual of Mental Disorders.

low IQ score, growing up in a city, cigarette smoking and poor social integration. In order to control for the possibility that cannabis use might be a consequence of prodromal manifestations of psychosis, the analyses were repeated on a subsample of individuals who developed schizophrenia only 5 years after conscription, and the findings obtained were similar to the ones with the entire cohort. The authors conclude that the findings are 'consistent with a causal relationship between cannabis use and schizophrenia'.

The Dutch NEMESIS sample

An analysis of the Netherlands Mental Health Survey and Incidence Study (NEMESIS: Van Os *et al.*, 2002) goes beyond the reliance on hospital discharge register data for outcomes and examines the effect of cannabis use on psychotic symptoms among the general population. In this study, 4045 psychosis-free and 59 subjects with self-reported symptoms of psychosis were assessed at baseline and were administered follow-up assessments 1 year later, and again 3 years after the baseline assessment. For those subjects who reported psychotic symptoms, an additional clinical interview was conducted by an experienced psychiatrist or psychologist (at baseline and at 3-year follow-up). Compared to non-users, individuals using cannabis at baseline were nearly three times more likely to manifest psychotic symptoms at follow-up. This risk remained significant after statistical adjustment for a range of factors including ethnic group, marital status, educational level, urbanicity and discrimination. The authors also found a dose–response relationship, with the highest risk (odds ratio $= 6.8$) being observed for the highest level of cannabis use. Further analysis revealed that lifetime history of cannabis use at baseline, as opposed to use of cannabis at follow-up, was a stronger predictor of psychosis 3 years later. This suggests that the association between cannabis use and psychosis is not merely the result of short-term effects of cannabis use leading to an acute psychotic episode. Use of other drugs did not explain the risk associated with cannabis use for later psychosis: although use of other drugs was associated with psychosis outcomes, the effects were not significant after taking into account cannabis use. In this study, the short time-lag between baseline and follow-up assessments tends to provide more support for an association between cannabis use and psychosis, rather than verifying temporal priority. The authors conclude that this study confirms 'that cannabis use is an independent risk factor for the emergence of psychosis in psychosis-free persons and that those with an established vulnerability to psychotic disorders are particularly sensitive to its effects, resulting in a poor outcome'.

The Dunedin birth cohort

The Dunedin Multidisciplinary Health and Development Study (Silva and Stanton, 1996) is a study of a general-population birth cohort of 1037 individuals born in

Dunedin, New Zealand, in 1972–1973 (96% follow-up rate at age 26). Although small, this study has several unique advantages: (1) it has information on self-reported psychotic symptoms at age 11, before the onset of cannabis use; (2) it allows the age of onset of cannabis use to be examined in relation to later outcome, as self-reports of cannabis use were obtained at ages 15 and 18; and (3) it does not rely on treatment data for outcomes as the entire cohort were assessed at age 26 using a standardized psychiatric interview schedule yielding *Diagnostic and Statistical Manual of Mental Disorders* (*DSM*-IV: American Psychiatric Association, 1994) diagnoses (Poulton *et al.*, 2000). This allowed the examination of schizophrenia outcome both as a continuum (by examination of symptoms) and as a disorder (*DSM*-IV schizophreniform disorder) in this population. Of note, in obtaining a schizophreniform diagnosis, the interview protocol ruled out psychotic symptoms occurring while under the influence of alcohol and drugs.

Those subjects using cannabis at ages 15 and 18 had higher rates of psychotic symptoms at age 26 compared to non-users. This remained significant after controlling for psychotic symptoms predating the onset of cannabis use (Arseneault *et al.*, 2002). The effect was stronger with earlier use. In addition, onset of cannabis use by age 15 was associated with an increased likelihood of meeting diagnostic criteria for schizophreniform disorder at age 26. Indeed, 10.3% of the age-15 cannabis users in this cohort were diagnosed with schizophreniform disorder at age 26, as opposed to 3% of the controls. After controlling for age-11 psychotic symptoms, the risk for adult schizophreniform disorder remained elevated (odds ratio = 3.1), though was no longer statistically significant, possibly due to power limitation.

Cannabis use by age 15 did not predict depressive outcomes at age 26 (indicating specificity of the outcome) and the use of other illicit drugs in adolescence did not predict schizophrenia outcomes over and above the effect of cannabis use (indicating specificity of the exposure). A significant exacerbation or interaction effect was found between cannabis use by age-18 and age-11 psychotic symptoms (Fig. 7.2). This effect indicates that age-18 cannabis users had elevated scores on the schizophrenia symptom scale only if they had reported psychotic symptoms at age 11. This study concludes that 'using cannabis in adolescence increases the likelihood of experiencing symptoms of schizophrenia in adulthood'.

Thus, the Dunedin study provides further support for the idea that cannabis use in adolescence is a risk factor for later schizophrenia outcomes, and adds several new pieces of evidence: (1) cannabis use in adolescence is a risk factor for experiencing symptoms of schizophrenia in adulthood, over and above psychotic symptoms prior to cannabis use; (2) there is a strong developmental effect in that early cannabis use (by age 15) is a stronger risk factor for schizophreniform disorder than later use (age 18); and (3) there is specificity of both exposure and outcome.

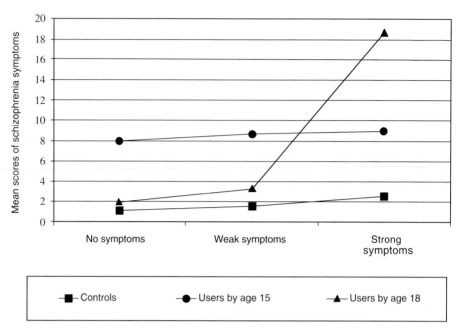

Figure 7.2   Interaction between cannabis use at age 18 and psychotic symptoms at age 11 in predicting adult schizophrenia symptoms

Methodological issues

Before coming to a conclusion about cannabis as a causal risk factor for schizophrenia based on the results of the studies from the three population-based samples discussed above, it is important to point out some methodological limitations.

First, various measures of schizophrenia outcome were used in these studies: hospital discharge, pathology-level of psychosis, psychotic symptoms and schizophreniform disorder. The heterogeneity of the outcome makes it difficult to draw a firm conclusion on schizophrenia from the findings reported by these studies. However, it is at least reassuring that all studies converge in showing an elevated risk for psychosis in later life amongst cannabis users.

Second, all measures of cannabis use were based on self-reports and were not supplemented by urine tests or hair analysis. In particular, the reliability of non-anonymous interviews with conscripts as a source of information about drug use may be questionable (underreporting could be conceivable in this situation). However, Andréasson *et al.* (1987) argued that this problem would create an underestimation of the risk associated with cannabis use for later schizophrenia. This is true only if participants underreport their cannabis use, regardless of whether they have schizophrenia or not. In the Dunedin study, members have learned after many years of involvement with the study that all information they provide remains strictly confidential and the answers are likely to provide a good estimate of actual levels of drug use in that population (Arseneault *et al.*, 2002).

Third, there is limited information on other illicit drug use. It would be informative to gather more precise information about other illicit drugs used by young people, to control more effectively for possible confounding effects of, for example, stimulant drug use.

Fourth, most studies were unable to establish whether prodromal manifestations of schizophrenia preceded cannabis use, leaving the possibility that cannabis use may be a consequence of emerging schizophrenia rather than a cause of it. Recent findings indicated that schizophrenia is typically preceded by psychological and behavioural changes years before the onset of diagnosed disease (Jones *et al.*, 1994; Cannon *et al.*, 1997; Malmberg *et al.*, 1998). It is, then, possible that cannabis use may be a consequence of early emerging schizophrenia rather than predisposing to its development. Thus, it has become crucial to control for these early signs of psychosis to establish clearly temporal priority between cannabis use and adult psychosis. To date, the Dunedin study is the only study to demonstrate temporal priority by showing that adolescent cannabis users are at increased risk of experiencing schizophrenic symptoms in adult life, even after taking into account childhood psychotic symptoms that preceded the onset of cannabis use.

Finally, there was limited statistical power in studies using self-reports of schizophrenia outcomes (in the NEMESIS and Dunedin studies) for examining such a rare outcome disorder. It will be important for future studies to examine larger population samples in order to assess a greater number of individuals with psychotic disorders.

Alternative explanations

One might speculate that cannabis is a 'gateway drug' for the use of harder drugs (Kazuo and Kandel, 1984) and that individuals who use cannabis heavily might also be using other substances such as amfetamines, phenylcyclidine and LSD, which are thought to be psychotogenic (Murray *et al.*, 2003). Support for this explanation is provided by recent findings showing that use of other drugs among young adults is almost always preceded by cannabis use (Fergusson and Horwood, 2000). This is especially true for heavy cannabis users (50 times or more per year) who were 140 times more likely to move on to other illicit drugs than people who did not use cannabis before. However, in the Dunedin, Dutch and Swedish studies, the association between cannabis and schizophrenia held even when adjusting for the use of other drugs (Arseneault *et al.*, 2002; Van Os *et al.*, 2002; Zammit *et al.*, 2002).

A second possibility is that individuals who use cannabis in adolescence continue to use this illicit substance in adulthood and, because cannabis use intoxication can be associated with transient psychotic symptoms (see Chapter 5), this could account for the observed association. The Dunedin study is the only study for which psychiatric interview explicitly ruled out schizophrenia symptoms if these occurred only following substance use.

A third possibility is that early-onset cannabis use is a proxy measure for poor pre-morbid adjustment which is known to be associated with schizophrenia (Cannon *et al.*, 1997; 2002). However, Arseneault *et al.* (2002) found that cannabis use was specifically related to schizophrenia outcomes, as opposed to depression, suggesting specificity in longitudinal association rather than general poor premorbid adjust-ment. Having said this, other evidence supports an association between cannabis use and depression (see Chapter 4).

Is cannabis a cause for schizophrenia?

We have shown that all the available prospective population-based studies on the issue have found that cannabis use is associated with later schizophrenia outcomes. All these studies support the concept of temporal priority by showing that cannabis use most probably preceded schizophrenia. These studies also provide evidence for direction by showing that the association between adolescent cannabis use and adult psychosis persists after controlling for many potential confounding variables, such as disturbed behaviour, low IQ, place of upbringing, cigarette smoking, poor social integration, sex, age, ethnic groups, level of education, unemployment, single marital status and psychotic symptoms prior to cannabis use. Further evidence for a causal relationship is provided by the presence of a dose–response relationship between cannabis use and schizophrenia (Andréasson *et al.*, 1987; Van Os *et al.*, 2002; Zammit *et al.*, 2002), specificity of exposure, i.e. cannabis use (Arseneault *et al.*, 2002; Van Os *et al.*, 2002; Zammit *et al.*, 2002) and specificity of the association to schizophrenia-related outcomes (Arseneault *et al.*, 2002).

What kind of cause is it?

We have shown that, based on the best evidence currently available, cannabis use is likely to play a causal role in regard to schizophrenia. However, further questions now arise. How strong is the causal effect and is cannabis use a *necessary* or *sufficient* cause of schizophrenia?

The studies reviewed earlier show that cannabis use is clearly not a *necessary* cause for the development of schizophrenia, by failing to show that all adults with schizophrenia used cannabis in adolescence. It is also clear that cannabis use is not a sufficient cause for later psychosis since the majority of adolescent cannabis users did not develop schizophrenia in adulthood. Therefore we can conclude that cannabis use is a component cause, among possibly many others, forming a causal constellation that leads to adult schizophrenia.

What might the other component causes be?

Unfortunately we get little insight on component causes other than cannabis from the studies reviewed in this chapter. Cannabis use appeared to increase the risk of schizophrenia outcomes primarily among those vulnerable individuals by virtue of psychotic symptoms prior to diagnosable schizophrenia outcome (Arseneault *et al.*, 2002; Van Os *et al.*, 2002). Verdoux and colleagues (see Chapter 5) have shown that, among cannabis users, adverse psychological effects were more common in those rated as 'psychosis-prone'. However the interaction is not a simple one.

High-risk studies

Two studies have explored the role of cannabis use in the development of psychotic symptoms in groups of young people considered to be at high risk of developing psychotic symptoms. An analysis of the Edinburgh High Risk Study found that both individuals at high genetic risk of schizophrenia (by virtue of two affected relatives) and individuals with no family history of schizophrenia were at increased risk of psychotic symptoms after cannabis use (Miller *et al.*, 2001). Also, an Australian study followed up a group of 100 individuals who presented to an early intervention service (Phillips *et al.*, 2002). Cannabis use or dependence at entry to the study was not associated with the development of psychotic illness (transition to psychosis) over a 12-month period of follow-up after entry to the study. However, the low level of reported cannabis use amongst the group could indicate that the sample may not be representative of the population of 'prodromal' individuals.

How strong is the causal effect?

Can we say anything about the strength of the causal effect of cannabis for schizophrenia? We are somewhat hampered in this endeavour, since the strength of any particular cause depends on the prevalence of the other component causes in the population (Rothman and Greenland, 1998). As we have discussed above, we do not know, at present, any other component causes in the 'schizophrenia constellation'. We can make some broad suggestions. A component cause, even if it is very common, will rarely cause a disorder if the other component causes in the causal constellation are rare. That will hold regardless of the prevalence of the component cause of interest in the population or its role in the pathophysiology of the disorder. On the other hand, the rarer a component cause relative to its partners in any sufficient cause, the stronger that component cause will appear. Since cannabis use is relatively common in the population but appears to cause schizophrenia rarely, it would follow that at least one of the other component causes in the causal constellation is rare. Indeed, as Table 7.2 shows, cannabis use appears to confer only

Table 7.2 Findings from epidemiological studies on cannabis use and schizophrenia

	Risk (OR, 95% CI)	Adjusted risk (OR, 95% CI)	Confounding variables controlled for	Dose–response relationship	Specificity of risk factor	Specificity of outcome
Swedish conscript cohort	1. 6.0 (4.0–8.9) for those who used cannabis > 50 times at 18	2.3 (1.0–5.3)	Psychiatric diagnosis at conscription Parents divorced	Yes	No	N/A
	1. 6.7 (4.5–10.0) for those who used cannabis > 50 times at age 18	3.1 (1.7–5.5)	Diagnosis at conscription IQ score Social integration Disturbed behaviour Cigarette smoking Place of upbringing	Yes	Yes	Yes
NEMESIS	1. 3.25 (1.5–7.2) 2. 28.54 (7.3–110.9) 3. 16.15 (3.6–72.5) for cannabis use at baseline (age 16–17)	2.76 (1.2–6.5) 24.17 (5.44–107.5) 12.01 (2.4–64.3)	Age Sex Ethnic group Single marital status Education Urbanicity Discrimination	Yes	Yes	N/A
Dunedin study	1. 6.91 (5.1–8.7) (B)[a] 2. 4.50 (1.1–18.2) Users by the age of 15 and continued at 18	6.56 (4.78–8.34)[a] 3.12 (0.7–13.3)	Sex Social class Psychotic symptoms prior to cannabis use	N/A	Yes	Yes

OR, odds ratio; CI, confidence interval; NEMESIS, Netherlands Mental Health Interview Survey and Incidence Study.
[a] Beta of multiple linear regression.

% who used in last 12 months

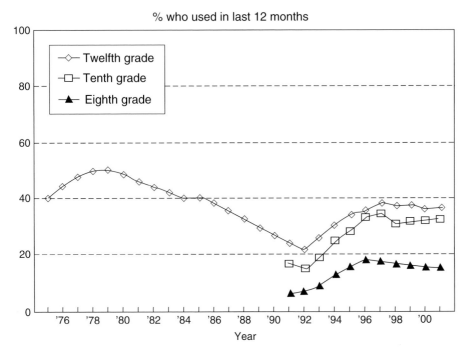

Figure 7.3   Trends in annual use of cannabis in the USA in 2001. (Adapted with permission from Johnston *et al.*, 2002.)

a two- or threefold increase in relative risk for schizophrenia. Does this mean that we should not worry about cannabis as a causal factor?

There is another way of looking at this issue. Once causality is assumed, the strength of a particular association from a public health point of view can be assessed with the population attributable fraction (PAF). This gives a measure of the number of cases of the disorder in the population that could be eliminated (i.e. would not occur) by removal of a harmful causal factor. The PAF for the Dunedin study is 8. In other words, removal of cannabis use from the New Zealand age-15 population would have led to an 8% reduction in the incidence of schizophrenia in that population. The NEMESIS group reported higher PAFs, possibly because the outcome measures they used did not exclusively include clinical psychosis cases (i.e. need for care). These are not insignificant figures from a public health point of view. However, the possibility of eliminating cannabis use totally from the population is rather remote and it may be advisable to concentrate on those for whom adverse outcomes are more common.

A further factor is that the Dunedin study showed that cannabis use in early adolescence (cf. first reported use at age 18) was associated with the strongest effects on schizophrenia outcomes. Trends of cannabis use among adolescents in the USA indicate that cannabis use under the age of 16 is a fairly new phenomenon that has only appeared since the early 1990s (Fig. 7.3: Johnston *et al.*, 2002). One would therefore predict an increase in rates of schizophrenia over the next 10 years. Although the majority of young people are able to use cannabis in adolescence without harm, a vulnerable minority experiences harmful outcomes. Epidemiological evidence suggests that cannabis use among psychologically vulnerable young adolescents should be strongly discouraged by parents, teachers and health practitioners alike. Findings also suggest that the youngest cannabis users are most at risk (Arseneault *et al.*, 2002) perhaps because their cannabis use became long-standing. This encourages policy- and law-makers to concentrate their effort on delaying onset of cannabis use. At the same time, research is required to estimate the long-term impact of frequent cannabis use that begins at an early age.

Conclusion

In this chapter, we have tried to determine whether cannabis is a cause of schizophrenia and, if so, whether it is a necessary or a sufficient cause. Recent empirical evidence suggests that cannabis is not a necessary cause for schizophrenia. Neither is it a sufficient cause. Cannabis use is rather a component cause and, as such, is a part of a complex constellation including other component causes, possibly some necessary ones such as genetic predisposition, leading to the development of schizophrenia. The other components of this causal constellation remain to be determined.

REFERENCES

American Psychiatric Association (1994). *Diagnostic and Statistical Manual of Mental Disorders*, 4th edition. Washington, DC: APA.

Andréasson, S., Allebeck, P., Engström, A. and Rydberg, U. (1987). Cannabis and schizophrenia: a longitudinal study of Swedish conscripts. *Lancet*, 11, 1483–1485.

Arseneault, L., Cannon, M., Poulton, R. *et al.* (2002). Cannabis use in adolescence and risk for adult psychosis: longitudinal prospective study. *Br. Med. J.*, **325**, 1212–1213.

Cannon, M., Jones, P., Gilvarry, C. *et al.* (1997). Premorbid social functioning in schizophrenia and bipolar disorder: similarities and differences. *Am. J. Psychiatry*, **154**, 1544–1550.

Cannon, M., Caspi, A., Moffitt, T. E. *et al.* (2002). Evidence for early-childhood, pan-developmental impairment specific to schizophreniform disorder: results from a longitudinal birth cohort. *Arch. Gen. Psychiatry*, **59**, 449–456.

Cantwell, R., Brewin, J., Glazebrook, C. *et al.* (1999). Prevalence of substance abuse in first-episode psychosis. *Br. J. Psychiatry*, **174**, 150–153.

Duke, P. J., Pantelis, C., McPhillips, M. A. and Barnes, T. R. E. (2001). Comorbid non-alcohol substance misuse among people with schizophrenia. *Br. J. Psychiatry*, **179**, 509–513.

Farrell, M., Howes, S., Taylor, C. *et al.* (1998). Substance misuse and psychiatric comorbidity: an overview of the OPCS National Psychiatric Comorbidity Survey. *Addict. Behavi.*, **23**, 909–918.

Fergusson, D. M. and Horwood, L. J. (2000). Does cannabis use encourage other forms of illicit drug use? *Addiction*, **95**, 505–520.

Grech, A., Takei, N. and Murray, R. (1998). Comparison of cannabis use in psychotic patients and controls in London and Malta. *Schizophr. Res.*, **29**, 22.

Hall, W. and Degenhardt, L. (2000). Cannabis use and psychosis: a review of clinical and epidemiological evidence. *Aust. NZ J. Psychiatry*, **34**, 26–34.

Hambrecht, M. and Hafner, H. (1996). Substance abuse and the onset of schizophrenia. *Biol. Psychiatry*, **40**, 1155–1163.

Hill, A. B. (1965). The environment and disease: association or causation? *Proc. R. Soc. Med.*, **58**, 295–300.

Johns, A. (2001). Psychiatric effects of cannabis. *Br. J. Psychiatry*, **178**, 116–122.

Johnston, L. D., O'Malley, P. M. and Bachman, J. G. (2002). Monitoring the future national results on adolescent drug use: overview of key findings 2001. NIH publication no. 02–5105. Bethesda, MD: National Institute on Drug Abuse.

Jones, P., Rodgers, B., Murray, R. and Marmot, M. (1994). Child developmental risk factors for adult schizophrenia in the British 1946 birth cohort. *Lancet*, **344**, 1398–1402.

Kazuo, Y. and Kandel, D. B. (1984). Patterns of drug use from adolescence to young adulthood: II. Sequences of progression. *Am. J. Public Health*, **74**, 668–672.

Malmberg, A., Lewis, G., David, A. and Allebeck, P. (1998). Premorbid adjustment and personality in people with schizophrenia. *Br. J. Psychiatry*, **172**, 308–313.

Mathers, D. C. and Ghodse, A. H. (1992). Cannabis and psychotic illness. *Br. J. Psychiatry*, **161**, 648–653.

McCreadie, R. G. (2002). Use of drugs, alcohol and tobacco by people with schizophrenia: case-control study. *Br. J. Psychiatry*, **181**, 321–323.

Meehl, P. (1977). Specific etiology and other forms of strong influence: some quantitative meanings. *J. Med. Phil.*, **2**, 33–53.

Menezes, P. R., Johnson, S., Thornicroft, G. *et al.* (1996). Drug and alcohol problems among individuals with severe mental illnesses in South London. *Br. J. Psychiatry*, **168**, 612–619.

Miller, P., Lawrie, S. M., Hodges, A. *et al.* (2001). Genetic liability, illicit drug use, life stress and psychotic symptoms: preliminary findings from the Edinburgh study of people at high risk for schizophrenia. *Soc. Psychiatry Psychiatric Epidemiol.*, **36**, 338–342.

Murray, R. M., Grech, A., Phillips, P. and Johnson, S. (2003). What is the relationship between substance abuse and schizophrenia? In *The Epidemiology of Schizophrenia*. ed. R. Murray, P. Jones, E. Susser, J. Van Os and M. Cannon, pp. 317–342. Cambridge, UK: Cambridge University Press.

Negrete, J. C., Knapp, W. P., Douglas, D. and Smith, W. B. (1986). Cannabis affects the severity of schizophrenia symptoms: results of a clinical survey. *Psychol. Med.*, **16**, 515–520.

Phillips, L. J., Curry, C., Yung, A. R. *et al.* (2002). Cannabis use is not associated with the development of psychosis in an 'ultra' high-risk group. *Aust. NZ J. Psychiatry*, **36**, 800–806.

Poulton, R., Caspi, A., Moffitt, T. E. *et al.* (2000). Children's self-reported psychotic symptoms and adult schizophreniform disorder: a 15-year longitudinal study. *Arch. Gen. Psychiatry*, **57**, 1053–1058.

Regier, D., Farmer, M. E., Rae, D. S. *et al.* (1990). Comorbidity of mental disorders with alcohol and other drug abuse: results from the epidemiologic catchment area (ECA) study. *J. A. M. A.*, **264**, 2511–2518.

Robins, L. N. and Regier, D. A. (1991). *Psychiatric Disorders in America: The Epidemiologic Catchment Area Study*. New York: The Free Press.

Rothman, K. J. and Greenland, S. (eds) (1998). *Modern Epidemiology*, 2nd edn. Philadelphia: Lippincott-Raven.

Silva, P. A. and Stanton, W. R. (eds) (1996). *From Child to Adult: The Dunedin Multidisciplinary Health and Development Study*. Auckland: Oxford University Press.

Susser, M. (1991). What is a cause and how do we know one? A grammar for pragmatic epidemiology. *Am. J. Epidemiol.*, **133**, 635–648.

Thornicroft, G. (1990). Cannabis and psychosis. *Br. J. Psychiatry*, **157**, 25–33.

Tien, A. Y. and Anthony, J. C. (1990). Epidemiological analysis of alcohol and drug use as risk factors for psychotic experiences. *J. Nerv. Ment. Dis.*, **178**, 473–480.

Van Os, J., Bak, M., Bijl, R. V., De Graaf, R. and Verdoux, H. (2002). Cannabis use and psychosis: a longitudinal population-based study. *Am. J. Epidemiol.*, **156**, 319–327.

Wheatley, M. (1998). The prevalence and relevance of substance use in detained schizophrenic patients. *J. Forensic Psychiatry*, **9**, 114–129.

World Health Organization (1992). *International Statistical Classification of Diseases and Related Health Problems*, 10th edn. Geneva: WHO.

Zammit, S., Allebeck, P., Andréasson, S., Lundberg, I. and Lewis, G. (2002). Self-reported cannabis use as a risk factor for schizophrenia: further analysis of the 1969 Swedish conscript cohort. *Br. Med. J.*, **325**, 1199–1201.

8

Cannabis abuse and the course of schizophrenia

Don Linszen, Bart Peters and Lieuwe de Haan

University of Amsterdam, The Netherlands

As detailed elsewhere in this book (Chapter 3), cannabis has been used for centuries to produce euphoria and relaxation as desired mental effects. However, adverse effects of intoxication with cannabis include anxiety and panic (Thomas, 1996; Reilly *et al.*, 1998), depression (Bovasso, 2001; Patton *et al.*, 2002: see Chapter 4), and impairment in certain domains of cognitive function (see Chapters 3 and 13). Psychosis, including paranoid delusions and hallucinations, has been found to be an effect of cannabis use in cohort studies from New Zealand (Thomas, 1996), Vietnam (Talbott and Teague, 1969), India (Chopra and Smith, 1974) and Pakistan (Chaudry *et al.*, 1991) (Chapter 6). This work suggests that cannabis, especially in high doses, can produce a toxic psychosis in people without mental disorders. Evidence for cannabis (and especially heavy abuse) as a causal risk factor for psychotic disorders comes from epidemiological studies of Swedish conscripts (Andreasson *et al.*, 1987; Zammit *et al.*, 2002), from the Dunedin study from New Zealand (Arsenault *et al.*, 2002), from a Dutch sample (Van Os *et al.*, 2002) and from a study of Israeli conscripts (Weiser *et al.*, 2001) (see Chapter 7).

Schizophrenia and related psychotic disorders are clinical syndromes with a wide variation in symptoms between individuals (Thaker and Carpenter, 2001). Factor-analytic studies of schizophrenia have revealed that the symptoms are best described by three dimensions or syndromes: reality distortion (hallucinations and delusions), psychomotor poverty (restriction of affect, loss of motivation and restricted emotional experience) and disorganization (disorganized thought, incongruity of affect and bizarre behaviour) (Liddle, 1987).

Our group (Van der Does *et al.*, 1995) found a fourth dimension with depression-related symptoms. Cognitive impairments have been established as central features of schizophrenia as well: deficits have been established in attention, short-term

Marijuana and Madness: Psychiatry and Neurobiology, ed. D. Castle and R. Murray. Published by Cambridge University Press. © Cambridge University Press 2004.

memory, verbal memory, concentration and planning and problem-solving tasks (Bilder *et al.*, 2000).

Given that cannabis use can cause a wide variety of effects that resemble the extensive and varied symptomatology of schizophrenia itself, questions arise such as: What is the impact of cannabis use on psychotic relapse and the symptomatic course of schizophrenia? Is there evidence for aggravation of the course of all symptom dimensions? or Do positive consequences such as relief of negative symptoms occur with cannabis use? This chapter reviews studies examining the effects of cannabis use on the course of schizophrenia. Studies that examined the relation of polydrug abuse and schizophrenia were excluded when they did not examine the independent effects of cannabis (Zisook *et al.*, 1992; Gupta *et al.*, 1996; Bersani *et al.*, 2002; Hunt *et al.*, 2002).

Cross-sectional and retrospective studies

Until the 1990s, studies examining the relationship between cannabis use and schizophrenia had consisted of case series, in which possible relationships between cannabis abuse and psychotic symptoms were difficult to test. In a few case-control studies, psychotic symptoms were evaluated retrospectively, using hospital files (Negrete *et al.*, 1986). Also, the observation period was typically of only a week's duration, and schizophrenic symptoms were evaluated once, on a cross-sectional basis (Peralta and Cuesta, 1992).

An increase in positive psychotic symptoms and disorganization in cannabis-abusing schizophrenia patients has been found repeatedly (Weil, 1970; Chopra and Smith, 1974; Treffert, 1978; Knudsen and Vilmar, 1984; Cleghorn *et al.*, 1991). Cleghorn *et al.* (1991), in a controlled study, reported that patients with schizophrenia and prominent cannabis abuse had significantly more hallucinations, delusions and thought disorder than controls. In terms of negative symptoms, Knudsen and Vilmar (1984) found negative symptoms overall, and affective flattening in particular, to be less pronounced in cannabis-abusing schizophrenia patients compared to those not using cannabis. Peralta and Cuesta (1992) found no aggravation of positive psychotic symptoms in patients with schizophrenia when exposed to cannabis, but an exacerbation of alogia as a negative symptom was established. In another case-control study (Dixon *et al.*, 1991), fewer positive and negative symptoms were found in a sample of drug-abusing patients with schizophrenia (cannabis being the drug of choice) compared to non-users. These cross-sectional and retrospective studies thus give somewhat conflicting results, perhaps reflecting the limitations of the methodology. Much more robust are prospective studies that allow the tracking of the effects of cannabis on psychotic symptoms over time.

Short-term prospective studies

The first large prospective cohort study that examined the relationship between cannabis abuse and the symptomatic course of recent-onset schizophrenia and related disorders (Linszen et al., 1994) was conducted over the course of a year using monthly assessments of psychotic symptoms with the Brief Psychiatric Rating Scale (BPRS). Twenty-four young cannabis-abusing patients were compared with 69 non-abusers. The mean age when they started cannabis abuse was 16 years, and the mean duration of abuse before admission was 3.9 years.

All but one of the cannabis-abusing patients started their habit at least 1 year prior to their first psychotic symptoms (mean 3 years, range 0–7 years). Within the group of 24 cannabis abusers, 13 heavy users (54%) could be identified, this group being defined as using more than one cigarette a day. The mild abusing group ($n = 11$) consumed between one cigarette a week and one a day. Hard drug abuse was rare (two patients used cocaine and ecstasy; one of these patients also used other drugs sporadically in combination with heavy cannabis abuse). The most relevant finding of this prospective study was the occurrence of significantly more, and earlier, psychotic relapses or exacerbations in the total group of cannabis-abusing patients over a 12-month period. When a distinction was made with respect to the intensity of abuse, the association became stronger: it appeared that particularly heavy cannabis-abusing patients relapsed more frequently and earlier. This finding was not confounded by exposure to alcohol and/or any other (psychoactive) drugs, or by differences in antipsychotic medication adherence and dosage. Two additional findings indicated a possible causal relationship between cannabis and psychotic relapse. First, 14 of the 24 cannabis-abusing patients reported an immediate increase in psychotic symptoms after cannabis exposure; 13 of these 14 patients were clinically in remission when they reported the evolution of psychotic symptoms. Six patients noted no such exacerbation of symptoms, whilst one further patient reported a decrease in psychotic symptoms when using cannabis.

In addition to psychotic relapse, we also examined the relationship between cannabis abuse and symptom dimensions over a 12-month period. Positive, negative, disorganization and depressive symptom dimensions were compared for the cannabis-abusing patients and non-abusers. No effect was found for the positive syndrome ($P = 0.43$), the negative syndrome ($P = 0.23$) or the depression syndrome ($P = 0.27$). In the mild abusing group, symptoms of anxiety and depression tended to be less prevalent than in the non- and heavy-abusing group, suggesting that those with mild cannabis abuse were using cannabis to 'self-medicate'. We could not confirm the existence of an amotivational syndrome, and there was no apparent exacerbation of negative symptoms in the cannabis-abusing group. However, in a re-analysis of the data, a main effect of cannabis abuse was found for the course of the symptoms of the disorganization dimension ($P = 0.01$), with the scores tending to increase over the 12-month period ($P < 0.01$) (Linszen *et al.*, 1995).

In a 1-year follow-up study from Spain (Martinez-Arevalo *et al.*, 1994), data were analysed from 62 young adults with schizophrenia who had suffered from at least one psychotic relapse. Cannabis consumption was found to be the best predictor of relapse and hospitalization over the follow-up period. However, patients had a history of psychoactive substance abuse before the study and misused alcohol during the follow-up period, potentially confounding the results.

A US study by Kovasznay *et al.* (1997) examined the relationship between substance use and psychotic disorders, and found that patients with schizophrenia reported significantly more cannabis use than patients with an affective psychotic disorder over a 6-month period. Enduring cannabis abuse was associated with exacerbation of overall symptoms scored on the BPRS.

Longer-term prospective studies

A shortcoming of the afore-mentioned prospective studies was the relative short follow-up period, given the long-term course of schizophrenia. A prospective case-control study from Germany (Caspari, 1999) followed a representative sample of 39 schizophrenia patients with cannabis use for 68 months after their first hospital admission. Patients with cannabis abuse showed a significantly higher rate of rehospitalization in the follow-up period and tended to have poorer psychosocial functioning than the non-abusing controls. They also had a higher score on the 'thought disturbance' and 'hostility' items on the BPRS. Shortcomings of this study included a lack of repeated measurements of the symptomatic course during the follow-up period (the BPRS was assessed only at the end of the study); thus, it remains uncertain whether aggravation of symptoms and rehospitalization were temporally related to cannabis exposure.

In a further German long-term case-control study of the effects of substance abuse in schizophrenia, Bühler *et al.* (2002) followed 115 first-episode patients over a 5-year period, with six assessments. The number of patients using cannabis alone was small ($n = 4$) and had to be combined with those who also used alcohol ($n = 12$) and those who used only alcohol ($n = 12$) for analysis. The comorbid patients were compared with 29 non-comorbid patients, matched for age and sex. At each assessment the substance-abusing group showed higher positive symptom scores than the non-abusers; there was a trend towards lower negative symptom scores (notably affective flattening) in the substance users. Subjects with substance abuse also exhibited poorer treatment adherence, lower utilization of rehabilitation services and a higher rate of unemployment than non-users after 5 years.

A methodological flaw in studies examining the influence of cannabis use on clinical samples of patients with psychotic disorders and schizophrenia is selection bias, for example from hospital-based recruitment. To avoid such bias, Van Os et al. (2002) used a population-based sample of individuals with a vulnerability to psychotic disorder, to establish whether alcohol and drug (cannabis) use influenced outcome. Of the 59 subjects with *Diagnostic and Statistical Manual of Mental Disorders* (*DSM*-III-R) (American Psychiatric Association, 1987) diagnosis of any psychosis at baseline for whom follow-up data were available, nine reported cannabis use. A strong additive interaction was found between cannabis use and established psychotic symptoms. The difference in risk of psychosis at follow-up between those who did and did not use cannabis was much stronger for those with an established vulnerability at baseline than those without one. The association was independent of use of other drugs at baseline, and over the follow-up period.

Conclusions

The most relevant finding of this review is that, in prospective studies of patients with schizophrenia and related disorders, cannabis abuse was an independent risk factor for more psychotic relapses and aggravation of psychotic and disorganization symptoms. When a distinction with respect to the intensity of abuse was made, it appeared that particularly heavy cannabis abusers suffered more relapses, and more florid psychotic and disorganization symptoms. In those studies that controlled for alcohol and other (psychoactive) substance use (Linszen et al., 1994; Van Os et al., 2002) these were not found to be confounding factors. Furthermore, antipsychotic medication dosage and adherence could not explain away the findings (Linszen et al., 1994).

These findings would be even more convincing had the studies included systematic laboratory confirmation of cannabinoid derivatives in urine. However, Martin et al. (1988) found that the information on use of 'soft' drugs given by patients is reliable. Moreover, evaluation in the Dutch study included reports of the patients and by experienced clinicians; also, personal use of cannabis is not illegal in the Netherlands.

Two additional findings in the Amsterdam study indicate a possible causal relationship between cannabis exposure and psychotic relapse. First, most of the cannabis-abusing patients reported an immediate exacerbation of psychotic symptoms after resuming cannabis abuse. Second, in all but one patient, cannabis abuse preceded the onset of the first psychotic episode by at least a year. This finding is congruent with the observations of epidemiological studies that consistently reveal cannabis abuse prior to illness onset to be an independent risk factor for schizophrenia (see Chapter 7).

Some support is given for the self-medication hypothesis of schizophrenia and cannabis (see Chapter 11), as schizophrenia patients successfully reduced their negative symptoms (Peralta and Cuesta, 1992), affective symptoms (Dixon *et al.*, 1991) or anxiety and depression with mild abuse (Linszen *et al.*, 1994). Knudsen and Vilmar (1984) also reported a reduction in level of side-effects of antipsychotic agents in patients using cannabis, though causal pathways are not clear.

A biological explanation for the demonstrated relation between psychotic symptoms and cannabis abuse may be found in recent pharmacological studies. Δ^9-Tetrahydrocannabinol (Δ^9-THC), the principal psychoactive constituent of cannabis, acts as a dopamine agonist in dopaminergic projections of the medial forebrain bundles (see Chapter 2). Dopaminergic hyperactivity is generally thought to relate to the presence of psychotic symptoms of schizophrenia, although other neurotransmitters may also be involved. An increase in dopamine could undo the dopamine receptor blockade of antipsychotic medication. In our study the intensity of abuse was correlated with an increase of psychotic relapses, suggesting that Δ^9-THC acts as a dopamine agonist in the projections of the medial forebrains of the patients as well. Future studies with brain-imaging techniques applied to heavy and non-abusing schizophrenia patients with standard antipsychotic medication may be indicated to reveal these differences in dopamine receptor blockade or in other neurotransmission systems. Cannabis abuse may also influence antipsychotic drug metabolism, lowering plasma levels of active metabolites. Thus, cannabis abusers could be relatively undertreated.

It is also possible that those persons who use cannabis regularly are more vulnerable to or have less effective coping mechanisms for dealing with intercurrent life events, because of their age or their personality structure. This same vulnerability to stress may produce a lower threshold for recurrence of the psychotic disorder, even if they discontinued cannabis use. A further interesting possibility is that there may be some common genetic basis for cannabis abuse, schizophrenia and underlying neuropsychological and neurobiological vulnerabilities of both disorders.

Further studies are needed to elucidate the relationship between cannabis abuse and psychotic symptoms in schizophrenia. These studies should include quantitative estimations of cannabis abuse repeated over time; laboratory confirmation of single- or poly-cannabis abuse; repeated assessments of dose–response effects; and repeated assessments of potential confounding variables, notably adherence with antipsychotic medication.

ACKNOWLEDGEMENTS

The cannabis study was funded in part by grants from the ZON/MW. The authors thank J. Verhoeff M.D. and J. B. van Borssum Waalkes M.D. for their support of the study.

REFERENCES

American Psychiatric Association (1987). *Diagnostic and Statistical Manual of Mental Disorders* (*DSM*-III-R), 3rd edn. Washington, DC: American Psychiatric Association.

Andreasson, S., Allebeck, P., Engström, A. and Rydberg, U. (1987). Cannabis and schizophrenia. A longitudinal study of Swedish conscripts. *Lancet,* **2,** 1483–1486.

Arseneault, L., Cannon, M., Poulton, R. *et al.* (2002). Cannabis use in adolescence and risk for adult psychosis; longitudinal prospective study. *Br. Med. J.,* **325,** 1212–1213.

Bersani, G., Orlandi, V., Kotzalidis, G. D. and Pancheri, P. (2002). Cannabis and schizophrenia: impact on onset, course, psychopathology and outcomes. *Eur. Arch. Psychiatry Clin. Neurosci.,* **252,** 86–92.

Bilder, R. M., Goldman, R. S., Robinson, D. *et al.* (2000). Neuropsychology of first-episode schizophrenia: initial characterization and clinical correlates. *Am. J. Psychiatry,* **157,** 549–559.

Bovasso, G. B. (2001). Cannabis abuse as a risk factor for depressive symptoms. *Am. J. Psychiatry,* **158,** 2033–2037.

Bühler, B., Hambrecht, M., Löffler, W., Heiden an der, W. and Häfner, H. (2002). Precipitation and determination of the onset and course of schizophrenia by substance abuse – a retrospective and prospective study of 232 population-based first illness episodes. *Schizophr. Res.,* **54,** 243–251.

Caspari, D. (1999). Cannabis and schizophrenia: results of a follow-up study. *Eur. Arch. Psychiatry Clin. Neurosci.,* **249,** 45–49.

Chaudry, H. R., Moss, H. B., Bashir, A. *et al.* (1991). Cannabis psychosis following bhang ingestion. *Br. J. Addict.,* **86,** 1075–1081.

Chopra, G. S. and Smith, J. W. (1974). Psychotic reactions following cannabis use in East Indians. *Arch. Gen. Psychiatry,* **30,** 24–27.

Cleghorn, J. M., Kaplan, R. D., Szechtman, B. *et al.* (1991). Cannabis abuse and schizophrenia: effect on symptoms but not on neurocognitive function. *J. Clin. Psychiatry,* **52,** 26–30.

Dixon, L., Haas, G., Weiden, P. J., Sweeney, J. and Frances A. J. (1991). Drug abuse in schizophrenic patients: clinical correlates and reasons for use. *Am. J. Psychiatry,* **148,** 224–230.

Gupta, S., Hendricks, S., Kenkel, A. M., Bhatia, S. C. and Haffke, E. A. (1996). Relapse in schizophrenia: is there a relationship to substance abuse? *Schizophr. Res.,* **20,** 153–156.

Hunt, G. E., Bergen, J. and Bashir, M. (2002). Medication compliance and comorbid substance abuse in schizophrenia: impact on community survival 4 years after a relapse. *Schizophr. Res.,* **54,** 253–264.

Knudsen, P. and Vilmar, T. (1984). Cannabis and neuroleptic agents in schizophrenia. *Acta Psychiatr. Scand.,* **69,** 162–174.

Kovasznay, B., Fleischer, J., Tanenberg-Karant, M. *et al.* (1997). Substance use disorder and the early course of illness in schizophrenia and affective psychosis. *Schizophr. Bull.,* **23,** 195–201.

Liddle, P. (1987). The symptoms of chronic schizophrenia. A re-examination of the positive–negative dichotomy. *Br. J. Psychiatry,* **151,** 145–151.

Linszen, D. H., Dingemans, P. M. and Lenior, M. E. (1994). Cannabis abuse and the course of recent-onset schizophrenic disorders. *Arch. Gen. Psychiatry,* **51,** 273–279.

Linszen, D. H., Dingemans, P. M. and Lenior, M. E. (1995). Symptom dimensions of schizophrenic and cannabis abuse: a longitudinal study. *Schizophr. Res.*, **15**, 16.

Martin, G. W., Wilkinson A. and Kapur B. M. (1988). Validation of self-reported cannabis use by urine analysis. *Addict. Behav.*, **13**, 147–150.

Martinez-Arevalo, M. J., Calcedo-Ordoñez, A. and Varo-Prieto, J. R. (1994). Cannabis consumption as prognostic factor in schizophrenia. *Br. J. Psychiatry*, **164**, 679–684.

Negrete, J. C., Knapp, W. P., Douglas, D. E. and Smith, B. (1986). Cannabis affects the severity of schizophrenic symptoms: results of a clinical survey. *Psychol. Med.*, **16**, 515–520.

Patton, G. C., Coffey, C., Carlin, J. B. *et al.* (2002). Cannabis use and mental health in young people: cohort study. *Br. Med. J.*, **325**, 1195–1198.

Peralta, V. and Cuesta, M. J. (1992). Influence of cannabis abuse on schizophrenic psychopathology. *Acta Psychiatr. Scand.*, **85**, 127–130.

Reilly, D., Didcott, R., Swift, W. *et al.* (1998). Longterm cannabis use: characteristics of users in Australian rural areas. *Addiction*, **93**, 837–846.

Talbott, J. A. and Teague, J. W. (1969). Marijuana psychosis. *J.A.M.A.*, **210**, 299–302.

Thaker, G. K. and Carpenter, W. T. (2001). Advances in schizophrenia. *Nature Med.*, **7**, 667–671.

Thomas, H. (1996). A community survey of adverse effects of cannabis use. *Drug Alcohol Depend.*, **42**, 201–207.

Treffert, D. A. (1978). Marijuana use in schizophrenia: a clear hazard. *Am. J. Psychiatry*, **135**, 1213–1215.

Van der Does A. J. W, Dingemans, P. M. A. J., Linszen, D. H., Nugter, M. A. and Scholte, W. F. (1995). Dimensions and subtypes of recent-onset schizophrenia: a longitudinal analysis. *J. Nerv. Ment. Dis.*, **183**, 681–687.

Van Os, J., Bak, M. *et al.* (2002). Cannabis use and psychosis: a longitudinal population-based study. *Am. J. Epidemiol.*, **156**, 4, 319–327.

Weil, A. T. (1970). Adverse reactions to marijuana, classification and suggested treatment. *N. Engl. J. Med.*, **282**, 997–1000.

Weiser, M., Weisenberg, A., Rabinowitz, J. *et al.* (2001). Association between nonpsychotic psychiatric diagnosis in adolescent males and subsequent onset of schizophrenia. *Arch. Gen. Psychiatry*, **58**, 959–964.

Zammit, S., Allebeck, P., Andreasson, S., Lundberg, I. and Lewis, G. (2002). Self reported cannabis use as a risk factor for schizophrenia in Swedish conscripts of 1969: historical cohort study. *Br. Med. J.*, **325**, 1199–1201.

Zisook, S., Heaton, R., Moranville, J. *et al.* (1992). Past substance abuse and clincal course of schizophrenia. *Am. J. Psychiatry*, **149**, 552–553.

9

The endogenous cannabinoid system in schizophrenia

Suresh Sundram, Brian Dean and David Copolov

Mental Health Research Institute, Victoria, Australia

The human endogenous cannabinoid system is an appealing target in the investigation of schizophrenia. This is both because of clinical studies supporting the association between cannabis use and schizophrenia as well as the capacity of Δ^9-tetrahydrocannabinol (Δ^9-THC) to induce psychotic symptoms in non-psychotic individuals (see Chapters 3–5). Only since the recent elucidation of the endogenous cannabinoid system have direct investigations into its potential role in schizophrenia and other neuropsychiatric disorders become possible. The endocannabinoid system contains the cannabinoid CB_1, CB_{1A} and CB_2 receptors; the endogenous cannabinoids (most importantly, anandamide, 2-arachidonylglycerol (2-AG) and palmitoylethanolamide), their respective synthetic and degradative enzymes and a transport process. This chapter provides an overview of the human endogenous cannabinoid system, focusing specifically on those aspects relevant to schizophrenia (see also Chapters 1 and 2 for a broader overview), and then reviews studies concerning this system in schizophrenia.

The human endogenous cannabinoid system

The cannabinoid CB_1 receptor in the brain

The first component of the human endogenous cannabinoid system to be identified was the CB_1 receptor (Herkenham et al., 1990). The gene for this receptor is located on region q14–q15 of chromosome 6 (Hoehe et al., 1991) and encodes for a 472-amino-acid protein (Matsuda et al., 1990). This receptor has seven trans-membrane-spanning domains and interacts with guanine nucleotide-binding proteins (G proteins) as part of its signal transduction mechanism, placing it within the superfamily of G protein-coupled receptors. There is a posttranscriptional splice variant of the CB_1 receptor, the CB_{1A} receptor, which contains 411 amino acids

Marijuana and Madness: Psychiatry and Neurobiology, ed. D. Castle and R. Murray. Published by Cambridge University Press. © Cambridge University Press 2004.

(Shire *et al.*, 1995). This splice variant does not appear to differ functionally from the CB_1 receptor (Matsuda, 1997).

The distribution of the CB_1 receptor has been mapped in the human brain (Fig. 9.1) (Herkenham *et al.*, 1990; Westlake *et al.*, 1994; Glass *et al.*, 1997). There is a very high density of CB_1 receptors in the globus pallidus, substantia nigra pars reticulata, subiculum, Ammon's horn and the molecular layers of the dentate gyrus in the hippocampus and cerebellum, with a dense but lower level of binding in the neocortex, the remainder of the hippocampus, entorhinal cortex, amygdaloid complex and striatum. Neocortical binding is laminated, with highest levels in laminae I, V and VI, a thin dense band in IV(b) and low binding in II, III and IV(a and c). The regional density of cortical CB_1 receptors also varies, with the densest binding being in the association areas of the frontal, temporal and limbic lobes and lowest densities in the primary motor and sensory cortices. Thalamic CB_1 receptor binding corresponds anatomically to cortical binding, with moderate binding in the mediodorsal and anterior complex nuclei that connect to cortical associational areas, and very low levels in the geniculate bodies, ventral posterior and ventrolateral nuclei that connect to the primary sensory and motor cortices. The hypothalamus, nucleus solitarius and central grey substance exhibit moderate levels of CB_1 receptor binding whilst there are minimal levels in the brainstem and area postrema.

In areas of very dense CB_1 receptor binding, levels are of the same order of magnitude as those of striatal dopamine, cortical benzodiazepine and whole-brain glutamate receptor densities (Herkenham *et al.*, 1990). These comparisons, however, need to be viewed in the light of the recent demonstration of physiological activity of the cannabinoid agonist, *R*-(+)-WIN55 212 in CB_1 knockout mice (Di Marzo *et al.*, 2000; Breivogel *et al.*, 2001). This has raised the possibility of non-CB_1 cannabinoid receptors in the central nervous system (CNS), which, although estimated to be small (Elphick and Egertova, 2001), may have confounded the initial estimates of CB_1 receptor density.

The distribution of mRNA for the CB_1 receptor follows a pattern of distribution closely paralleling that of CB_1 receptor binding (Mailleux *et al.*, 1992; Westlake *et al.*, 1994). The localization of the mRNA in the cortex is densest in laminae I and II, and in the deep laminae IV, V and VI, with variation between cortical regions. However, both in the hippocampus and cerebral cortex, the mRNA is extremely dense in some neurons surrounded by low to moderate densities in the majority of cells. This contrasts with other regions, for example the cerebellum, where mRNA distribution is relatively uniform across neurons. Equivalent levels of mRNA and binding are not maintained in the molecular layer of the hippocampal dentate gyrus, globus pallidus, substantia nigra and entopeduncular nucleus, where binding is high with minimal levels of mRNA; and conversely in the dentate hilus

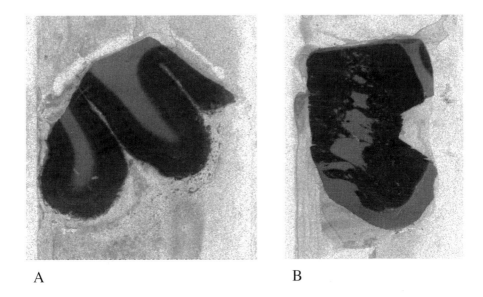

A   B

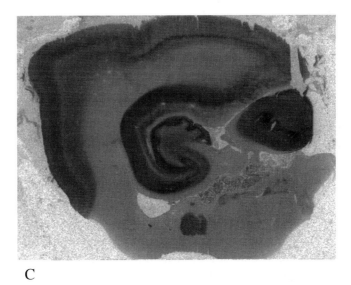

C

Figure 9.1   Representative autoradiograms showing the pattern of distribution of the cannabinoid CB_1 receptor in (A) the dorsolateral prefrontal cortex, (B) caudate putamen and (C) hippocampus and surrounding entorhinal cortex from postmortem human brain as demonstrated by the total binding of the tritium-labelled cannabinoid CB_1 receptor antagonist, $[^3H]CP55\ 940$.

and medial habenula with high mRNA signal and low binding levels. These differences between mRNA and binding levels may indicate gene transcription of the CB_1 receptor in a cell body remote from the receptor's terminal axonal location.

Relative to the density of the mRNA for the CB_1 receptor, the mRNA for the CB_{1A} receptor shows a variable pattern of brain regional densities (between 1 and 20% of the CB_1 receptor) (Shire *et al.*, 1995). The physiological significance of this variable difference between the distributions of the mRNA for the CB_1 and CB_{1A} receptors remains to be determined (Matsuda, 1997; Elphick and Egertova, 2001).

Endogenous cannabinoid receptor ligands

As detailed in Chapters 1 and 2, there are two major known endogenous cannabinoid ligands, anandamide (Devane *et al.*, 1992) and 2-AG, both derived from arachidonic acid (Stella *et al.*, 1997). These are not the only endogenous cannabinoid ligands, but are predominant in the CNS and their concentrations exhibit regional CNS and species variation. The only study to date in human brain has demonstrated high levels of anandamide not only in regions of high CB_1 receptor density, the hippocampus, striatum, cortex and cerebellum, but also in regions of low density such as the thalamus (Felder *et al.*, 1996). This discrepancy between the distribution of anandamide and the CB_1 receptor has raised speculation of another CNS cannabinoid receptor (Howlett *et al.*, 2002). In addition, there is a substantial mismatch between the reported whole-brain concentration of anandamide and CB_1 receptor density. Anandamide is present at a concentration similar to that of the monoamine neurotransmitters and about one-tenth that of γ-aminobutyric acid (GABA) and glutamate (Felder *et al.*, 1996). This contrasts with a CB_1 receptor density similar to GABA and glutamate receptors (see above). 2-AG is less well characterized than anandamide but has been variously estimated (depending upon the measurement method used) to be present in the CNS at a concentration 170 times greater (Stella *et al.*, 1997) or at a level less (Bisogno *et al.*, 1999) than that of anandamide. It is thus premature to speculate whether 2-AG levels could help account for the high CB_1 receptor densities.

The synthesis of both endocannabinoids requires cleavage from the membrane phospholipid pool, anandamide by N-acyltransferase then phospholipase D, and 2-AG by phospholipase C, then sn-1-diacylglycerol lipase (Elphick and Egertova, 2001). Inactivation of both anandamide and 2-AG is likely to be through enzymatic hydrolysis by fatty-acid amide hydrolase (FAAH) for both anandamide (Cravatt *et al.*, 1996) and 2-AG (Goparaju *et al.*, 1998), and by a recently identified monoglyceride lipase for 2-AG (Dinh *et al.*, 2002). A neuronal transporter for anandamide that is rapid, saturable and temperature-dependent has been characterized (Di Marzo *et al.*, 1994), but is yet to be isolated or cloned. 2-AG and Δ^9-THC inhibit anandamide transport, suggesting these may also be substrates for the transporter

(Rakhshan *et al.*, 2000). Competitive blockade of transport of anandamide by *N*-(4-hydroxyphenyl)-arachidonamide (AM404) in rat cortical neurons augments anandamide-induced CB_1 receptor-mediated effects (Beltramo *et al.*, 1997). However, the physiological significance of this transport process in the human CNS remains to be determined.

Investigations of the human endogenous cannabinoid system in schizophrenia

The known functions of the endogenous cannabinoid system and the effects of exogenous agonists, in particular Δ^9-THC, are detailed in Chapters 1 and 2. There is some overlap between these latter effects and the clinical syndrome of schizophrenia. In particular, similarities in perceptual disturbance, mood changes, anhedonia and amotivation, cognitive impairment and frank psychosis are discussed in Chapters 3 and 5 and point to some potential commonality of mechanism compatible with involvement of the endocannabinoid system in schizophrenia. Investigations of this have included:

- Assessment of perceptual disturbances in patients with schizophrenia, compared to non-psychiatric controls under the influence of cannabis
- Measurement of the endogenous cannabinoids in cerebrospinal fluid (CSF)
- Measurement of CB_1 receptor density and related studies in postmortem human CNS tissue
- Association studies of CB_1 receptor gene polymorphisms

These will be reviewed in turn.

Perceptual disturbances in patients with schizophrenia, compared to non-psychiatric controls under the influence of cannabis

A particular form of perceptual disturbance that has relevance to studying models pertinent to schizophrenia is that of binocular depth inversion (Schneider *et al.*, 2002). This is a visual illusion that occurs when stereoscopically presented images which are concave appear convex; this is greater with images of high contextual relevance (for example, images of faces). When this occurs, binocular disparity is assumed to be overridden by higher cognitive processes (Emrich *et al.*, 1997).

Emrich *et al.* (1997) investigated binocular depth inversion in subjects with schizophrenia and normal controls. Healthy control subjects, before and after consuming cannabis resin, were compared with actively psychotic (mean Brief Psychiatric Rating Scale (BPRS) score of 39) subjects with schizophrenia who were not given cannabis. Subjects with schizophrenia scored significantly worse than control subjects with both familiar ($P < 0.001$) and unfamiliar ($P < 0.05$) objects. Control subjects scored significantly worse postcannabis consumption, and maximal impairment correlated with highest plasma Δ^9-THC levels (Emrich *et al.*, 1997). This finding was replicated in a larger group of control subjects given synthetic Δ^9-THC (dronabinol) (Leweke *et al.*, 1999a). This effect, however, is not specific for cannabis intoxication, also having been reported in alcohol withdrawal (Schneider *et al.*, 1996).

Human CSF studies

In an initial study, Leweke *et al.* (1999b) measured CSF levels of anandamide, 2-AG, palmitoylethanolamide (PEA) and a non-cannabinoid acylethanolamide, oleylethanolamide (OEA) (as a positive control) using high-pressure liquid chromatography (HPLC) and gas chromatography/mass spectroscopy (GC/MS) techniques in people with schizophrenia and normal controls. Mean anandamide and PEA levels were approximately twofold higher in the schizophrenia cohort ($n = 10$) versus normal controls ($n = 11$), whilst OEA levels were not different and 2-AG levels were not detectable in either group (Leweke *et al.*, 1999b). No subjects met criteria for substance dependence, and age and gender did not correlate with CSF levels (Leweke *et al.*, 1999b). Overall, medication status did not correlate with CSF levels although, as five subjects with schizophrenia were neuroleptic-naive and five had been or were on antipsychotic medication at the time of the studies, it was not possible fully to exclude any medication effect.

In a subsequent larger study, for which only preliminary data have been reported, the same group (Leweke, 2002) measured, using HPLC/MS, CSF anandamide levels in medication-naive ($n = 19$) and neuroleptic-treated ($n = 34$) subjects with schizophrenia; subjects with affective disorders ($n = 11$); subjects with dementia ($n = 6$); and age- and gender-matched healthy controls ($n = 76$). There was an 8.5-fold increase in CSF anandamide levels in medication-naive subjects with schizophrenia compared to controls, whereas there were no differences in the other patient groups compared to the control group (Leweke, 2002). The difference between medication-naive and medicated subjects with schizophrenia may reflect either psychotic symptom intensity or an antipsychotic medication effect. Interestingly, although overall the mean anandamide level in the treated schizophrenia group did not differ from the control group, those subjects taking atypical antipsychotic medications had a mean anandamide level significantly higher than both control subjects and schizophrenia subjects treated with typical antipsychotics (Leweke, 2002).

A number of factors need to be considered when interpreting these CSF studies. First, anandamide has a very short half-life when synaptically released (Ameri, 1999) due to its rapid transport and hydrolysis by FAAH (Wilson and Nicoll, 2002). Therefore, even small differences in collection and processing of samples could result in variations in findings between groups. Also, measurements of endogenous cannabinoids are technically difficult given their lipophilicity requiring solvent extraction and the possible introduction of systematic error (Yang *et al.*, 1999; Porter and Felder, 2001). Second, CSF anandamide levels represent the dynamic equilibrium between biosynthesis, release and degradation; therefore, a change may reflect disturbance in any or all of the components involved in these processes, which are both neuronal and glial (Beltramo *et al.*, 1997). Third, non-neuronal sources of endogenous cannabinoids, such as the cerebrovascular endothelium and circulating cells, including platelets and macrophages (Hillard, 2000), may be contributing to the measured total. Fourth, CSF levels can only give an indication of global CNS change without the capacity to determine regional specificity. Finally, the use of exogenous cannabinoids is markedly increased in subjects in the prodromal and established phases of schizophrenia compared to healthy controls (Hambrecht and Hafner, 2000; Buhler *et al.*, 2002; and see Chapter 11). Although it may be feasible to exclude acute cannabis intoxication by plasma or urine drug-screening of subjects, this does not eliminate the possibility of persisting effects of cannabis use on the endogenous cannabinoid system biasing results in this group.

These caveats aside, dopamine D2 receptor signalling increases anandamide release, at least in the dorsal striatum in rats, an effect blocked by the antipsychotic raclopride (Giuffrida *et al.*, 1999). Therefore, the human CSF anandamide data would support increased dopamine D2 signalling in neuroleptic-naive schizophrenia and its reversal in those treated with dopamine D2 antagonists, consistent with the dopamine hypothesis of schizophrenia (Meltzer and Stahl, 1976).

Postmortem human brain studies

Radioligand binding and quantitative autoradiography of the CB_1 receptor using postmortem human CNS tissue addresses some of the limitations affecting CSF studies. In particular, it allows clear regional localization of changes and measures a stable component of the endogenous cannabinoid system. This methodology has demonstrated in Huntington's disease a dramatic loss of CB_1 receptor binding in the substantia nigra and globus pallidus, consistent with loss of striatal GABA projection neurons (Glass *et al.*, 1993; 2000). We are aware of only one published study examining CB_1 receptor changes in schizophrenia (Dean *et al.*, 2001).

This study (Dean *et al.*, 2001) compared binding of [^{3}H]CP55 940 in the dorsolateral prefrontal cortex (DLPFC), Brodmann's area 9, caudate putamen (C-P) and hippocampal formation from tissue obtained postmortem from 14 subjects with schizophrenia and 14 non-psychiatrically ill controls. Some subjects from both groups had consumed cannabis prior to death, allowing a comparison between recent cannabis users and those who were abstinent. The methodology and concentration of [^{3}H]CP55 940 used were previously shown to provide a good measure of the density of the CB_1 receptor (Herkenham *et al.*, 1990). When all subjects with schizophrenia were compared with all control subjects, the mean CB_1 receptor density was increased by approximately 19% only in the DLPFC ($P < 0.05$). There were no significant differences between the groups in receptor density in C-P or hippocampal formation. In subjects who had recently consumed cannabis (as determined by GC/MS of postmortem plasma), there was a 23% increase in CB_1 receptor density in the C-P compared to non-users, independent of schizophrenia ($P < 0.05$); in this comparison there were no significant differences in the DLPFC nor, again, in the hippocampus. The differences in the DLPFC between control and schizophrenia subjects and in the C-P between users and non-users could not be accounted for by postmortem interval, brain pH, age or gender. There were also no significant correlations between [^{3}H]CP55 940 binding and duration of illness or final recorded antipsychotic drug dose in those with schizophrenia or with plasma Δ^9-THC levels in the cannabis users.

A number of factors need to be considered in interpreting these data, including the small number of subjects. In addition, changes in CB_1 receptor binding seen in the DLPFC in schizophrenia may be due to long-term antipsychotic medication effects, although a study of chronic antipsychotic drug treatment in rats did not show changes in CB_1 receptor binding in the cerebral cortex, C-P or hippocampus (Sundram *et al.*, 2000). It is also not possible to determine whether changes in CB_1 receptor binding correlate with particular psychosis symptom clusters. This would be of particular interest given the cognitive disorganization and working-memory deficits of schizophrenia which have been associated with the DLPFC by some (Perlstein *et al.*, 2001) and the effects of exogenous cannabinoids on these processes (Pistis *et al.*, 2001; see Chapter 2).

The changes in CB_1 receptor binding observed in this study are modest compared to those described in Huntington's disease (97.5% decrease in the substantia nigra pars reticulata) (Glass *et al.*, 1993). However, the loss in Huntington's disease is due to the specific degeneration of striatonigral terminals (Glass *et al.*, 1993) with no analogous pathology identified in schizophrenia (Harrison, 1999). In contrast, CB_1 receptor binding decreases seen in Alzheimer's disease (37–45% in the hippocampus and 49% in the caudate) did not correlate with neuropathology but did correlate with age and were seen in other cortical disorders (Westlake *et al.*, 1994). Given that the CB_1 receptor density in schizophrenia was increased and did not correlate with age, it would seem unlikely that the changes in schizophrenia were a non-specific marker of cortical pathology or degeneration.

For the most part, CB_1 receptors are located on presynaptic neurons (Egertova and Elphick, 2000) and, when stimulated, possibly by retrograde passage of anandamide (Wilson and Nicoll, 2001), inhibit neurotransmitter release through inhibition of voltage-dependent Ca^{2+} channels (Hoffman and Lupica, 2000) and possibly other mechanisms (for review, see Schlicker and Kathmann (2001)). In rodent models, this endocannabinoid signalling in the hippocampus and cerebral cortex may play a role in cognition and learning (for review see Wilson and Nicoll (2002)). However, to date, no studies have been conducted on the physiological effects of CB_1 receptor stimulation in either the human DLPFC or C-P. Therefore, as with the CSF studies, it is too early to ascribe pathophysiological effects to the increases in CB_1 receptor density in schizophrenia or in association with cannabis use.

A subsequent study (Dean et al., 2003), using tissue from the same control and schizophrenia subjects, examined levels of the dopamine transporter (DAT) and tyrosine hydroxylase (TH) in the C-P in subjects who were (1) non-cannabis users ($n = 19$) or (2) cannabis users ($n = 9$) at time of death. The rationale for this study was that a number of animal studies have shown facilitating effects of cannabinoids on dopamine activity (reviewed in Chapter 10). These included the observations that Δ^9-THC acutely decreased dopamine uptake into rat striatal synaptosomes, increased dopamine release from striatal slices (Sakurai-Yamashita et al., 1989) and increased activity and expression of TH in vivo (Bonnin et al., 1996; Hernandez et al., 1997). The hypothesis was that if Δ^9-THC effects in animals reflected human CNS effects, then cannabis use in humans would increase extraneuronal dopamine through stimulation of TH and inhibitory effects on DAT (Dean et al., 2003).

The mean DAT level, as measured by [^{3}H]mazindol binding, was significantly decreased (by 19%; $P = 0.01$) in non-using subjects with schizophrenia ($n = 9$) compared to the non-using controls ($n = 10$). This difference was not apparent between the two cannabis-using groups, nor were these groups significantly different from the non-using control group. TH levels did not vary across any of the groups (Dean et al., 2003). The DAT is the most important regulator of synaptic dopamine (Amara and Kuhar, 1993) and, therefore, a mean decrease in the DAT level may functionally lead to an increase in synaptic dopamine. Again, this would be consistent with the dopamine hypothesis of schizophrenia (Meltzer and Stahl, 1976). Although cannabis use did not affect DAT levels in control users, in schizophrenia it may act to upregulate or increase DAT towards control levels (Dean et al., 2003), consistent with the idea of cannabis use being a form of self-medication in schizophrenia (Khantzian, 1997; see Chapter 11). Nevertheless, given the small number of subjects, these data should be viewed as preliminary.

This finding of differences in DAT levels in postmortem C-P in schizophrenia contingent upon cannabis abstinence (Dean et al., 2003) is intriguing in the light of a case reporting a schizophrenia subject scanned using single-photon emission computed tomography (SPECT) both before and after cannabis use (Voruganti et al., 2001). The postcannabis scan showed a 20% decrease in striatal dopamine D^2 receptor binding, with a clinical effect of worsening psychotic symptoms following an initial anxiolytic effect (Voruganti *et al.*, 2001). The decrease in binding was postulated to represent increased synaptic dopamine transmission but it is not possible from this type of study to establish whether this was due to increased release or decreased reuptake of synaptic dopamine (Voruganti *et al.*, 2001). The SPECT data are, however, consistent with the hypothesis that repeated cannabis use, through initially increasing synaptic dopamine, could entrain a homeostatic upregulation of the DAT in the C-P of subjects with schizophrenia, as observed in the postmortem study described above (Dean *et al.*, 2003). This would result in lower baseline synaptic dopamine levels through increased clearance (Amara and Kuhar, 1993). Such upregulation, especially if more widespread through the CNS, could result in long-term modulation of hyperdopaminergic-related symptoms providing a neurobiological framework for the self-medication hypothesis of cannabis use in schizophrenia (Khantzian, 1997).

CB$_1$ receptor gene polymorphisms in schizophrenia

The investigation of endocannabinoid trait markers in schizophrenia has focused upon the gene for the CB$_1$ receptor. Two polymorphisms for the CB$_1$ receptor gene have been identified, a triplet repeat $(AAT)_n$ in the 3′ flanking region (Dawson, 1995) and a biallelic silent mutation of 1359 G-to-A at the 453 codon in the coding exon (Gadzicki *et al.*, 1999). The first investigation of the triplet repeat in schizophrenia, using linkage analysis, a transmission disequilibrium test and an association study, failed to demonstrate a significant association in 135 schizophrenia subjects compared to 101 controls (Dawson, 1995). Further, an association study comparing 127 subjects with schizophrenia and 146 control subjects in a Han Chinese population also failed to show a significant association between the triplet repeat frequency and schizophrenia (Tsai *et al.*, 2000). In contrast, a Japanese study of 296 control and 242 schizophrenia subjects revealed significant differences in the distribution of the allelic triplet repeat frequency between the two groups ($P = 0.046$) (Ujike *et al.*, 2002). This difference was most robust in the hebephrenic subgroup ($n = 128$; $P < 0.003$) but not apparent in the paranoid subgroup. If this association is confirmed, it may support CB$_1$ receptor involvement in hebephrenic schizophrenia, or alternatively may represent a marker for other genes close to the allele. However, the distribution of allele frequency was markedly different between Caucasian (Comings *et al.*, 1997) and Japanese (Ujike *et al.*, 2002) populations, suggesting that similar future studies in Caucasian populations will need to account for this in calculating sample size and subgroup composition of patients with schizophrenia. To date, the functional effect of this triplet repeat on the CB$_1$ receptor gene transcription rate has not been elucidated.

The first investigation of the 1359 A/G polymorphism was conducted in a French Caucasian sample of 102 subjects with schizophrenia and 63 healthy controls (Leroy *et al.*, 2001). Overall there were no significant differences between the two groups either in allele frequency or genotype distribution. Dividing the patient group into substance-using ($n = 42$) and non-using, however, revealed a significant decrease in homozygosity for the G allele in non-users compared to users ($P < 0.04$) (Leroy *et al.*, 2001). As for the triplet repeat, the 1359 A/G polymorphism does not result in a known functional outcome but may be a marker of a nearby, unknown functional genetic variation (Leroy *et al.*, 2001). When this polymorphism was investigated in the same Japanese sample used for the study of the triplet repeats (Ujike *et al.*, 2002), there were no significant differences in allelic or genotypic distribution between schizophrenia and control groups. This cohort of subjects had no known history of substance use disorders so it was not possible to examine for any effect of such use. Again, however, allelic and genotypic frequencies markedly differed between Caucasian (Gadzicki *et al.*, 1999; Leroy *et al.*, 2001) and Japanese (Ujike *et al.*, 2002) populations, limiting the capacity to compare between studies of different ethnic groups.

One final study (Sipe *et al.*, 2002) did not examine for a CB_1 receptor gene polymorphism but for a polymorphism within the gene encoding for FAAH, which is primarily responsible for clearing anandamide from the synaptic cleft (see above). This missense mutation codes for the conversion of cytosine 385 to adenosine ($385C \rightarrow A$), which results in a proline residue at position 129 being converted to threonine (Sipe *et al.*, 2002). This produces a less stable enzyme, potentially leading to increased levels of synaptic anandamide (Sipe *et al.*, 2002). The study describes a significant association only with problem drug use, and not with a variety of other neuropsychiatric disorders including schizophrenia (Sipe *et al.*, 2002). The sample of people with schizophrenia was relatively small ($n = 48$) and it was not clear whether any subjects were comorbid for problem drug use. Thus, it will be of value to explore associations for this functional polymorphism in larger populations of people with schizophrenia, especially comparing substance-using and non-using subgroups.

Although the CB_1 receptor gene association studies cited above have not demonstrated significant overall differences between schizophrenia and control populations, they have indicated that polymorphisms may be significantly associated with particular patient subgroups. This argues for study populations to be sufficiently large to allow characterization of patient subpopulations, especially for substance use disorders and ethnicity.

Conclusions

The enhanced understanding of the endogenous cannabinoid system provides substantial scope for investigation of its potential dysfunction in schizophrenia. The initial studies in this area offer evidence of changes in a number of components of this system, namely CSF endocannabinoid levels, CB_1 receptor density and potentially gene polymorphisms for the CB_1 receptor and other components of the endo-cannabinoid system. These, however, await confirmation and should be viewed as preliminary. Moreover, the changes remain associational in nature, requiring demonstration of any functional effects. Similarly, it is not possible, as yet, to determine whether the changes described in the endogenous cannabinoid system in schizophrenia are primary due to the disease pathology; reflect secondary or compensatory effects; or are responses to exogenous cannabinoids or antipsychotic or other medications. However, the further exploration of this system in schizophrenia could enhance our understanding of the pathology of this disorder and ultimately inform the development of novel therapies.

REFERENCES

Amara, S. G. and Kuhar, M. J. (1993). Neurotransmitter transporters: recent progress. *Annu. Rev. Neurosci.*, **16**, 73–93.

Ameri, A. (1999). The effects of cannabinoids on the brain. *Progr. Neurobiol.*, **58**, 315–348.

Beltramo, M., Stella, N., Calignano, A. *et al.* (1997). Functional role of high-affinity anandamide transport, as revealed by selective inhibition. *Science*, **277**, 1094–1097.

Bisogno, T., Berrendero, F., Ambrosino, G. *et al.* (1999). Brain regional distribution of endo-cannabinoids: implications for their biosynthesis and biological function. *Biochem. Biophys. Res. Commun.*, **256**, 377–380.

Bonnin, A., de Miguel, R., Castro, J. G., Ramos, J. A. and Fernandez-Ruiz, J. J. (1996). Effects of perinatal exposure to delta 9-tetrahydrocannabinol on the fetal and early postnatal development of tyrosine hydroxylase- containing neurons in rat brain. *J. Mol. Neurosci.*, **7**, 291–308.

Breivogel, C. S., Griffin, G., Di, M. V. and Martin, B. R. (2001). Evidence for a new G protein-coupled cannabinoid receptor in mouse brain. *Mol. Pharmacol.*, **60**, 155–163.

Buhler, B., Hambrecht, M., Loffler, W., an der, H. W. and Hafner, H. (2002). Precipitation and determination of the onset and course of schizophrenia by substance abuse – a retrospective and prospective study of 232 population-based first illness episodes. *Schizophr. Res.*, **54**, 243–251.

Comings, D. E., Muhleman, D., Gade, R. *et al.* (1997). Cannabinoid receptor gene (CNR1): association with i.v. drug use. *Mol. Psychiatry*, **2**, 161–168.

Cravatt, B. F., Giang, D. K., Mayfield, S. P. *et al.* (1996). Molecular characterization of an enzyme that degrades neuromodulatory fatty-acid amides. *Nature*, **384**, 83–87.

Dawson, E. (1995). Identification of a polymorphic triplet marker for the brain cannabinoid receptor gene: use in linkage and association studies of schizophrenia. *Psych. Gen.*, **5**, s50–s51.

Dean, B., Sundram, S., Bradbury, R., Scarr, E. and Copolov, D. (2001). Studies on [3H]CP-55940 binding in the human central nervous system: regional specific changes in density of cannabinoid-1 receptors associated with schizophrenia and cannabis use. *Neuroscience*, **103**, 9–15.

Dean, B., Bradbury, R. and Copolov, D. L. (2003). Cannabis-sensitive dopaminergic markers in postmortem CNS: changes in schizophrenia. *Biol. Psychiatry*, **53**, 585–592.

Devane, W. A., Hanus, L., Breuer, A. *et al.* (1992). Isolation and structure of a brain constituent that binds to the cannabinoid receptor. *Science*, **258**, 1946–1949.

Di Marzo, V., Fontana, A., Cadas, H. *et al.* (1994). Formation and inactivation of endogenous cannabinoid anandamide in central neurons. *Nature*, **372**, 686–691.

Di Marzo, V., Breivogel, C. S., Tao, Q. *et al.* (2000). Levels, metabolism, and pharmacological activity of anandamide in CB(1) cannabinoid receptor knockout mice: evidence for non-CB(1), non-CB(2) receptor-mediated actions of anandamide in mouse brain. *J. Neurochem.*, **75**, 2434–2444.

Dinh, T. P., Carpenter, D., Leslie, F. M. *et al.* (2002). Brain monoglyceride lipase participating in endocannabinoid inactivation. *Proc. Natl Acad. Sci. USA*, **99**, 10819–10824.

Egertova, M. and Elphick, M. R. (2000). Localisation of cannabinoid receptors in the rat brain using antibodies to the intracellular C-terminal tail of CB. *J. Comp. Neurol.*, **422**, 159–171.

Elphick, M. R. and Egertova, M. (2001). The neurobiology and evolution of cannabinoid signalling. *Philos. Trans. R. Soc. Lond. B Biol. Sci.*, **356**, 381–408.

Emrich, H. M., Leweke, F. M. and Schneider, U. (1997). Towards a cannabinoid hypothesis of schizophrenia: cognitive impairments due to dysregulation of the endogenous cannabinoid system. *Pharmacol. Biochem. Behav.*, **56**, 803–807.

Felder, C. C., Nielsen, A., Briley, E. M. *et al.* (1996). Isolation and measurement of the endogenous cannabinoid receptor agonist, anandamide, in brain and peripheral tissues of human and rat. *FEBS Lett.*, **393**, 231–235.

Gadzicki, D., Muller-Vahl, K. and Stuhrmann, M. (1999). A frequent polymorphism in the coding exon of the human cannabinoid receptor (CNR1) gene. *Mol. Cell Probes*, **13**, 321–323.

Giuffrida, A., Parsons, L. H., Kerr, T. M. *et al.* (1999). Dopamine activation of endogenous cannabinoid signaling in dorsal striatum. *Nature Neurosci.*, **2**, 358–363.

Glass, M., Faull, R. L. and Dragunow, M. (1993). Loss of cannabinoid receptors in the substantia nigra in Huntington's disease. *Neuroscience*, **56**, 523–527.

Glass, M., Dragunow, M. and Faull, R. L. (1997). Cannabinoid receptors in the human brain: a detailed anatomical and quantitative autoradiographic study in the foetal, neonatal and adult human brain. *Neuroscience*, **77**, 299–318.

Glass, M., Dragunow, M. and Faull, R. L. (2000). The pattern of neurodegeneration in Huntington's disease: a comparative study of cannabinoid, dopamine, adenosine and GABA(A) receptor alterations in the human basal ganglia in Huntington's disease. *Neuroscience*, **97**, 505–519.

Goparaju, S. K., Ueda, N., Yamaguchi, H. and Yamamoto, S. (1998). Anandamide amidohydrolase reacting with 2-arachidonoylglycerol, another cannabinoid receptor ligand. *FEBS Lett.*, **422**, 69–73.

Hambrecht, M. and Hafner, H. (2000). Cannabis, vulnerability, and the onset of schizophrenia: an epidemiological perspective. *Aust. NZ J. Psychiatry*, **34**, 468–475.

Harrison, P. J. (1999). The neuropathology of schizophrenia. A critical review of the data and their interpretation. *Brain*, **122** (Pt 4), 593–624.

Herkenham, M., Lynn, A. B., Little, M. D. *et al.* (1990). Cannabinoid receptor localization in brain. *Proc. Natl Acad. Sci. USA*, **87**, 1932–1936.

Hernandez, M. L., Garcia-Gil, L., Berrendero, F., Ramos, J. A. and Fernandez-Ruiz, J. J. (1997). Delta 9-tetrahydrocannabinol increases activity of tyrosine hydroxylase in cultured fetal mesencephalic neurons. *J. Mol. Neurosci.*, **8**, 83–91.

Hillard, C. J. (2000). Endocannabinoids and vascular function. *J. Pharmacol. Exp. Ther.*, **294**, 27–32.

Hoehe, M. R., Caenazzo, L., Martinez, M. M. *et al.* (1991). Genetic and physical mapping of the human cannabinoid receptor gene to chromosome 6q14–q15. *New Biol.*, **3**, 880–885.

Hoffman, A. F. and Lupica, C. R. (2000). Mechanisms of cannabinoid inhibition of GABA(A) synaptic transmission in the hippocampus. *J. Neurosci.*, **20**, 2470–2479.

Howlett, A. C., Barth, F., Bonner, T. I. *et al.* (2002). International Union of Pharmacology. XXVII. Classification of cannabinoid receptors. *Pharmacol. Rev.*, **54**, 161–202.

Khantzian, E. J. (1997). The self-medication hypothesis of substance use disorders: a reconsideration and recent applications. *Harvard Rev. Psychiatry*, **4**, 231–244.

Leroy, S., Griffon, N., Bourdel, M. C. *et al.* (2001). Schizophrenia and the cannabinoid receptor type 1 (CB$_1$): association study using a single-base polymorphism in coding exon 1. *Am. J. Med. Genet.*, **105**, 749–752.

Leweke, F. M. (2002). Elevated CSF endocannabinoid levels in schizophrenic patients versus controls. *Int. J. Neuropsychopharmacol.*, **5**[S1], s47.

Leweke, F. M., Schneider, U., Thies, M., Munte, T. F. and Emrich, H. M. (1999a). Effects of synthetic delta9-tetrahydrocannabinol on binocular depth inversion of natural and artificial objects in man. *Psychopharmacology (Berl.)*, **142**, 230–235.

Leweke, F. M., Giuffrida, A., Wurster, U., Emrich, H. M. and Piomelli, D. (1999b). Elevated endogenous cannabinoids in schizophrenia. *Neuroreport*, **10**, 1665–1669.

Mailleux, P., Parmentier, M. and Vanderhaeghen, J. J. (1992). Distribution of cannabinoid receptor messenger RNA in the human brain: an in situ hybridization histochemistry with oligonucleotides. *Neurosci. Lett.*, **143**, 200–204.

Matsuda, L. (1997). Molecular aspects of cannabinoid receptors. *Crit. Rev. Neurobiol.*, **11**, 143–166.

Matsuda, L. A., Lolait, S. J., Brownstein, M. J., Young, A. C. and Bonner, T. I. (1990). Structure of a cannabinoid receptor and functional expression of the cloned cDNA. *Nature*, **346**, 561–564.

Meltzer, H. Y. and Stahl, S. M. (1976). The dopamine hypothesis of schizophrenia: a review. *Schizophr. Bull.*, **2**, 19–76.

Perlstein, W. M., Carter, C. S., Noll, D. C. and Cohen, J. D. (2001). Relation of prefrontal cortex dysfunction to working memory and symptoms in schizophrenia. *Am. J. Psychiatry*, **158**, 1105–1113.

Pistis, M., Porcu, G., Melis, M., Diana, M. and Gessa, G. L. (2001). Effects of cannabinoids on prefrontal neuronal responses to ventral tegmental area stimulation. *Eur. J. Neurosci.*, **14**, 96–102.

Porter, A. C. and Felder, C. C. (2001). The endocannabinoid nervous system: unique opportunities for therapeutic intervention. *Pharmacol. Ther.*, **90**, 45–60.

Rakhshan, F., Day, T. A., Blakely, R. D. and Barker, E.L. (2000). Carrier-mediated uptake of the endogenous cannabinoid anandamide in RBL- 2H3 cells. *J. Pharmacol. Exp. Ther.*, **292**, 960–967.

Sakurai-Yamashita, Y., Kataoka, Y., Fujiwara, M., Mine, K. and Ueki, S. (1989). Delta 9-tetrahydrocannabinol facilitates striatal dopaminergic transmission. *Pharmacol. Biochem. Behav.*, **33**, 397–400.

Schlicker, E. and Kathmann, M. (2001). Modulation of transmitter release via presynaptic cannabinoid receptors. *Trends Pharmacol. Sci.*, **22**, 565–572.

Schneider, U., Leweke, F. M., Niemcyzk, W. *et al.* (1996). Impaired binocular depth inversion in patients with alcohol withdrawal. *J. Psychiatr. Res.*, **30**, 469–474.

Schneider, U., Borsutzky, M. *et al.* (2002). Reduced binocular depth inversion in schizophrenic patients. *Schizophr. Res.*, **53**, 101–108.

Shire, D., Carillon, C., Kaghad, M. *et al.* (1995). An amino-terminal variant of the central cannabinoid receptor resulting from alternative splicing. *J. Biol. Chem.*, **270**, 3726–3731.

Sipe, J. C., Chiang, K., Gerber, A. L., Beutler, E. and Cravatt, B. F. (2002). A missense mutation in human fatty acid amide hydrolase associated with problem drug use. *Proc. Natl Acad. Sci. USA*, **99**, 8394–8399.

Stella, N., Schweitzer, P. and Piomelli, D. (1997). A second endogenous cannabinoid that modulates long-term potentiation. *Nature*, **388**, 773–778.

Sundram, S., Bradbury, R., Copolov, D. L. and Dean, B. (2000). Clozapine differentially and reversibly alters cannabinoid CB_1 receptor binding in the rat nucleus accumbens. *Int. J. Neuropsychopharmacol.*, **3**[S1], S132.

Tsai, S. J., Wang, Y. C. and Hong, C. J. (2000). Association study of a cannabinoid receptor gene (CNR1) polymorphism and schizophrenia. *Psychiatr. Genet.*, **10**, 149–151.

Ujike, H., Takaki, M., Nakata, K. *et al.* (2002). CNR1, central cannabinoid receptor gene, associated with susceptibility to hebephrenic schizophrenia. *Mol. Psychiatry*, **7**, 515–518.

Voruganti, L. N., Slomka, P., Zabel, P., Mattar, A. and Awad, A. G. (2001). Cannabis induced dopamine release: an in-vivo SPECT study. *Psychiatry Res.*, **107**, 173–177.

Westlake, T. M., Howlett, A. C., Bonner, T. I., Matsuda, L. A. and Herkenham, M. (1994). Cannabinoid receptor binding and messenger RNA expression in human brain: an in vitro receptor autoradiography and in situ hybridization histochemistry study of normal aged and Alzheimer's brains. *Neuroscience*, **63**, 637–652.

Wilson, R. I. and Nicoll, R. A. (2001). Endogenous cannabinoids mediate retrograde signalling at hippocampal synapses. *Nature*, **410**, 588–592.

Wilson, R. I. and Nicoll, R. A. (2002). Endocannabinoid signaling in the brain. *Science*, **296**, 678–682.

Yang, H. Y., Karoum, F., Felder, C. *et al.* (1999). GC/MS analysis of anandamide and quantification of N-arachidonoylphosphatidylethanolamides in various brain regions, spinal cord, testis, and spleen of the rat. *J. Neurochem.*, **72**, 1959–1968.

10

Cannabinoid 'model' psychosis, dopamine–cannabinoid interactions and implications for schizophrenia

D. Cyril D'Souza, Hyun-Sang Cho, Edward B. Perry and
John H. Krystal

Yale University School of Medicine, USA

Hypotheses relating to the association between cannabis and psychosis may be divided into two groups. The *exogenous* hypothesis, which has received far greater attention, suggests that the consumption of cannabinoid compounds produces psychotic disorders by mechanisms that are extrinsic to the pathophysiology of naturally occurring psychoses. As discussed elsewhere in this book, converging evidence from epidemiological, genetic, neurochemical, pharmacological and postmortem studies have provided support for an association between 'cannabis and madness' (see Chapters 3, 6, 8 and 9). These data also suggest a second, relatively nascent *endogenous* hypothesis, according to which cannabinoid (CB_1) receptor dysfunction may contribute to the pathophysiology of psychosis and/or schizophrenia, and further, that the putative CB_1 receptor dysfunction may be unrelated to the consumption of cannabinoid compounds.

This chapter addresses the exogenous hypothesis of cannabis consumption and psychosis. First, we review studies from a number of sources, supporting an association between cannabis consumption and the manifestation of psychotic symptoms in humans (the interested reader is referred to Chapters 3 and 5 for a more detailed exposition). We then detail a recent pharmacological study that assessed the effects of exposure to the principal psychoactive constituent of cannabis, Δ^9- tetrahydrocannabinol (Δ^9-THC) in patients with schizophrenia and normal controls. We conclude by suggesting possible mechanisms by which cannabis may induce psychosis and articulate the implications of these findings for a potential endocannabinoid contribution to the pathophysiology of schizophrenia.

Marijuana and Madness: Psychiatry and Neurobiology, ed. D. Castle and R. Murray. Published by Cambridge University Press. © Cambridge University Press 2004.

Review of published studies

Naturalistic epidemiological studies have attempted to establish a causal link between cannabis consumption and psychoses such as schizophrenia (see Chapters 6 and 7). However, these studies have some limitations. First, the large majority of these studies are retrospective. A significant limitation of retrospective studies is the difficulty in establishing whether a drug such as cannabis unmasks a latent psychosis or precipitates a *new* psychosis. Second, since individuals who use or abuse cannabis might also use or abuse other potentially psychotogenic drugs such as amfetamines, phencyclidine and LSD, it is difficult to link causality to any one drug. Third, naturalistic data provide relatively crude information about dose–response relationships. Herbal cannabis preparations contain varying amounts of over 60 cannabinoid compounds (reviewed in Ashton, 2001) which can modulate to varying degrees the principal psychoactive constituent of cannabis, Δ^9-THC. Further, we now know that the Δ^9-THC content of cannabis has changed over the years as a result of cloning high-yield plants and better growing techniques. Thus, it is difficult to estimate a Δ^9-THC dose from the number of 'joints' smoked or from the number of times an individual has used cannabis as the Δ^9-THC content of cannabis varies significantly (Baker *et al.*, 1981). Even if the amount of cannabis a person consumes is estimated accurately, because of factors such as dead space, depth of breath, vital capacity and amount of breath-holding, it is difficult to estimate the amount of Δ^9-THC that actually reaches the cannabinoid receptor (Azorlosa *et al.*, 1992). Fourth, retrospective self-reports of psychosis or psychotic symptoms in such studies may be inaccurate. Finally, schizophrenia is conceptualized as a syndrome of positive, negative and cognitive symptoms but most published reports are restricted to positive symptoms, thus limiting their relevance to the syndrome of schizophrenia.

Controlled laboratory-based pharmacological studies address some of the limitations of naturalistic epidemiological studies. There are several reports of pharmacological studies with cannabis or Δ^9-THC in humans. However, there are few controlled studies that specifically examined the psychotogenic effects of cannabis. In a study of healthy individuals who were administered 20 mg smoked or 40 mg oral Δ^9-THC, Jones (1971) did not observe robust psychotogenic effects, However, a few subjects reported ideas of reference, and delusions that the researcher was using secret (unexplained) tests and hidden recording devices. At doses higher than 20 mg smoked or 40 mg orally, psychotogenic effects, including delusions, loosening of associations and marked illusions, began to emerge. In studies performed under the auspices of the LaGuardia Committee on Marihuana, 12.5% of subjects experienced 'psychotic reactions' with doses of about 30–50 mg (oral) and 8–30 mg (smoked) Δ^9-THC (Mayors Committee On Marijuana, 1944). However, the sample was recruited from a prison population and possibly included individuals with established psychiatric disorders. In a study of medical housestaff studied with unassayed oral doses of cannabis, several subjects reported psychotic symptoms, including dissociation between thoughts and action, delusions of the presence of hidden recorders, hallucinations, fear of being hypnotized, fears of being subjected to electroconvulsive therapy (ECT) and *fears of developing schizophrenia* (Ames, 1958). Isbell *et al.* (1967) reported that Δ^9-THC (300–480 µg/kg orally and 200–250 µg/kg smoked) produced auditory and visual hallucinations in former opiate addicts. At higher doses a 'toxic psychosis' marked by delusions, catatonia and dissociative symptoms was observed. Taken collectively, these data suggest that the psychotogenic effects of cannabis or Δ^9-THC are dose-related; this conclusion is compatible with epidemiological data. However, these studies had several limitations, including the absence of placebo/control, lack of a double-blind, the inclusion of psychiatrically ill individuals and the lack of standardized measures of psychosis.

Leweke *et al.* (1999) reported the effects of synthetic Δ^9-THC in 17 healthy individuals under controlled laboratory conditions (see also Chapter 9). The study included subjects with past experience but no recent consumption of cannabinoids. The overall lifetime consumption of cannabinoids was limited to 10 times to exclude the long-term effects of cannabis use. Subjects with a history of recurrent abuse of illicit drugs other than cannabinoids or other psychiatric disorders were excluded. The primary outcome measure was binocular depth perception described as a model of illusionary perception. Subjects received oral 120 µg dronabinol (Marinol) per kg body weight. The study was not placebo-controlled; subjects were told that they might receive a placebo or active drug but in fact they always received active drug. Subjective reactions ranged from mild euphoria to more pronounced reactions, including feelings of loss of self-control and body distortion suggestive of psychotic-like symptoms. One subject experienced a transient psychotic episode described as 'a paranoid psychotic state with persecutory delusions, delusions of thought insertion, attentional irritability, fear, and – to some extent – verbal aggressive behavior'. These symptoms resolved spontaneously within minutes to hours. Such findings provided evidence suggesting that, at certain doses, Δ^9-THC can induce transient psychotic-like symptoms even in healthy individuals. However, the study was limited by the lack of a placebo control, double-blind and standardized behavioural assessments of psychosis.

The current study

More recently, D'Souza *et al.* (unpublished data) reported on the behavioural and cognitive effects of Δ^9-THC in a double-blind, placebo-controlled study of schizophrenia patients and healthy controls. Only stable, medicated (antipsychotic-treated) patients were included. The study included subjects with past cannabis experience but without lifetime cannabis abuse or dependence. Subjects with a history of current abuse of drugs other than nicotine were excluded. Healthy subjects with a family history of any *Diagnostic and Statistical Manual of Mental Disorders* (*DSM*: American Psychiatric Association, 1994) axis I disorder were excluded. Healthy subjects also underwent a structured clinical interview for *DSM*-IV (healthy) and were excluded if they had any significant psychiatric disorder. Subjects received in random order 5 or 2.5 mg of Δ^9-THC, or vehicle (ethanol 2 ml) by intravenous route over 2 min. Standardized assessments of psychosis (Positive and Negative Syndrome Scale (PANSS): Kay and Opler, 1986), perception (Clinician Administered Dissociative Symptoms Scale: Bremner *et al.*, 1998), and mood states (Visual Analog Scale: 'high', 'calm and relaxed', 'anxious') were assessed before drug administration and several times after. Neuropsychological tests sensitive to frontal and temporal cortical function were also assessed on each test day. These tests included verbal fluency, working memory, vigilance and distractibility, selective attention, immediate recall (learning) and delayed recall. Several safeguards were instituted, as outlined by D'Souza *et al.* (unpublished data).

Data were analysed using Statistical Analysis Software (SAS) Proc Mixed. Random-effects models with a random subject effect were fitted. Separate unstructured variance–covariance matrices were estimated for patients and healthy controls because of different variability over time and between groups. First, complete models with main effects and two-way and three-way interactions of dose, group and time were considered. The final models were obtained using backwards elimination, deleting effects with *P*-values larger than 0.05. Covariates included previous dose (order effects) and baseline scores (for group, interindividual and intraindividual differences). Additional *post-hoc* contrasts were conducted and Bonferroni correction was applied to control overall alpha.

Δ^9-THC transiently increased positive symptoms in medicated schizophrenia patients and induced transient positive symptoms in matched healthy controls (dose, time and dose × time: $P < 0.0001$). These effects were dose-related, occurred 10–20 min after drug administration and resolved by the end of the observation period (4 h). While the magnitude of increases in positive symptoms was modest (mean peak increase 5 points on the positive symptoms subscale of the PANSS), there were differences between schizophrenia patients and controls (group $P < 0.025$; Figs. 10.1 and 10.2).

Using a threshold score (three points) on the measure of positive symptoms to define clinically significant positive symptoms, schizophrenia patients appeared to be more sensitive to the psychotogenic effects of Δ^9-THC (group $P < 0.006$). Whereas 80% of the schizophrenia group had suprathreshold responses to 2.5 mg Δ^9-THC, only 35% of controls had a suprathreshold response. Similarly, whereas

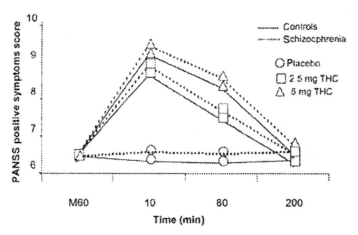

Figure 10.1 Δ⁹-Tetrahydrocannabinol (Δ⁹-THC)-induced positive symptoms of psychosis. PANSS, Positive and Negative Syndrome Scale.

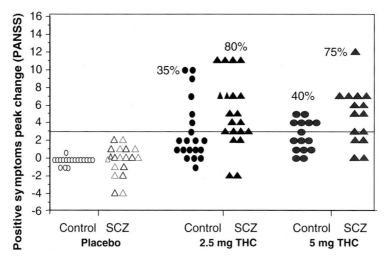

Figure 10.2 Δ⁹-Tetrahydrocannabinol (Δ⁹-THC)-induced positive symptoms of psychosis. PANSS, Positive and Negative Syndrome Scale; SCZ, schizophrenia.

75% of schizophrenia patients had a suprathreshold response to 5 mg Δ⁹-THC, only 40% of controls had a suprathreshold response.

Schizophrenia patients tended to report increases in positive symptoms unique to their individual condition (e.g. patients with predominantly paranoid symptoms reported more paranoid symptoms following Δ⁹-THC administration). Healthy controls reported a full range of schizophrenia-like positive symptoms. In this regard, some of the effects reported by controls were very similar to the positive symptoms associated with schizophrenia. For example, healthy controls reported

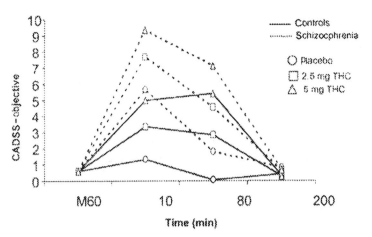

Figure 10.3 Δ⁹-Tetrahydrocannabinol (Δ⁹-THC)-induced perceptual alterations. CADSS, Clinician Administered Dissociative Symptoms Scale.

suspiciousness such as 'I thought you all were *trying to trick me* by changing the rules of the tests to make me fail. I thought you were turning the clock back to confuse me', or 'I thought that this was real . . . I was convinced this wasn't an experiment', or 'I thought you all were giving me THC through the BP [blood pressure] machine and the sheets'. Healthy controls also reported conceptual disorganization such as 'I couldn't keep track of my thoughts . . . they'd suddenly disappear', or 'It seemed as if all the questions were coming to me at once . . . everything was happening in staccato', or 'my thoughts were fragmented . . . the past, present and future all seemed to be happening at once'. Healthy subjects also reported unusual thoughts such as 'I thought you could read my mind, that's why I didn't answer . . . I felt as if my mind was nude', or 'I felt I could see into the future . . . I thought I was God'. These effects reported by carefully screened healthy subjects appear to be remarkably similar to the kinds of psychotic symptoms reported by patients with schizophrenia.

Perceptual alterations were captured by the Clinician Administered Dissociative Symptoms Scale (CADSS; Figs. 10.3 and 10.4). These quasipsychotic perceptual alterations did not meet the threshold of capture on the PANSS. The scale includes a subject-rated component that measures alterations in time perception, external perception, body perception, feelings of unreality and altered memory. There is also a clinician-rated component that measures whether subjects were 'spaced out', looked 'separated or detached', if they said or did 'something bizarre', or if they needed redirection. Δ⁹-THC transiently but robustly induced a full range of subject-rated (dose $P < 0.007$, time $P < 0.0001$, dose × time $P < 0.0013$) and clinician-rated (dose $P < 0.0057$, time $P < 0.0001$, dose × time $P < 0.003$) perceptual alterations in

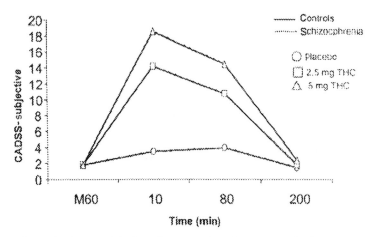

Figure 10.4 Δ^9-Tetrahydrocannabinol (Δ^9-THC)-induced perceptual alterations. CADSS, Clinician Administered Dissociative Symptoms Scale.

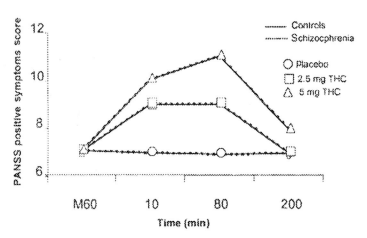

Figure 10.5 Δ^9-Tetrahydrocannabinol (Δ^9-THC)-induced negative symptoms and euphoria. PANSS, Positive and Negative Syndrome Scale.

a dose-related manner. The clinician-rated scores suggested that the schizophrenia group were more vulnerable to these symptoms (group $P < 0.0068$, group × time $P < 0.01$), but these differences were not statistically significant (group × dose × time).

Δ^9-THC also transiently induced schizophrenia-like negative symptoms, including blunted affect and emotional withdrawal (dose, time, dose × time $P < 0.0001$). These effects were small, dose-related and not different between the two groups (Figs. 10.5 and 10.6). These schizophrenia-like negative symptoms may have been confounded by the known cataleptic and sedating effects of Δ^9-THC.

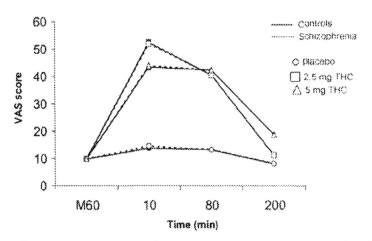

Figure 10.6 Δ^9-Tetrahydrocannabinol (Δ^9-THC)-induced negative symptoms and euphoria, as self-rated on the Visual Analog Scale (VAS).

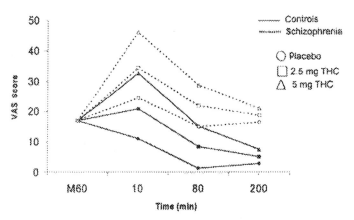

Figure 10.7 Δ^9-Tetrahydrocannabinol (Δ^9-THC)-induced anxiety and 'panic' as assessed on the Visual Analog Scale (VAS).

As expected, both groups of subjects reported dose-related increases in 'high' measured by the Visual Analog Scale (0–100 scale) but there were no differences between the groups. However, inconsistent with the known anxiolytic effects of cannabis, both groups of subjects also reported dose-related anxiogenic effects with Δ^9-THC (group $P < 0.0006$, dose $P < 0.0008$, time $P < 0.0001$, dose $\times$ time $P < 0.02$: Figs. 10.7 and 10.8). This inconsistency between the known anxiolytic effects of cannabis consumption and the anxiogenic effects of Δ^9-THC seen in this study is probably a dose-related issue. Thus, cannabis may have an inverted U-shaped dose–response curve where low doses are anxiolytic but at higher doses anxiogenic effects emerge (see Chapter 3). Furthermore, consistent with reports of

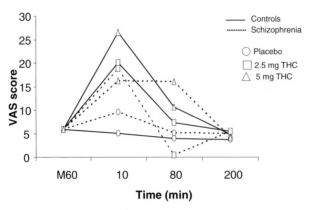

Figure 10.8 Δ⁹-Tetrahydrocannabinol (Δ⁹-THC)-induced anxiety and 'panic' as assessed on the Visual Analog Scale (VAS).

panic attacks induced by consumption of herbal cannabis products, both groups reported feeling 'panicky' following Δ^9-THC administration (dose $P < 0.03$, time $P < 0.002$, group $\times$ dose $\times$ time $P < 0.015$). This is most likely related to the dose of Δ^9-THC, route of administration (intravenous) and rate of administration (2 min).

The effects of Δ^9-THC on a variety of tests of frontal and temporal cortical function were also studied. Learning was assessed using immediate recall of a 12-word list. Subjects were asked to recall the list immediately after presentation and this was repeated three times (learning). Thirty minutes after the initial presentation, subjects were asked to recall the list (delayed recall). Subjects were then provided with cues and asked to recall the list. Finally, the 12-word list along with words not belonging to the original list were presented, and subjects were asked to identify the words that were presented from the original list (recognition recall). For none of these tasks were subjects told whether their recall was correct (Figs. 10.9 and 10.10).

Δ^9-THC disrupted learning (immediate recall) in a dose-related manner in both schizophrenia patients and controls. The group ($P < 0.0001$), dose ($P < 0.0001$), trial ($P < 0.0001$), dose $\times$ trial ($P < 0.04$), group $\times$ trial (NS) and group $\times$ dose $\times$ trial ($P < 0.05$) were statistically significant. The dose-related effects of Δ^9-THC on learning and immediate recall were particularly robust in healthy controls. In schizophrenia patients there were small differences between the 2.5 and 5 mg Δ^9-THC conditions, most likely related to a 'floor' effect. Δ^9-THC 5 mg appeared to disrupt learning and recall in the subjects with schizophrenia. Further, 5 mg Δ^9-THC disrupted learning and recall in healthy controls down to the same level as the performance of schizophrenia patients under the placebo (vehicle) condition. Δ^9-THC also disrupted delayed recall in a dose-dependent manner in both groups (group $P < 0.0001$, dose $P < 0.0001$). Despite being provided with cues

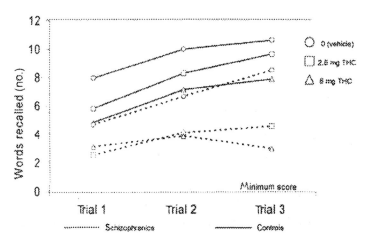

Figure 10.9 Δ^9-Tetrahydrocannabinol (Δ^9-THC)-impaired immediate recall (learning) and delayed recall using the Hopkins Verbal Learning Test.

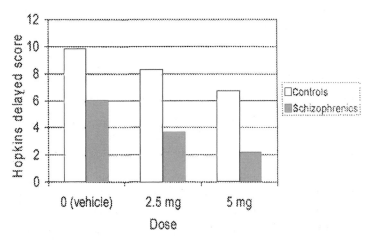

Figure 10.10 Δ^9-Tetrahydrocannabinol (Δ^9-THC)-impaired immediate recall (learning) and delayed recall.

(cued recall), both groups had difficulties recalling the list under the influence of Δ^9-THC (group $P < 0.0001$, dose $P < 0.0002$). Further, Δ^9-THC disrupted recognition of the word list (recognition recall) in a dose-dependent manner in both groups (group $P < 0.02$, dose $P < 0.002$). Finally, Δ^9-THC also increased the number of false-positive responses during recall in both groups and in a dose-dependent manner (dose $P < 0.0003$). These data illustrate the robust amnestic effects of Δ^9-THC on learning and memory in both healthy individuals and in schizophrenia patients, who already have such deficits as a consequence of their disorder (Figs. 10.11 and 10.12). The effects of Δ^9-THC in healthy individuals are consistent

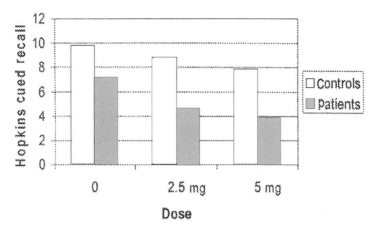

Figure 10.11 Δ^9-Tetrahydrocannabinol (Δ^9-THC)-impaired cued and recognition recall using the Hopkins Verbal Learning Test.

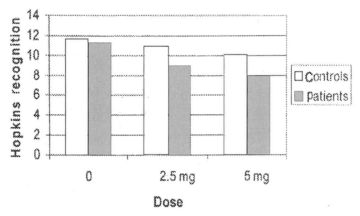

Figure 10.12 Δ^9-Tetrahydrocannabinol (Δ^9-THC)-impaired cued and recognition recall using the Hopkins Verbal Learning Test.

with other studies in humans showing that cannabis acutely impairs performance on short-term memory tasks (Miller and Branconnier, 1983; Miller, 1984; Chait and Pierri, 1992; and see Chapter 3). The disruption in recall appears to be related to difficulties in both encoding and retrieval.

In healthy individuals, Δ^9-THC did not impair performance on verbal fluency, a task sensitive to frontal cortical performance (Fig. 10.13). However, there were group differences ($P < 0.002$) and a suggestion of dose-related impairments in the schizophrenic patients. Δ^9-THC did not increase the number of perseverations on this task in healthy individuals, but there were group differences ($P < 0.03$) and a suggestion of dose-related impairments in those with schizophrenia.

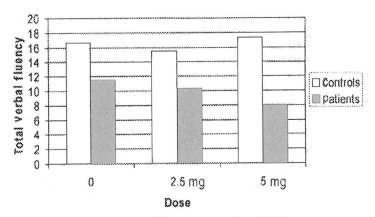

Figure 10.13 Δ^9-Tetrahydrocannabinol (Δ^9-THC)-impaired verbal fluency.

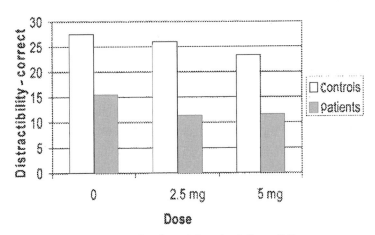

Figure 10.14 Δ^9-Tetrahydrocannabinol (Δ^9-THC)-impaired distractibility.

Distractibility and vigilance to visual stimuli were measured using a continuous performance task in which subjects attended to numbers presented sequentially on a screen (Fig. 10.14). The subject pushed a button to signal when a '9' was preceded by a '1'. The distractibility task was identical to the vigilance task with the exception that numbers were presented sequentially in three contiguous columns. Subjects had to attend to the middle column and ignore the numbers presented in the outer two columns. Δ^9-THC reduced the number of correct responses in both groups (dose $P < 0.005$, group $P < 0.0001$). Further, Δ^9-THC increased the tendency for omissions (dose $P < 0.005$, group $P < 0.0001$) but had no significant effect on the number of commissions (group < 0.002, dose $P = $ NS). The distractibility task places greater demands on attention than the vigilance task.

The effects of participation in this study on the course of schizophrenia (number of hospitalizations, number of emergency room visits, number of admissions to crisis programmes or day programmes, changes in medication treatment, PANSS scores) and cannabis consumption were studied 1, 3 and 6 months after study participation. There was no evidence that participation in this study was associated with a negative impact on the course of schizophrenia or cannabis consumption. Similarly, healthy subjects were tracked 1, 3 and 6 months after study participation to detect any effects on cannabis consumption or the emergence of psychiatric problems. There was no evidence that study participation had any negative impact on cannabis consumption or development of psychiatric problems.

In summary, data from this controlled pharmacological laboratory paradigm demonstrate that, at certain doses, Δ^9-THC can induce a spectrum of schizophrenia-like symptoms in carefully selected healthy individuals without any obvious predisposition for schizophrenia. The transient schizophrenia-like symptoms observed in healthy individuals included positive symptoms, negative symptoms and cognitive deficits. These symptoms occurred without any alteration in sensorium, dispelling the notion of a 'toxic' delirium/psychosis that has been reported to occur with cannabis consumption. However, not all healthy subjects experienced psychotic-like symptoms, provoking interest in what factors might predispose individuals to the psychotogenic effects of Δ^9-THC.

Δ^9-THC also induced transient increases in positive symptoms, negative symptoms and cognitive deficits in clinically stable schizophrenic patients treated with a dopamine D2 receptor antagonist. Schizophrenia patients appeared to be more sensitive to some, though not all, effects of Δ^9-THC; they appeared particularly sensitive to positive symptoms and some cognitive deficits. These differences occurred despite the fact that the schizophrenia subjects were in a stable phase of their illness and were receiving treatment with dopamine D2 receptor antagonists. While speculative, it is tempting to hypothesize that the vulnerability to the effects of Δ^9-THC may have been greater if the patients had been in an unstable phase of their illness, or were unmedicated. However, ethical considerations precluded study of schizophrenic patients in either an unmedicated state or during an unstable phase of their illness. At the doses used, there were no data from the current study to support the 'self-medication' hypothesis that has often been cited as a reason why schizophrenia patients use cannabis (see Chapter 11).

Some important issues need to be considered in interpreting and in generalizing these findings. The doses of Δ^9-THC employed were higher than those typically consumed in herbal cannabis preparations. The rate of administration (over 2 min) was significantly faster than the manner in which people typically consume cannabis. The route of administration (intravenous) is not how cannabis is usually taken. These factors may have resulted in faster delivery and higher doses of

Δ^9-THC than is typically smoked by recreational users. Finally, while only Δ^9-THC was administered in this study, the effects of cannabis are a composite of several (up to 40) cannabis compounds that may have synergistic and antagonistic effects. The clinical contribution of cannabidiol and other cannabinoids, terpenoids and flavonoids to clinical cannabis effects has been proposed as an 'entourage effect' (Mechoulam and Ben-Shabat, 1999; reviewed in detail in McPartland and Russo, 2001). For example, cannabidiol, a major component of cannabis, is reported to have anxiolytic effects (Zuardi *et al.*, 1982) and also antipsychotic-like effects (Zuardi *et al.*, 1995). Thus, cannabidiol, which was not administered in this study, may offset the psychotogenic and anxiogenic effects of Δ^9-THC. Briefly summarized, cannabidiol has antianxiety effects (Zuardi *et al.*, 1982), antipsychotic benefits (Zuardi *et al.*, 1995), modulates the metabolism of THC by blocking its conversion to the more psychoactive 11-hydroxy-THC (Bornheim and Grillo, 1998), prevents glutamate excitotoxicity and serves as a powerful antioxidant (Hampson *et al.*, 2000). These factors raise questions about the social relevance and generalizibility of the study's findings. However, these data may be consistent with the observation that most studies associating cannabis and psychosis/schizophrenia suggest that negative consequences occur with heavy proloned cannabis use (see Chapters 3–5).

A cannabinoid 'model' psychosis

The observation that Δ^9-THC induced transient schizophrenia-like symptoms in healthy individuals provides preliminary support for a laboratory-based cannabinoid 'model' psychosis. This adds to the small list of other drugs, including dopaminergic stimulants (amfetamine), serotonergic agents (LSD and psylocibin) and glutamatergic antagonists (ketamine) that have been studied as laboratory-based models of endogenous psychotic disorders. These laboratory-based 'model psychoses' have important potential uses in the study of the pathophysiology and treatment of schizophrenia and related psychoses. These paradigms can also be used to study potential pharmacotherapies.

There are, however, some limitations to laboratory-based paradigms of schizophrenia. First, schizophrenia or perhaps certain types of schizophrenia have a neurodevelopmental basis. Further, schizophrenia has a course that evolves over time, and the phenomenology of schizophrenia also evolves over time. Thus, positive symptoms may be more prominent early in the course of the disorder while negative symptoms and cognitive decline may be more prominent with progression of the disorder. Further, certain symptoms may be episodic in nature and only present during decompensation. As a result, some model psychoses may apply to specific subgroups of symptoms or specific phases of the disorder. Second, schizophrenia is a disorder of abnormal brain morphology. Discrepancies between the impact of structural abnormalities in schizophrenic brain and drug effects in a healthy brain could reflect the incomplete overlap of associated behaviours or symptoms. Third, schizophrenia is a heterogeneous disorder and hence a specific pharmacological model may be relevant to some, though not all, subtypes. Finally, the symptoms of schizophrenia are not exclusive to this disorder and hence the effects of a drug in a model psychosis may be relevant to psychosis in general and not limited to the psychosis of schizophrenia. Nevertheless, the effects of Δ^9-THC in this laboratory paradigm may provide a laboratory-based 'model' to study the contributions of CB_1 receptor function to psychotic disorders.

What mechanisms might underlie the capacity of Δ^9-THC to induce psychosis? The endocannabinoid system has been shown to modulate neurotransmitter systems including dopaminergic, glutamatergic, GABAergic and cholinergic systems. Thus, the obvious mechanisms to consider would be those receptor systems that have already been implicated in the pathophysiology of psychotic disorders, namely dopamine, glutamate and γ-aminobutyric acid (GABA).

Behavioural, biochemical and electrophysiological data demonstrate the involvement of dopaminergic systems in some of the actions of cannabinoids. Cannabinoids increase the activity and expression of tyrosine hydroxylase (Bonnin *et al.*, 1996; Hernandez *et al.*, 1997). Consistent with this, Bloom (1982) and Maitre *et al.* (1970) have demonstrated that THC increases the synthesis of dopamine. THC has also been shown to inhibit dopamine uptake (Banerjee *et al.*, 1975; Johnson *et al.*, 1976; Hershkowitz *et al.*, 1977), and Poddar and Dewey (1980) demonstrated that THC inhibits the dopamine transporter.

In common with other euphoriant drugs, Δ^9-THC has been shown to enhance neuronal firing of mesolimbic dopamine projections from the ventral tegmental area (VTA) to nucleus accumbens (NAc) (French *et al.*, 1997; Gessa *et al.*, 1998; Wu and French, 2000). Δ^9-THC has also been shown to increase the release of dopamine in the shell of the NAc (Chen *et al.*, 1990; 1991; Tanda *et al.*, 1997), an effect that is also seen with heroin, cocaine, *d*-amfetamine and nicotine. The release of dopamine in the NAc following systemic administration of Δ^9-THC may result from local actions at or near the dopamine terminal projections in the NAc (Chen *et al.*, 1993). Consistent with electrophysiological studies, CB_1 receptor agonists have been shown to induce immediate early gene c-*fos*, a marker of increased neuronal excitation, in the NAc (Miyamoto *et al.*, 1996), and mesocorticolimbic dopaminergic cells within VTA (Patel and Hillard, 2003). It is of note that the effects of Δ^9-THC on *fos* expression are blocked by dopamine antagonists (Miyamoto *et al.*, 1996). These data suggest that dopamine may play a role in cannabinoid psychomimetic actions. Szabo *et al.* (2002) suggest that CB_1 receptor activation inhibits GABAergic neurotransmission in the VTA by a presynaptic mechanism. Depression of the GABAergic inhibitory effect on dopaminergic neurons would increase their firing rate in vivo, with a resultant increase in dopamine in the NAc, a principal projection of dopaminergic VTA neurons. The effect of cannabinoids on increasing mesolimbic dopaminergic activity may provide one explanation for the positive psychotic symptoms induced by Δ^9-THC. If so, then dopamine D2 receptor antagonists should be effective in treating the positive psychotic symptoms induced by Δ^9-THC.

In the pharmacological study discussed above, Δ^9-THC increased positive symptoms in schizophrenia patients despite long-term treatment with dopamine D2 receptor antagonists. In contrast, the dopamine D2 receptor antagonists olanzapine and haloperidol appear to be equally effective in the treatment of cannabis-induced psychotic disorder (Berk et al., 1998). The effects of haloperidol (0.05 mg/kg) pretreatment on Δ^9-THC (2.5 mg IV) are being studied in an ongoing protocol at our centre. Healthy subjects carefully screened for any psychiatric disorder completed 2 days of testing, during which they received haloperidol or placebo followed 90 min later by placebo, and 180 min later by active Δ^9-THC. Preliminary data suggest that, consistent with our above-mentioned work, Δ^9-THC induced a full spectrum of schizophrenia-like symptoms in healthy individuals (see also Chapter 5). However, haloperidol pretreatment (3.5 mg in a 70-kg individual) did not attenuate Δ^9-THC-induced positive psychotic symptoms. These preliminary data suggest that dopaminergic systems may not contribute significantly to the pathophysiology of cannabinoid-induced psychosis. Further, haloperidol pretreatment does not appear to have any effects on the euphoric or cognitive effects of Δ^9-THC. Finally, haloperidol and Δ^9-THC may interact to produce more extrapyramidal, sedating and anxiogenic effects. Pretreatment of rats with Δ^9-THC has been shown to potentiate the hypokinesia produced by haloperidol. Thus, at doses which do not produce catalepsy when administered alone, cannabinoids have been shown to enhance the catalepsy produced by dopamine D1 and D2 receptor antagonists (Anderson et al., 1996), and, conversely, D1 and D2 receptors attenuate the motor dysfunction caused by cannabinoids in rats (Meschler et al., 2000; Fig. 10.15).

In contrast to the evidence suggesting that cannabinoids facilitate dopaminergic neurotransmission, there is evidence that cannabinoids inhibit dopaminergic neurotransmission. For example, cannabinoids reduce motor activity, induce catalepsy (Rodriguez de Fonseca et al., 1998) and inhibit amphetamine- and cocaine-induced motor activity (Ferrari et al., 1999; Gorriti et al., 1999), similar to neuroleptics. The activation of D2 receptors enhances anandamide release in the striatum (Giuffrida et al., 1999) and the antagonism of CB_1 receptors potentiates the effects of dopamine D2 agonists (Giuffrida et al., 1999; Masserano et al., 1999). This behavioural and biochemical evidence supports a reciprocal interaction between

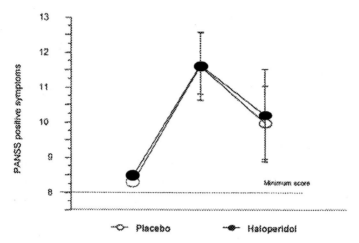

Figure 10.15 Dopamine antagonists do not antagonize Δ⁹-Tetrahydrocannabinol-induced psychosis. PANSS, Positive and Negative Syndrome Scale.

endogenous cannabinoids and dopamine transmission in the striatum, suggesting that the endocannabinoid system may act as an inhibitory feedback mechanism to 'brake' dopamine-induced facilitation of motor activity (Giuffrida *et al.*, 1999; Meschler *et al.*, 2000).

The effects of cannabinoids on dopaminergic neurotransmission in the prefrontal cortex (PFC) may explain some of the cognitive symptoms induced by these compounds. The PFC is implicated in several cognitive processes, including working memory and executive function, and is of further interest as the cognitive disorganization and working-memory deficits of schizophrenia are associated with the dorsolateral PFC (Goldman-Rakic, 1987; Perlstein *et al.*, 2001). Stimulation of cannabinoid CB_1 receptors stimulates the activity of mesoprefrontal dopaminergic transmission in terms of both firing rate and burst firing (Diana *et al.*, 1998). An inverted U-shape between dopaminergic tone and cognitive performance has been proposed whereby reduced or enhanced dopaminergic activity would interfere with optimal working memory performance (Dolan *et al.*, 1995). Given that supranormal stimulation of D1 dopamine receptors in the PFC has been shown to impair working memory, the deficits in working memory produced by cannabinoids may be related to their capacity to enhance dopaminergic neurotransmission in the PFC. Further, the activity of pyramidal neurons, the major efferents of the PFC, is regulated by complex interactions between dopaminergic and GABAergic neurons arising from the VTA, glutamatergic cortical and hippocampal efferents and an extensive network of GABAergic interneurons. The mesocortical dopamine system exerts significant inhibitory control on the activity of PFC pyramidal neurons (Pirot *et al.*, 1992; Gioanni *et al.*, 1998) by releasing GABA from GABAergic interneurons in the PFC (Gellman and Aghajanian, 1993; Grobin and Deutch, 1998). The PFC has a high density of CB_1 receptors and cannabinoids have been demonstrated to modulate neuronal inputs impinging on PFC neurons. By suppressing GABAergic and dopaminergic inhibitory neurotransmission, cannabinoids might lead to non-specific activation of the PFC which in turn may disrupt normal signal processing and result in poor integration of transcortical inputs (Pistis *et al.*, 2001). Systemically administered cannabinoids may also enhance excitatory inputs to the PFC arising from other brain regions, such as the hippocampus or other cortical areas, disrupting cognitive processes. Finally, cannabinoids have been shown to influence glutamatergic synaptic transmission and plasticity in the PFC, resulting in favouring long-term depression at the expense of long-term potentiation (Auclair *et al.*, 2000).

Finally, some of the cognitive effects of cannabinoids are mediated by actions of CB_1 receptors in the hippocampus. CB_1 receptors are capable of modulating both inhibitory and excitatory neurotransmitter release in the hippocampus and thereby effecting synaptic plasticity. CB_1 receptors are expressed at especially high density in the dentate gyrus, CA1, and CA3 regions of the hippocampus (Herkenham *et al.*, 1990; 1991; Matsuda *et al.*, 1990; Tsou *et al.*, 1998). Long-term potentiation (LTP) and long-term depression (LTD) of CA3–CA1 synaptic transmission in the hippocampus are two in vitro models for learning and memory. CB_1 receptor activation blocks LTP in the CA1 region (Nowicky *et al.*, 1987; Collins *et al.*, 1994; 1995; Terranova *et al.*, 1995; Misner and Sullivan, 1999) and has also been shown to inhibit hippocampal LTD in the CA1 region (Misner and Sullivan, 1999). Hippocampal LTP and LTD require depolarization of the postsynaptic membrane to relieve magnesium blockade of *N*-methyl-*D*-aspartate (NMDA) receptors and allow entry of calcium (Nicoll and Malenka, 1995). Cannabinoid receptors are present on the presynaptic terminals of glutamatergic synapses in the hippocampus (Pettit *et al.*, 1998) and their activation is associated with a reduction of glutamate release (Piomelli *et al.*, 2000). Cannabinoids also reduce glutamate release through a G protein-mediated inhibition of the calcium channels responsible for neurotransmitter release (Sullivan, 1999; Wilson and Nicoll, 2001). Cannabinoids, by reducing neurotransmitter release, could impair long-term synaptic plasticity in the hippocampus by failing to depolarize the postsynaptic CA1 membrane to a level that relieves magnesium block.

CB_1 cannabinoid receptors are primarily located on GABAergic interneurons in hippocampus (Marsicano and Lutz, 1999; Tsou *et al.*, 1999). Interneurons are necessary for synchronization of the large principal cell populations underlying memory consolidation and for the precise association of external inputs. Cannabinoids reduce GABA release from hippocampal interneurons (Sullivan, 1999) and this might result in an increase in excitability of hippocampal pyramidal cells.

GABAergic interneurons are believed to orchestrate fast synchronous oscillations in the gamma range. This plays a role in synchronizing pyramidal cell activity (Hoffman and Lupica, 2000). Gamma oscillations are synchronized over long distances in the brain and are hypothesized to bind together sensory perceptions and to play a role in cognition (reviewed in Wilson and Nicoll, 2002). CB$_1$ agonists decrease the power of such oscillations in hippocampal slices (Hájos *et al.*, 2000) and may thus disrupt the synchronous activity of pyramidal cells, thereby interfering with memory consolidation and internal representations in humans. These mechanisms may underlie the amnestic and other cognitive effects of cannabinoids but clearly warrant further study.

Conclusions

In conclusion, pharmacological studies address some of the limitations of other approaches that attempted to clarify the association between cannabis and 'madness'. Controlled pharmacological studies demonstrate that Δ^9-THC can induce a full range of *transient* schizophrenia-like positive psychotic symptoms, negative symptoms and cognitive deficits, amongst other behavioural effects. Taken together with other supporting data from epidemiological, neurochemical, genetic, electrophysiological and postmortem approaches, these data from pharmacological studies suggest that cannabinoid receptor dysfunction may contribute to the pathophysiology of schizophrenia. Thus, there is tentative support for both the exogenous and endogenous hypotheses.

While preclinical data suggest that dopaminergic systems may play an important role in the psychotogenic effects of cannabinoids, preliminary clinical data do not support this. The mechanisms underlying the capacity of cannabinoids to induce psychosis are unclear and warrant further study. Understanding the mechanisms may in addition provide novel therapeutic strategies for the treatment of psychoses.

REFERENCES

American Psychiatric Association (1994). *Diagnostic and Statistical Manual of Mental Disorders,* 4th edn. Washington, DC: American Psychiatric Association.

Ames, F. (1958). A clinical and metabolic study of acute intoxication with *Cannabis sativa* and its role in model psychoses. *J. Mental Sci.,* **104**, 972–999.

Anderson, J. J., Kask, A. M. and Chase, T. N. (1996). Effects of cannabinoid receptor stimulation and blockade on catalepsy produced by dopamine receptor antagonists. *Eur. J. Pharmacol.,* **295**, 163–168.

Ashton, C. H. (2001). Pharmacology and effects of cannabis: a brief review. *Br. J. Psychiatry,* **179**, 270–271.

Auclair, N., Otani, S., Soubrie, P. and Crepel. F. (2000). Cannabinoids modulate synaptic strength and plasticity at glutamatergic synapses of rat prefrontal cortex pyramidal neurons. *J. Neurophysiol.*, **83**, 3287–3293.

Azorlosa, J. L., Heishman, S. J., Stitzer, M. L. and Mahaffey, J. M. (1992). Marijuana smoking: effect of varying delta 9-tetrahydrocannabinolcontent and number of puffs. *J. Pharmacol. Exp. Ther.*, **261**, 114–122.

Baker, P. B., Taylor, B. J. and Gough, T. A. (1981). The tetrahydrocannabinol and tetrahydro-cannabinolic acid content of cannabis products. *J. Pharm. Pharmacol.*, **33**, 369–372.

Banerjee, S. P., Snyder, S. H. and Mechoulam, R. (1975). Cannabinoids: influence on neurotrans-mitter uptake in rat brain. *J. Pharmacol. Exp. Ther.*, **194**, 74–81.

Berk, M., Brook, S. and Trandafir, A. I. (1998). A comparison of olanzapine with haloperi-dol in cannabis-induced psychotic: a double-blind randomized controlled trial. *Int. Clin. Psychopharmacol.*, **14**, 177–180.

Bloom, A. S. (1982). Effect of delta-9-tetrahydrocannabinol on the synthesis of dopamine and norepinephrine in mouse brain synaptosomes. *J. Pharmacol. Exp. Ther.*, **221**, 97–103.

Bonnin, A., de-Miguel, R., Castro, J. G., Raos, J. A. and Fernadez-Ruiz, J. J. (1996). Effects of perinatal exposure to delta-9-THC on the fetal and early postnatal development of tyrosine hydroxylase-containing neurons in rat brain. *J. Mol. Neurosci.*, **7**, 291–308.

Bornheim, L. M. and Grillo, M. P. (1998). Characterization of cytochrome P450 3A inactivation by cannabidiol: possible involvement of cannabidiol-hydroxyquinone as a P450 inactivator. *Chem. Res. Toxicol.*, **11**, 1209–1216.

Bremner, J. D., Krystal, J. H., Putnam, F. W. *et al.* (1998). Measurement of dissociative states with the Clinician-Administered Dissociative States Scale (CADSS). *J. Trauma Stress* **11**, 125–136.

Chait, L. D. and Perry, J. L. (1992). Factors influencing self-administration of, and subjective response to, placebo marijuana, *Behav. Pharmacol.*, **3**, 545–552.

Chen, J., Paredes, W., Lowinson, J. H. and Gardner, E. L. (1990). Delta-9-tetrahydrocannabinol enhances presynaptic dopamine efflux in the medial prefrontal cortex. *Eur. J. Pharmacol.*, **190**, 259–262.

Chen, J., Paredes, W., Lowinson, J. H. and Gardner, E. L. (1991). Strain specific facilitation of dopamine efflux by delta-9-tetrahydrocannabinol in the nucleus accumbens of the rats: an in vivo microdialysis study. *Neurosci. Lett.*, **129**, 136–140.

Chen, J., Marmur, R., Pulles, A., Paredes, W. and Gardner, E. L. (1993). Ventral tegmental microinjection of delta 9-tetrahydrocannabinol enhances ventral tegmental somatoden-dritic dopamine levels but not forebrain dopamine levels: evidence for local neural action by marijuana's psychoactive ingredient. *Brain Res.*, **621**, 65–70.

Collins, D. R., Pertwee, R. G. and Davies, S. N. (1994). The action of synthetic cannabinoids on the induction of long-term potentiation in the rat hippocampal slice. *Eur. J. Pharmacol.*, **259**, R7–R8.

Collins, D. R., Pertwee, R. G. and Davies, S. N. (1995). Prevention by the cannabinoid antago-nist, SR141716A, of cannabinoid-mediated blockade of long-term potentiation in the rat hippocampal slice. *Br. J. Pharmacol.*, **115**, 869–870.

Diana, M., Melis, M. and Gessa, G. L. (1998). Increase in meso-prefrontal dopaminergic activity after stimulation of CB1 receptors by cannabinoids, *Eur. J. Neurosci.*, **10**, 2825–2830.

Dolan, R. J., Fletcher, P., Frith, C. D. *et al.* (1995). Dopaminergic modulation of impaired cognitive activation in the anterior cingulate cortex in schizophrenia. *Nature*, **378**, 180–182.

Ferrari, F., Ottani, A. and Giuliani, D. (1999). Influence of the cannabinoid agonist HU 210 on cocaine- and CQP 201-403-induced behavioural effects in rat. *Life Sci.*, **65**, 823–831.

French, E. D., Dillon, K. and Wu, X. (1997). Cannabinoids excite dopamine neurons in the ventral tegmentum and substantia nigra. *Neuroreport*, **8**, 649–652.

Gellman, R. L. and Aghajanian, G. K. (1993). Pyramidal cells in piriform cortex receive a convergence of inputs from monoamine activated GABAergic interneurons. *Brain Res.*, **600**, 63–73.

Gessa, G. L., Melis, M., Muntoni, A. L. and Diana, M. (1998). Cannabinoids activate mesolimbic dopamine neurons by an action on cannabinoid CB1 receptors. *Eur. J. Pharmacol.*, **341**, 39–44.

Gioanni, Y., Thierry, A. M., Glowinski, J. and Tassin, J. P. (1998). Alpha$_1$-adrenergic, D1, and D2 receptors interactions in the prefrontal cortex: implication for modality of action of different types of neuroleptics. *Synapse*, **30**, 362–370.

Giuffrida, A., Parsons, L. H., Kerr, T. M. *et al.* (1999). Dopamine activation of endogenous cannabinoid signaling in dorsal striatum. *Nature Neurosci.*, **2**, 358–363.

Goldman-Rakic, P. S. (1987). The circuitry of primate prefrontal cortex and the regulation of behavior by representational memory. In *Handbook of Physiology: The Nervous System*, ed. V. M. Mountcastle, pp. 373–417. Bethesda, MD: American Physiological Society.

Gorriti, M. A., Rodriguez de Fonseca, F., Navarro, M. and Palomo, T. (1999) Chronic (–)-delta9-tetrahydrocannabinol treatment induces sensitization to the psychomotor effects of amphetamine in rats. *Eur. J. Pharmacol.*, **365**, 33–42.

Grobin, A. C. and Deutch, A. Y. (1998). Dopaminergic regulation of extracellular gamma-aminobutyric acid levels in the prefrontal cortex. *J. Pharmacol. Exp. Ther.*, **285**, 350–357.

Hájos, N., Katona, I., Naiem, S. S. *et al.* (2000). Cannabinoids inhibit hippocampal GABAergic transmission and network oscillations. *Eur. J. Neurosci.*, **12**, 3239–3249.

Hampson, A. J., Grimaldi, M., Lolic, M. *et al.* (2000). Neuroprotective antioxidants from marijuana, *Ann. NY Acad. Sci.*, **899**, 274–282.

Herkenham, M., Lynn, A. B., Little, M. D. *et al.* (1990). Cannabinoid receptor localization in brain. *Proc. Natl Acad. Sci.*, **87**, 1932–1936.

Herkenham, M., Lynn, A. B., Johnson, M. R. *et al.* (1991). Characterization and localization of cannabinoid receptors in rat brain: a quantitative in vitro autoradiographic study. *J. Neurosci.*, **11**, 563–583.

Hernandez, M. L., Garcia-Gil, L., Berrendro, F., Ramos, J. A. and Fernandez-Ruiz, J. J. (1997). δ-9-tetrahydrocannabinol increases the activity of tyrosine hydroxylase in cultured fetal mesencephalic neurons. *J. Mol. Neurosci.*, **8**, 83–91.

Hershkowitz, M., Goldman, R. and Raz, A. (1977). Effect of cannabinoids on neurotransmitter uptake. ATPase activity and morphology of mouse brain synaptosomes. *Biochem. Pharmacol.*, **26**, 1327–1331.

Hoffman, A. F. and Lupica, C. R. (2000). Mechanisms of cannabinoid inhibition of GABA(A) synaptic transmission in the hippocampus. *J. Neurosci.*, **20**, 2470–2479.

Isbell, H., Gorodetsky, C. W., Jasinski, D. R. *et al.* (1967). Effects of delta-9-transhydrocannabinol in man. *Psychopharmacologia*, **11**, 184–188.

Johnson, K. M., Ho, B. T. and Dewey, W. L. (1976). Effects of delta9-tetrahydrocannabinol on neurotransmitter accumulation and release mechanisms in rat forebrain synaptosomes. *Life Sci.*, **19**, 347–356.

Jones, R. T. (1971). Tetrahydrocannabinol and the marijuana-induced social "high," or the effects of the mind on marijuana. *Ann. NY Acad. Sci.*, **191**, 155–165.

Kay, S. R. and Opler, L. A. (1986). *Positive and Negative Symptoms Scale (PANSS) Rating Manual.* Bronx, New York: Albert Einstein College of Medicine, Department of Psychiatry.

Leweke, F. M., Schneider, U., Thies, M., Munte, T. F. and Emrich, H. M. (1999). Effects of synthetic delta-9-tetrahydrocannabinol on binocular depth inversion of natural and artificial objects in man. *Psychopharmacologia*, **142**, 230–235.

Maitre, L., Staehelin, M. and Bein, H. J. (1970). Effect of an extract of cannabis and of some cannabinols on catecholamine metabolism in rat brain and heart. *Agents Actions*, **1**, 136–143.

Marsicano, G. and Lutz, B. (1999). Expression of the cannabinoid receptor CB1 in distinct neuronal subpopulations in the adult mouse forebrain. *Eur. J. Neurosci.* **11**, 4213–4225.

Masserano, J. M., Karoum, F. and Wyatt, R. J. (1999). SR 141716A, a CB1 cannabinoid receptor antagonist, potentiates the locomotor stimulant effects of amphetamine and apomorphine. *Behav. Pharmacol.*, **10**, 429–432.

Matsuda, L. A., Lolait, S. J., Brownstein, M. J., Young, A. C. and Bonner, T. I. (1990). Structure of a cannabinoid receptor and functional expression of the cloned cDNA. *Nature*, **346**, 561–564.

Mayor's Committee On Marijuana (1944). *The Marijuana Problem in the City of New York.* Lancaster, PA: Jacques Catell Press.

McPartland, J. M. and Russo, E. B. (2001). Cannabis and cannabis extracts: greater than the sum of their parts? *J. Cannabis Ther.*, **1**, 103–132.

Mechoulam, R. and Ben-Shabat, S. (1999). From gan-zi-gun-nu to anandamide and 2-arachidonoylglycerol: the ongoing story of cannabis. *Nature Prod. Rep.*, **16**, 131–143.

Meschler, J. P., Conley, T. J. and Howlett, A. C. (2000). Cannabinoid and dopamine interaction in rodent brain: effects on locomotor activity. *Pharmacol. Biochem. Behav.*, **67**, 567–573.

Miller, L. L. (1984). Marijuana: acute effects on human memory. In *The Cannabinoids: Chemical, Pharmacological and Therapeutic Aspects*, ed. S. Agurell, W. L. Dewey and R. E. Willette, pp. 21–46. New York, NY: Academic Press.

Miller, L. and Branconnier, R. J. (1983). Cannabis: effects on memory and the cholinergic limbic system. *Psychol. Bull.*, **99**, 441–456.

Misner, D. L. and Sullivan, J. M. (1999). Mechanism of cannabinoid effects on long-term potentiation and depression in hippocampal CA1 neurons. *J. Neurosci.*, **19**, 6795–6805.

Miyamoto, A., Yamamoto, T., Ohno, M. *et al.* (1996). Roles of dopamine D1 receptors in delta 9-tetrahydrocannabinol-induced expression of Fos protein in the rat brain. *Brain Res.*, **710**, 234–240.

Nicoll, R. A. and Malenka, R. C. (1995). Contrasting properties of two forms of long-term potentiation in the hippocampus. *Nature*, **377**, 115–118.

Nowicky, A. V., Teyler, T. J. and Vardaris, R. M. (1987). The modulation of long-term potentiation by delta-9-tetrahydrocannabinol in the rat hippocampus, in vitro. *Brain Res. Bull.*, **19**, 663–672.

Patel, S. and Hillard, C. J. (2003). Cannabinoid-induced Fos expression within A10 dopaminergic neurons. Cannabinoid CB(1) receptor agonists produce cerebellar dysfunction in mice. *J. Pharmacol. Exp. Ther.*, **297**, 629–637.

Perlstein, W. M., Carter, C. S., Noll, D. C. and Cohen, J. D. (2001). Relation of prefrontal cortex dysfunction to working memory and symptoms in schizophrenia. *Am. J. Psychiatry*, **158**, 1105–1113.

Pettit, D. A., Harrison, M. P., Olson, J. M., Spencer, R. F. and Cabral, G. A. (1998). Immuno-histochemical localization of the neural cannabinoid receptor in rat brain. *J. Neurosci. Res.*, **51**, 391–402.

Piomelli, D., Giuffrida, A., Calignano, A. and Rodriguez de Fonseca, F. (2000). The endocannabi-noid system as a target for therapeutic drugs. *Trends Pharmacol. Sci.*, **21**, 218–224.

Pirot, S., Godbout, R., Mantz, J. *et al.* (1992). Inhibitory effects of ventral tegmental area stim-ulation on the activity of prefrontal cortical neurons: evidence for the involvement of both dopaminergic and GABAergic components. *Neuroscience*, **49**, 857–865.

Pistis, M., Porcu, G., Melis, M., Diana, M. and Gessa, G. L. (2001). Effects of cannabinoids on prefrontal neuronal responses to ventral tegmental area stimulation. *Eur. J. Neurosci.*, **14**, 96–102.

Poddar, M. K. and Dewey, W. L. (1980). Effects of cannabinoids of catecholamine uptake and release in hypothalmic and striatal synaptosomes. *J. Pharmacol. Exp. Ther.*, **214**, 63–67.

Rodriguez de Fonseca, F., Del Arco, I., Martin-Calderon, J. L., Gorriti, M. A. and Navarro, M. (1998). Role of the endogenous cannabinoid system in the regulation of motor activity. *Neurobiol. Dis.*, **5**, 483–501.

Sullivan, J. M. (1999). Mechanisms of cannabinoid-receptor-mediated inhibition of synaptic transmission in cultured hippocampal pyramidal neurons. *J. Neurophysiol.*, **82**, 1286–1294.

Szabo, B., Siemes, S. and Wallmichrath, I. (2002). Inhibition of GABAergic neurotransmission in the ventral tegmental area by cannabinoids. *Eur. J. Neurosci.*, **5**, 2057–2061.

Tanda, G., Pontieri, F. E. and Di Chiara, G. (1997). Cannabinoid and heroin activation of meso-limbic dopamine transmission by a common mu1 opioid receptor mechanism. *Science*, **276**, 2048–2050.

Terranova, J. P., Michaud, J. C., Le Fur, G. and Soubrie, P. (1995). Inhibition of long-term potenti-ation in rat hippocampal slices by anandamide and WIN55212-2: reversal by SR141716 A, a selective antagonist of CB1 cannabinoid receptors. *Naunyn-Schmiedebergs Arch. Pharmakol.*, **352**, 576–579.

Tsou, K., Brown, S., Sanudo-Pena, M. C., Mackie, K. and Walker, J. M. (1998). Immuno-histochemical distribution of cannabinoid CB1 receptors in the rat central nervous system. *Neuroscience*, **83**, 393–411.

Tsou, K., Mackie, K., Sanudo-Pena, M. C. and Walker, J. M. (1999). Cannabinoid CB1 receptors are localized primarily on cholecystokinin-containing GABAergic interneurons in the rat hippocampal formation. *Neuroscience*, **93**, 969–975.

Wilson, R. I. and Nicoll, R. A. (2001). Endogenous cannabinoids mediate retrograde signaling at hippocampal synapses. *Nature*, **410**, 588–592.

Wilson, R. I. and Nicoll, R. A. (2002). Endocannabinoid signalling in the brain. *Science*, **296**, 678–682.

Wu, X. and French, E. D. (2000). Effects of chronic delta9-tetrahydrocannabinol on rat midbrain dopamine neurons: an electrophysiological assessment. *Neuropharmacologia*, **39**, 391–398.

Zuardi A. W., Shirakawa, I., Finkelfarb, E. and Karniol. I. G. (1982). Action of cannabidiol on the anxiety and other effects produced by delta 9-THC in normal subjects. *Psychopharmalogia*, **76**, 245–250.

Zuardi, A. W., Morais, S. L., Guimaraes, F. S. and Mechoulam, R. (1995). Antipsychotic effect of cannabidiol. *J. Clin. Psychiatry*, **56**, 485–486.

11

Motives that maintain cannabis use among individuals with psychotic disorders

Catherine Spencer

c/o University of Melbourne, Australia

Rather than attempt to explain fully the complex relationship between cannabis and psychosis, this chapter focuses on what drives people with psychotic disorders to continue their cannabis use. Regardless of what precipitated the cannabis use, it is important to understand what maintains it or why individuals with psychotic disorders continue to use it, despite the negative impact that cannabis use may be having on their mental state. Understanding the motivation for cannabis use may provide insight into the circumstances in which the individual will use substances, the amount consumed, possible consequences and ideal strategies for behaviour change (Simons *et al.*, 1998). This insight can inform psychological treatments that attempt to reduce that use, as well as adjunctive pharmacological treatment and other aspects of psychiatric rehabilitation.

There are various factors to be considered in understanding why people with psychotic disorders continue to use cannabis. These include: (1) level of insight into both their mental illness and the effects of cannabis on symptoms; (2) biological drives for cannabis use (e.g. dopaminergic); (3) genetic or learned family influences; (4) sociocultural influences; (5) impact of affective/psychotic symptoms; (6) personality variables and coping strategies; and (7) addiction. It is argued, however, that the final common pathway or motivation to use cannabis is (8) the expectations of the direct and indirect effects cannabis use will have on affect. These expectations of use/reasons for use/cognitive motivations have been comprehensively researched among the general population, including adolescent, college student, community and substance abusing and dependent samples (Newcomb *et al.*, 1988; Schafer and Brown, 1991; Cooper *et al.*, 1992; Cooper, 1994: Stewart *et al.*, 1996; Simons *et al.*, 1998). This has led to the development of scales that assess a variety of reasons and expectancies related to substance use (Schafer and Brown, 1991; Cooper, 1994) as well as to motivational models of substance

Marijuana and Madness: Psychiatry and Neurobiology, ed. D. Castle and R. Murray. Published by Cambridge University Press. © Cambridge University Press 2004.

use (Cox and Klinger, 1988; Cooper, 1994). These theories have in turn informed treatments (Marlatt and Gordon, 1985; Miller and Rollnick, 1991).

Self-reported reasons for cannabis and other drug use have also been researched both qualitatively and quantitatively among people with psychotic disorders. This chapter reviews this research and seeks to establish whether reasons for cannabis use among people with psychotic disorders differ from reasons for cannabis use among the general population. Self-reported reasons for cannabis use among individuals with psychotic disorders have been criticized as *post-hoc* rationalizations (Miller *et al.*, 1994). However, this chapter will demonstrate that the replication of motives across numerous studies, the influence those motives have on patterns of use and the relationship with symptoms indicates the validity of these motives and their role in maintaining cannabis use. Cognitive motivational models do not exclude biological, genetic and sociocultural perspectives. On the contrary, they complement them (Marlatt and Gordon, 1985; Cox and Klinger, 1988; Schafer and Brown, 1991; Khantzian, 1997; Graham, 1998). They provide an understanding of motivations for cannabis use of which individuals are consciously aware. To the individual they represent the final common pathway to cannabis use and to the clinician they represent a starting point for assessment and tailoring treatment.

Reasons for substance use

Investigations of reasons for substance use among people with psychotic disorders were initially exploratory and qualitative (Test *et al.*, 1989; Dixon *et al.*, 1991; Warner *et al.*, 1994; Addington and Duchak, 1997). A number of structured interviews were developed (Test *et al.*, 1989; Dixon *et al.*, 1991), with participants generally selecting from a list of statements those that represent their perceived reasons for use. The lists generally included reasons which represent using drugs to (1) socialize, for example 'something to do with friends' (Test *et al.*, 1989); (2) enhance or improve mood, for example 'to feel less anxious, more relaxed' and 'to relieve boredom' (Test *et al.*, 1989); and (3) reduce symptoms and medication side-effects, for example 'to decrease hallucinations' and 'to make side effects more tolerable' (Test *et al.*, 1989).

Findings are similar across studies. For example, Test *et al.* (1989) interviewed 29 individuals with psychotic disorders in the USA, who were significant users of alcohol, and cannabis and other street drugs. The items 'relieve boredom', 'something to do with friends', and 'feel less anxious, more relaxed', were selected as the most important reasons driving substance use by more than 40% of the sample. Patients were also asked to select, from a list of feelings, how they felt before and after their last episode of drug use. Feelings reported prior to use were consistent with the reasons for use. However, the sample size was too small to examine differences in reasons for use between substances.

These findings were confirmed by Warner *et al.* (1994), using the same protocol with 55 psychotic outpatients. The reasons most important to participants were social interaction, relief of unpleasant affective states, relief of boredom and improved self-esteem. The results also established some differences in reasons for use between different substances. Relief of boredom and reduction of anxiety were reasons mostly associated with cannabis use and these participants were less likely to have structured daily activities. Most participants recognized that substance use worsened, or at least did not improve, paranoia or hallucinations.

Dixon *et al.* (1991) conducted structured interviews with 83 psychotic inpatients (48% substance-dependent) about their substance use, using a list of statements similar to those of Test *et al.* (1989). The authors added items that they believed probe for negative symptom relief, including 'to increase pleasure', 'to feel more emotions' and 'to talk more'. Arguably, these could equally represent efforts to enhance affect or facilitate social interaction. Motivations representing relief of positive symptoms and medication side-effects were also added. Again, results indicated that social affiliation, the enhancement of positive affect and now reduction of negative affect were key motivations. A smaller proportion of subjects (less than 20%) endorsed items representing relief of positive symptoms or medication side-effects. No differences in reasons for use were apparent across substances. However, whilst both alcohol and cannabis were used to decrease depression and anxiety, subjects were significantly more likely to rate cannabis as increasing suspiciousness and hallucinations. Cannabis and cocaine were significantly more likely than alcohol subjectively to 'increase energy'.

Addington and Duchak (1997) replicated this study with 41 psychotic outpatients meeting (*Diagnostic and Statistical Manual of Mental Disorders* (*DSM*-III-R: American Psychiatric Association, 1987) criteria for substance abuse or dependence. Again, reasons for use were reported for both alcohol and cannabis, with 95% of participants reporting using cannabis to 'increase pleasure' and 'get high', compared to 74% endorsing these reasons for alcohol use. The same pattern was apparent for using to relieve depression and 'to be more sociable'. Using cannabis to relieve side-effects of medication and to decrease hallucinations was endorsed by 40% of respondents; this is higher than in earlier studies, perhaps because the entire sample met criteria for abuse and dependence compared to only 48% of the Dixon *et al.* (1991) sample. Research in the general substance-using population indicates that experienced users will have more well-established reasons for use and discriminate in their reasons for use across different substances (Simons *et al.*, 2000).

Two Australian studies investigating reasons for use amongst people with psychosis are particularly important because they asked open-ended questions about reasons for use (Baigent *et al.*, 1995; Fowler *et al.*, 1998), as opposed to the 'forced choice' method of previous studies (Test *et al.*, 1989; Dixon *et al.*, 1991). Despite this difference in methodology, the results are similar. Baigent *et al.* (1995) interviewed 63 schizophrenia patients using the self-report Brief Symptom Inventory (BSI; Derogatis, 1993) and a substance abuse interview schedule designed by the authors. Reasons for use did not vary across substances. Participants reported the initial reasons for starting their substance use as peer pressure (54%), relief of dysphoria, depression or anxiety (31%) and experimentation (13%). Reasons for continuing use fell into two groups: (1) to relieve dysphoria, depression and anxiety (80%); and (2) as a fundamental aspect of social interaction (20%). This result is validated by subjects' responses regarding their most troublesome mental health problems, which were significantly positively correlated with the Global Severity Index of the BSI (Baigent *et al.*, 1995). These were hallucinations/delusions (38%), depression/anxiety (24%) and social fears/deficits (20%). The authors concluded that since all drugs had a subjective positive effect on the latter two symptoms, it is understandable that subjects used them mainly for this purpose. The amount of cannabis smoked in the previous 2 months was significantly positively correlated with self-reported social life ratings, highlighting the social aspect of participants' cannabis use.

Subjects were aware that the drugs could exacerbate their psychotic symptoms. Thus, the subjective effects of substances were elicited using 10 five-point interval scales measuring mood, anxiety, energy, hostility, suspicion, thought clarity, distractibility, group attachment and positive and negative symptoms. Participants reported that both negative and positive symptoms were slightly elevated by cannabis. Alcohol also exacerbated negative, but not positive symptoms. The perceived enhancing functions fulfilled by alcohol and cannabis use appeared to outweigh the perceived problems associated with their use (Baigent *et al.*, 1995).

In a later Australian study, Fowler *et al.* (1998) interviewed 194 schizophrenia outpatients, asking open-ended questions about reasons for use for each category of substance they had used during the preceding 6 months. Sixty per cent of participants had a lifetime diagnosis of substance abuse or dependence (*DSM-III-R* criteria) and 30% met such criteria at the time of the study. Their responses were grouped into four main categories, through item analysis. *Drug intoxication effects* included statements such as 'to feel good', 'to get high', 'to enhance things'. *Dysphoria relief* included statements such as 'to relax' and 'to take bad feelings away'. *Social effects* included 'to be sociable' and 'to face people better'. The last category, *illness- and medication-related effects*, included statements such as 'to get away from the voices' and 'relieve the feeling of ill health'. Dysphoria relief and drug intoxication effects were rated most highly in cannabis use (62% and 41% respectively). Ratings for social reasons were not reported. There were minimal differences between substance users and substance abusers in their reasons for using alcohol, cannabis and amfetamines. However, as in previous studies (Addington and Duchak, 1997) cannabis abusers were more likely than mere users to nominate illness- and medication-related reasons for substance use (16% versus 0%).

Hypotheses generated

The reasons for use given in the six studies reviewed above vary very little across substances, with cannabis being used for similar reasons to alcohol despite differences in subjective effects. Most authors conclude that reasons for cannabis and other substance use among individuals with psychotic disorders are similar to the reasons for use by young people in the general population; that is, to enjoy the experience of intoxication, to escape from emotional distress and to take part in social activity (Test et al., 1989; Dixon et al., 1991; Warner et al., 1994; Baigent et al., 1995; Addington and Duchak, 1997; Fowler et al., 1998). A minority of subjects interviewed, perhaps those with heavier use, used cannabis or other drugs to attempt to reduce negative or positive symptoms and medication side-effects.

Although mental health clinicians see symptom exacerbation or amotivational consequences of substance use, some patients clearly perceive their substance use as functional. These functions (intoxication, relief of dysphoria and social affiliation) may not differ from the reasons non-mentally ill persons cite for their substance use. Test et al. (1989) suggest that these reasons have great salience for persons with schizophrenic disorders who often have little daily structure, are uncomfortable with symptoms or side-effects and may experience serious problems with social relationships.

Warner et al. (1994) conclude, as did Test et al. (1989), that individuals with psychotic disorders may calculate the most advantageous benefit-to-cost ratio in their substance use. They may tailor drug use to improve affective symptoms with minimal increase in positive symptoms.

Some authors hypothesize that dysphoria may be the key to substance use, and suggest that schizophrenia patients use alcohol and cannabis to relieve or self-medicate a variety of psychotic and non-psychotic experiences (Dixon et al., 1991; Addington and Duchak, 1997). In this sense psychotic individuals may not differ from the general population in using substances to regulate affect or to self-medicate.

The self-medication hypothesis

The self-medication theory of substance use was first proposed by Khantzian in 1985, and rearticulated in 1997. Based on his experience of treating drug addicts among the general population with psychodynamic therapy, Khantzian (1985) observed that persons with substance use disorders suffer in the extreme with their feelings. They are either overwhelmed by painful affects or do not feel enough emotions. Individuals select and abuse substances which help them relieve painful affects or to experience or control emotions when they are absent or confusing. This theory would appear to encompass the self-medicating of a variety of primary and secondary symptoms of psychosis. Thus, Khantzian (1997) proposed that individuals will select the drug that has the desired effect on their inner state.

The self-medication hypothesis is disputed by Mueser and colleagues (1995), who suggest that psychotic patients' drug choice has more to do with availability of a particular substance, and that findings that non-users do not have worse symptoms discount self-medication as a major motive. Khantzian (1997) acknowledges that availability may limit choice and that tolerance may reduce the original effects, but argues that correlational studies of symptoms and substance use may not highlight patterns of self-medication unless symptoms and reasons for use are self-reported. The individuals' subjective experience of painful affect may not be evident to mental health staff and may escape objective diagnostic measures. Subjective states of distress, rather than psychiatric disorders, may be the important operatives that govern self-medication (Khantzian, 1997).

The more recently proposed Affect Regulation Model (Blanchard *et al.*, 2000) differs from the self-medication model. Unlike the self-medication model, which proposes that substance use attempts to modulate acute symptomatology in a manner that matches pharmacological properties of substances to alleviate the symptom, the affect regulation model proposes that individual differences in personality traits and coping skills underlie the use of substances to regulate affect.

Other authors have hypothesized that psychotic individuals use substances for social affiliation purposes (Baigent *et al.*, 1995; Gearon and Bellack, 1999). These authors suggest that interpersonal factors are more primary for psychotic patients than using drugs to control emotions. However, Khantzian argues that social affiliation would have an indirect effect on affect (1997). Overall, it appears that the use of substances to modify affect and for social purposes are both important factors for many people with psychotic illnesses.

Motivational models of substance use

The findings and hypotheses generated from the studies outlined above fit with motivational models of substance use which have been generated from research with the general population (Cox and Klinger, 1988; Cooper, 1994); they also have the potential to inform cognitive-behavioural treatments. Motivational models suggest that individuals use substances to achieve desired effects, and can encompass affect regulation and social affiliation as motivators for use. The motivational model was established through Cox and Klinger's (1988) research into alcohol use, which demonstrated that people are motivated to drink by their expectations about the affective changes that will occur. Cox and Klinger (1988) propose that biochemical reactivity, sociocultural and environmental influences, past reinforcement from drinking and conditioned reactions to alcohol are all involved in the decision to drink or not to drink. Contextual factors such as availability and the physical setting (for example, others encouraging the person to drink) are also important. However, the final common pathway to alcohol use is mediated by cognitive processes. These include thoughts, memories and perceptions that determine a person's expectations about the direct and indirect effects that drinking will have on their affect. This can be an enhancement of positive affect or a reduction in negative affect. The direct influence on affect would be the improvement in mood that comes from the direct chemical effect of alcohol. An indirect effect would be enhancement of positive affect through the approval drinking may bring from peers. This model also argues that people's expectations of changes in affect in response to alcohol use are potentially a more potent source of change than the pharmacological action of alcohol itself. Cox and Klinger (1988) also provide a cognitive explanation of why the expected effects may not correspond to the actual effects of drinking. Thus, an individual may place too much emphasis on the positive, immediate effects while discounting the delayed negative effects. For example, an individual with a psychotic disorder may use cannabis to affiliate with a group of friends, but later finds that he feels more suspicious and paranoid around them.

Cox and Klinger (1988) also argue that the decision to drink involves weighing up the advantages and disadvantages of drinking. If a person does not have satisfying positive incentives to pursue, or is not making satisfactory progress to achieving goals, weight will be added to his or her expectations that he or she can enhance positive affect by drinking. A person without work, financial goals or significant relationships that can be impaired through drinking has less to lose. Such factors are also likely to be pertinent for people with psychotic disorders.

Although originally developed to explain alcohol use, much empirical support has been established for this motivational model in explaining the use of both alcohol and cannabis in the general population. Johnston and O'Malley (1986) examined the reasons for substance use in 3500 adolescents a year, over a period of 10 years. The most highly ranked items across all substances were 'having fun with friends', 'getting high' and 'to relax or relieve tension'. Factor analysis identified that all reasons were represented by two factors, namely *social and recreational use* (e.g. 'to get high', 'have a good time with friends', 'because of boredom', 'to fit in with a group I like' and 'to experiment') and *coping with negative affect* (e.g. 'to relax', 'to get away from my problems' and 'because of anger or frustration'). Frequent users endorsed a greater number of reasons for use and were more likely to use alcohol and cannabis for psychological coping – that is, to cope with negative affect, boredom and, for stimulant users, to gain more energy.

Similarly, research by Newcomb and colleagues (1988) generated 15 items to assess various motivations for use of alcohol and cannabis in the general population. Exploratory factor analysis revealed an underlying four-factor structure that included *reduce negative affect* ('stop boredom', 'get rid of anxiety and tension', 'feeling sad, blue or depressed'), *enhance positive affect and creativity* ('enjoy what I am doing more', 'feel better about myself'), *social cohesion* ('feel good around people', 'friends pressure me into doing it') and *addiction* ('helps me get through the day', 'feel bad when I don't use it'). Reduce negative affect and social cohesion were the most commonly endorsed factors (Newcomb *et al.*, 1988). The same factor structure was confirmed for alcohol and cannabis. Thus, it appears that alcohol and cannabis use among the general population represent attempts to influence affect, either directly through using to reduce negative affect or enhance positive affect, or indirectly through enhancement of social affiliation.

Cooper and colleagues (1992) developed the Drinking Motives Questionnaire (DMQ), containing a list of statements specifying reasons for use and measuring the relative frequency of drinking for these motives. Factor analysis generated three categories of motives similar to those in the previous general population studies outlined above (Johnston and O'Malley, 1986; Newcomb *et al.*, 1988) as well as those established in the psychosis literature (Fowler *et al.*, 1998). These are as follows:

1. *coping motives* (to reduce and/or avoid negative emotional states) which include 'to relax', 'to forget your worries', 'because you feel more self confident or sure of yourself', 'because it helps when you are feeling nervous or depressed' and 'to cheer you up when you are in a bad mood'
2. *social motives* (to affiliate with others) which include 'as a way to celebrate', 'to be sociable', 'because it makes a social gathering more enjoyable', 'because it's what most of your friends do when you get together'
3. *enhancement motives* (to facilitate positive emotions) which include 'because you like the feeling', 'because it makes you feel good', 'to get high', 'because it is fun', 'because it's exciting'

A conformity motive (e.g. 'to be part of a group') was added by Cooper in a study using the DMQ with adolescents (1994) and a four-factor structure confirmed with factor analysis.

Cooper (1994) proposes a two-dimensional motivational model, where reasons for use are either internally or externally generated and either positively or negatively reinforcing. Direct effects were hypothesized to be through the *enhancement* (internally generated, positive reinforcement) and *coping motives* (internally generated, negative reinforcement), whilst *social* (externally generated, positive

reinforcement) and *conformity motives* (externally generated, negative reinforcement) were proposed as indirect enhancers of affect. Simons *et al.* (1998) examined
reasons for cannabis and alcohol use among 161 college students. To Cooper's four-
factor drinking motives measure (DMQ: Cooper, 1994), they added a fifth factor
(labelled 'expansion') representing use of cannabis for perceptual and cognitive
enhancement or expanded experiential awareness; this motive had been identified
in previous work with cannabis users (Schafer and Brown, 1991). Items included 'so
I can know myself better', 'so I can understand things differently', 'because it helps
me be more creative and original', 'so I can expand my awareness' and 'to be more
open to experiences'. In accordance with Cooper's model (1994), this represents
an additional internally generated, positive reinforcement motive. All five motivational factors demonstrated good internal consistency, discriminant and concurrent
validity. This factor structure was invariant across a range of experiences with the
drug. Cannabis was reportedly most commonly used for enhancement purposes,
followed by social purposes, expansion, coping and conformity, whilst alcohol was
most likely used for enhancement, followed by social purposes, coping, conformity
and expansion.

In a further study, Simons *et al.* (2000) examined the intraindividual motivational
differences between alcohol and cannabis among 46 experienced users (college
students who had used cannabis or alcohol 60 or more times in their lifetime).
Enhancement, coping and conformity motives did not differ across drugs, leading
the authors to conclude that these are common anticipated effects from alcohol
and cannabis, and that they represent individual strategies for affect regulation that
are not drug-specific. Social motives were more highly endorsed for alcohol and
expansion motives for cannabis. Thus, experienced users can discriminate in their
reasons for using these two drugs in terms of certain domains.

These similarities between alcohol and cannabis motives provide support for the
motivational models of substance use articulated by Cox and Klinger (1988) (see
above), in that, despite different pharmacological effects and variations in social
context, the final common pathway to substance use is the expectations about the
direct and indirect influence on affect. The factor structure of the DMQ is also
invariant across both alcohol and cannabis, and appears to be independent of the
degree of experience with the particular drug.

Overall, the reasons for cannabis use among the general population (Johnston
and O'Malley, 1986; Newcomb *et al.*, 1988; Schafer and Brown, 1991; Simons *et al.*,
1998) appear to be similar to reasons established in the qualitative studies among
the psychotic disordered population (Test *et al.*, 1989; Dixon *et al.*, 1991; Warner
et al., 1994; Baigent *et al.*, 1995; Addington and Duchak, 1997; Fowler *et al.*, 1998).
That is, to enhance affect, cope with negative affect (including psychotic symptoms)
and affiliate socially. Do these motives predict or maintain use?

Studies supporting a motivational model of cannabis use among individuals with psychotic disorders

Two studies have quantitatively examined the validity of motivational models in explaining cannabis use among individuals with psychotic disorders. Mueser *et al.* (1995) and Spencer *et al.* (2002) used validated self-report instruments, generated from the motivation and expectancy literature, with psychotic populations.

Mueser *et al.* (1995) used the earlier version of Cooper's Drinking Motives Measure (DMM: Cooper *et al.*, 1992) that included enhancement, coping and social motives but not conformity or expansion motives (Drug Use Motives Measure: DUMM). They also used the Alcohol Expectancy Questionnaire (AEQ), the Marijuana Effects Expectancy Questionnaire (MEEQ) and the Cocaine Effects Expectancy Questionnaire (CEEQ) (Schafer and Brown, 1991). These questionnaires were administered to 70 in- and outpatients with a diagnosis of schizophrenia or schizoaffective disorder who had used an illicit drug at least once in their lifetime.

A history of alcohol use disorder was present in 51% of the sample and drug use disorder in 50%; only 16% gave a history of use of only one substance. Recent alcohol use disorder was present in 29% of the sample and 26% had recent drug use disorder (cannabis or cocaine). Internal reliabilities of subscales within the DMM and the DUMM ranged from 0.74 (socialization motive on DMM) to 0.91 (enhancement motive of DUMM); these are comparable to those reported for the general population (Cooper *et al.*, 1992).

Examination of the relationship between alcohol or drug use disorder and motives revealed that subjects with a history of alcohol or drug use disorder scored higher on motive subscales. As reported by Cooper (1994), the coping motive was most strongly related to a history of substance abuse. Each subscale of the DMM or DUMM correlated with the scale which measured problems from drug use. Multiple analysis of variance between scores on the AEQ, MEEQ and CEEQ and measures of substance use indicated that patients with a history of drug use disorder tended to have higher expectancies than did patients with no such history. These findings are consistent with studies on persons with primary substance use disorder (Schafer and Brown, 1991; Cooper, 1994).

Mueser *et al.* (1995) concluded that the relationship between substance use disorder and expectancies and motives lends support to the validity of these measures in people with schizophrenia and related disorders. They also hypothesized that motives are the driving explanation underlying substance use.

More recently, Spencer and colleagues (2002) confirmed and extended the above findings. They quantitatively examined reasons for alcohol and cannabis use among 69 patients with psychotic disorders who had used alcohol or other drugs in the previous year. Up to a third of the sample had recently (in the previous 3 months) used problematic quantities of substances (mostly alcohol and cannabis) and/or reported psychological dependence on their substance of choice.

This study employed Cooper's DMQ (1994), including the conformity items developed for the adolescent population as these have particular relevance in psychosis, where social development is often arrested (Jackson et al., 1996) and social anxiety is highly comorbid (Heinssen and Glass, 1990; Penn et al., 1994); but excluding the 'expansion' motive of Simons et al. (1998). Spencer et al. (2002) also added additional items to the DMQ, to explore the putative use of substances to alleviate psychotic symptoms (positive and negative) as well as sequelae of the disorder (including social anxiety, isolation and medication side-effects). Table 11.1 shows both Cooper's items (1994) and the additional items that were shown to be unambiguous during interviewing and where the full range of responses (1 = never/almost never to 5 = always/almost always) were endorsed.

Factor analysis identified five motivational factors (Table 11.2). All four of Cooper's factors (coping, conformity, social and enhancement) were intact, with the majority of additional items loading on to these. The majority of additional items loaded with the coping items of the DMQ; this factor was labelled 'coping with unpleasant affect' (37% of variance). These additional items ('to decrease restlessness', 'to make it easier to sleep' and 'to slow down racing thoughts') were included to represent relief of positive symptoms, but could equally be seen as decreasing general anxiety or negative affect. Items representing use of substances to improve social confidence and social networks loaded with the conformity items of the DMQ; this was labelled 'conformity/acceptance' (8% of variance). The additional items which specifically included symptom labels such as 'voices' or 'paranoia' or 'medication side-effects' loaded on a separate factor, labelled 'relief of positive symptoms and medication side-effects' (6% of variance). The two other factors were consistent with Cooper's enhancement and social motives (accounting for 10% of variance).

Patients may not be aware of the distinction between primary dysphoria and dysphoria secondary to positive or negative psychotic symptoms and medication side-effects (Dixon et al., 1991; Earnst and Kring, 1997). This could explain why items representing use of substances to relieve mental health symptoms clustered into two separate factors. Items which obviously represented positive symptoms and side-effects such as 'to get away from the voices' and 'to reduce medication side-effects', represent one underlying motive for the psychotic participants in this study, and items describing the relief of general unpleasant affect represent a separate motive. The relatively infrequent use of cannabis or alcohol for the former motive indicate that the use of alcohol or cannabis to cope with general unpleasant affect is more common than their use to relieve positive symptoms or medication side-effects.

Table 11.1 Items from the Drinking Motives Questionnaire (DMQ) of Cooper *et al.* (1992)

Subscale	Items
Enhancement motives	9. Because it's exciting
	10. To get high
	14. Because it's fun
	34. Because it makes you feel good
Coping motives	6. To relax
	13. To forget your worries
	19. Because you feel more self-confident or sure of yourself
	20. To cheer you up when you are in a bad mood
	21. Because it helps you when you are feeling nervous
	31. Because it helps when you are feeling depressed
Social motives	23. As a way to celebrate
	22. Because it's what most of your friends do when you get together
	5. To be sociable
	16. Because it makes a social gathering more enjoyable
Conformity motives	28. Because your friends pressure you to do it
	29. To be liked
	30. So you won't feel left out

Additional items based on previous research with psychotic population

Coping with psychotic symptoms and sequelae	3. To make it easier to sleep
	11. To feel less suspicious or paranoid
	18. To get away from the voices
	15. To reduce side-effects of medication
	33. To feel more motivated
	1. To relieve boredom
	17. To help you talk to others
	4. To slow down racing thoughts
	7. To be part of a group
	24. To decrease restlessness
	26. To help me concentrate

(Reproduced, with permission, from Spencer *et al.* (2002).)

Table 11.2 Means, standard deviations (SD) and reliability coefficients (α) for motive subscales

Subscale	Rating		
	Mean	SD	α
Enhancement Because it makes you feel good Because it's fun To get high	2.69	1.19	0.75
Social motive It's what most of your friends do when you get together Because it makes a social gathering more enjoyable As a way to celebrate To be sociable	2.47	1.02	0.76
Coping with unpleasant affect Because it helps when you feel nervous It helps when you feel depressed To forget your worries To feel more motivated To make it easier to sleep To help me concentrate Because you feel more self-confident/sure of yourself To relieve boredom To decrease restlessness To slow down racing thoughts	2.08	0.94	0.92
Conformity and acceptance So you won't feel left out To be liked To help you talk to others To be part of a group Because your friends pressure you to do it	1.74	0.79	0.78
Relief of positive symptoms and medication side-effects To get away from the voices To reduce side-effects of medication To decrease suspiciousness and paranoia	1.59	0.99	0.41

(Reproduced, with permission, from Spencer *et al.* (2002).)

Thus, additional reasons for use specific to individuals with psychotic disorders can be incorporated into the four motive dimensions of coping, enhancement, social and conformity. Factor analysis indicates that psychotic individuals have similar reasons for substance use to the general population, with the possibility of an additional motive (relief of positive symptoms and medication side-effects). The factor analysis supports a cognitive motivational model of both alcohol and cannabis use (Cox and Klinger, 1988; Cooper, 1994). The fifth motive of relief of positive symptoms and medication side-effects suggests an additional use of drugs for internally generated negative reinforcement purposes among individuals with psychotic disorders.

In terms of cannabis specifically, participants in Spencer *et al.*'s (2002) study were most likely to use cannabis for enhancement purposes, followed by social and coping purposes, as indicated by mean subscale scores. They were less likely to use for conformity purposes and rarely for relief of positive symptoms and medication side-effects. Analysis of variance showed that mean scores for cannabis users were higher across all motives subscales, and significantly higher for enhancement, coping with unpleasant affect and conformity/acceptance.

Cannabis was therefore used more frequently than alcohol for these reasons. The higher frequency of use for the two latter motives indicates that cannabis users are just as likely to use for negative reinforcement such as coping with negative affect as for positive reinforcement (e.g. social and enhancement). Alcohol users were less likely to use for negative reinforcement, that is to cope with unpleasant affect or to conform/be accepted by a group.

Thus, the cognitive motivational model has validity in understanding reasons for cannabis use in the psychotic disordered population. The low frequency of cannabis and alcohol use for the motive reduce positive symptoms and medication side-effects could indicate that it is not as important in understanding the use of these substances by persons with psychotic disorders as has been hypothesized by previous authors (Dixon *et al.*, 1991; Addington and Duchak, 1997; Khantzian, 1997). Perhaps the expectation that cannabis will modify the general distress caused by the illness or other psychosocial factors is more important in understanding cannabis use in this population.

Spencer *et al.*'s study (2002) demonstrates that motives for cannabis and alcohol use play a significant role in maintaining use and associated problems. A multiple linear regression analysis indicated that participants' motives for using their substance of choice (alcohol or cannabis) predicted: (1) the amount consumed over the previous month (accounting for 35% of the variance); (2) the context in which they use that substance (accounting for 30–37% of the variance); (3) the problems associated with using that substance (47% of variance); and (4) the psychological dependence on that substance (57% of variance). Using alcohol or cannabis to cope with unpleasant affect or for enhancement purposes predicted heavier use. Using for these reasons also predicted more associated problems (i.e. social, personal and interpersonal problems) as measured by a self-report problem scale (Kavanagh *et al.*, 1998). The social motive did not predict problems or heavy use and appears to represent normative, socially acceptable and socially cued reasons for use (Cooper, 1994). Similarly, the conformity/acceptance motive does not appear to be related to heavy or problematic use amongst these participants.

Perhaps the most important finding of Spencer *et al.* (2002) is that using substances to cope with unpleasant affect and to relieve psychotic symptoms and medication side-effects led to stronger dependence on that substance as measured by Severity of Dependence Scale (Gossop *et al.*, 1995). This establishes the importance of these motives in the development of psychological dependence on cannabis or alcohol.

Motivational models of cannabis use in psychosis

Overall, the results examined thus far favour the hypothesis that reasons for cannabis use among individuals with psychotic disorders are not significantly different from those among the general population. Why, then, are people with psychotic disorders such as schizophrenia so likely to use cannabis? Why does the presence of psychotic symptoms increase the likelihood of cannabis dependence (Degenhardt and Hall, 2001)? And how do motivations for use mediate the association between symptoms and use itself?

Previous studies have indicated that there is a significant relationship between symptoms, reasons for use and substance use disorders (Baigent *et al.*, 1995; Fowler *et al.*, 1998). Spencer *et al.* (2002) examined this relationship further. Their motivational model proposed that reasons for use would mediate any relationship between symptoms and substance use, as the final pathway to substance use is the expectation of the direct or indirect effect on affect. Therefore motives are the mechanism through which symptoms lead to substance use. This is shown in Figure 11.1.

This mediational model was tested through multiple linear regression. Due to sample size constraints, alcohol and cannabis dependence could not be examined separately. Symptoms alone, as measured by the self-report BSI (Derogatis, 1993) and negative symptom total of the Positive and Negative Syndrome Scale (PANSS: Kay *et al.*, 1992) accounted for only 19% of the variance in substance dependence. However, addition of the five motive subscales from the Substance use Scale for Psychosis (SUSP) (Table 11.2) increased the proportion of variance explained to 47%. Furthermore, the effect of symptoms on variance was insignificant when motives were controlled for. This demonstrates that increases in symptoms led to increases in motives for use which in turn led to increased dependence on substances

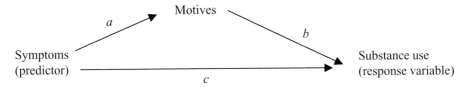

Figure 11.1 Mediational model.

(alcohol or cannabis). These findings apply across the range of quantities of alcohol and cannabis used, irrespective of whether the user met diagnostic criteria for substance abuse or dependence.

These findings provide support for the cognitive motivational model of alcohol and cannabis use (Cox and Klinger, 1988; Cooper, 1994; Simons *et al.*, 1998) which specifies that the final common pathway to substance use is the expectations people have about the effect that substance use will have on their affect. Symptoms or subjective distress alone do not lead to cannabis dependence. Rather, if individuals expect cannabis to have a direct or indirect effect on their affect, they will be more dependent on it. If psychotic individuals are distressed by symptoms (psychotic or otherwise) and have the expectation that cannabis use may reduce this distress or help them cope, their decision to use will be strengthened and the risk of dependence increased.

Adapting to symptoms of psychosis and sequelae of the illness can be very diffi-cult. Sequelae can involve feelings of loss, trauma, depression, anxiety, social anxiety, social stigma, impaired family and other social relationships, damage to self-esteem and self-concept and side-effects of medications (Strakowski *et al.*, 1994; Jackson *et al.*, 1996; Earnst and Kring, 1997). Developmentally, psychotic disorders tend to interrupt early adulthood or adolescence (Jackson *et al.*, 1996). Consequently, rewarding experiences such as career development, academic achievement and inti-mate relationships are not realized by these people. Thus development of self-worth, self-concept and goals for the future are significantly hampered. Cox and Klinger (1988) suggested that if people have less immediate or long-term negative con-sequences from their substance abuse, they are more likely to make the decision to use. The motivation to enhance affect will be strengthened by boredom and a lack of daily structure or meaningful activities. Coping motives will be reinforced by the negative affect that can arise from symptoms and their sequelae, notably their impact on self-concept and resulting hopelessness. Conformity and accep-tance motives will be reinforced by the reduction in opportunities to socialize, lack of accepting peer groups and the discomfort experienced in social situations. The mediational role of motives in the relationship between distress from symptoms and substance dependence disputes the hypothesis that self-reported reasons for use are merely *post-hoc* rationalizations (Miller *et al.*, 1994). Clearly they are important to an understanding of psychotic disordered individuals' substance use, which in turn can inform effective treatments. However, not all individuals with psychotic disorders use cannabis. How do these motivations or expectations develop in some individuals with psychotic disorders and not in others? In addition to biological, genetic, familial and sociocultural influences, individual personality and early learning experiences may lead to the development of cannabis dependence. Blanchard and colleagues (1999, 2000) argue that research examining reasons for comorbid substance use and psychotic disorders requires more of a focus on enduring individual differences in personality, stress and coping rather than transitory features of the illness, such as psychotic symptoms. Reasons for substance use may be readily identifiable at the level of traits as it has been among populations with primary substance use disorders. They propose that schizophrenia or vulnerability to the illness has been found to be associated with (1) trait negative affect, impulsivity, antisocial behaviour; (2) deficits in social skills, problem-solving or other effective coping strategies; and (3) reactivity to stress, thus placing these individuals at a higher risk to using substances to regulate affect. Their study (Blanchard *et al.*, 1999) with 39 schizophrenic and schizoaffective outpatients demonstrated that trait negative affect and the use of drugs and alcohol to cope predicted the severity of substance use problems. These results are consistent with previous findings indicating that substance use in psychosis is motivated by the expectation that negative emotions can be coped with through drug use, leading to drug-related problems (Mueser *et al.*, 1995; Spencer *et al.*, 2002). It extends the motive of coping with negative affect from the level of symptoms to that of personality.

This is consonant with Graham's argument (1998) that links reasons for use to early dysfunctional beliefs and positive drug experiences at significant developmental periods. Psychotic people may initially use substances to change affect, achieve a cognitive state or to facilitate social contact. They then develop dysfunctional substance-related beliefs about the substance use, for example, 'if I don't use cannabis, I will be unable to cope'.

Similarly, Khantzian's (1997) psychodynamic, developmental perspective argues that individuals learn that drugs and alcohol can relieve or change troubling and extreme emotional states. Khantzian believes that the long prodromal phase of a psychotic disorder which can involve much pain, suffering and social maladaptation may predispose the individual to drug and alcohol use at that time. He hypothesizes that substance-dependent persons self-medicate not only because they do not know how to tolerate or express their feelings, but also because they cannot regulate their self-esteem, relationships or self-care. Overall, these motivational models provide further understanding of why psychotic disordered individuals have higher rates of cannabis dependence than the general population and why they continue to use despite the detrimental effects on the course of their illness.

Conclusions

Both qualitative and quantitative research that examines self-reported reasons for cannabis use among individuals with psychotic disorders provide empirical support for a motivational model of psychotic individuals' cannabis use. The final common pathway to their substance use is the expectation that substances will have a direct or indirect impact on their affect. The main motives for use are to enhance affect, to cope with negative affect (whether it be primary or secondary to their psychotic illness), to enhance social affiliation/acceptance and (less commonly) to cope with positive symptoms or medication side-effects. With the exception of the latter motive, these are similar reasons for cannabis use among people without psychotic disorders. Using cannabis to cope with negative affect or to enhance affect has been demonstrated to predict problems with use and cannabis dependence.

Thus motives for use are not *post-hoc* rationalizations. Rather, they maintain use and are the generative mechanism through which distress from psychiatric symptoms influences cannabis use. In other words, for those individuals with clear expectations or beliefs about the effects cannabis will have on their affect, worsening psychiatric symptoms or distress will lead to a worsening of cannabis dependence. Reasons for use and substance-related beliefs or coping strategies can usefully be explored in both assessment and treatment of individuals with psychotic disorders who use cannabis to harmful levels. Therefore, both biological and psychosocial treatments should incorporate the individual's motives for cannabis use.

REFERENCES

Addington, J. and Duchak, V. (1997). Reasons for substance use in schizophrenia. *Acta Psychiatr. Scand.*, **96**, 329–333.

American Psychiatric Association (1987). *Diagnostic and Statistical Manual of Mental Disorders*, 3rd edn revised. Washington, DC: American Psychiatric Association.

Baigent, M., Holme, G. and Hafner, R. J. (1995). Self reports of the interaction between substance abuse and schizophrenia. *Aust. NZ J. Psychiatry*, **29**, 69–74.

Blanchard, J. J., Squires, D., Henry, T. *et al.* (1999). Examining an affect regulation model of substance abuse in schizophrenia: the role of traits and coping. *J. Nerv. Ment. Dis.*, **187**, 72–79.

Blanchard, J. J., Brown, S. A., Horan, W. P. and Sherwood, A. R. (2000). Substance use disorders in schizophrenia: review, integration and a proposed model. *Clin. Psychol. Rev.*, **20**, 207–234.

Cooper, M. L. (1994). Motivations for alcohol use among adolescents: development and validation of a four factor model. *Psychol. Assessment*, **6**, 117–128.

Cooper, M. L., Russel, M., Skinner, J. B. and Windle, M. (1992). Development and validation of a three-dimensional measure of drinking motives. *Psychol. Assessment*, **4**, 123–132.

Cox, W. M. and Klinger, E. (1988). A motivational model of alcohol use. *J. Abnormal Psychol.*, **97**, 168–180.

Degenhardt, L. and Hall, W. (2001). The association between psychosis and problematic drug use among Australian adults: findings from the National Survey of Mental Health and Well-being. *Psychol. Med.*, **31**, 659–668.

Derogatis, L. R. (1993). *Brief Symptom Inventory (BSI)*. Minneapolis: National Computer Systems.

Dixon, L., Haas, G., Weiden, P. J., Sweeney, J. and Frances, A. J. (1991). Drug abuse in schizophrenic patients: clinical correlates and reasons for use. *Am. J. Psychiatry*, **148**, 224.

Earnst, K. S. and Kring, A. M. (1997). Construct validity of negative symptoms: an empirical overview. *Clin. Psychol. Rev.*, **17**, 167–189.

Fowler, I. L., Carr, V. J., Carter, N. T. and Lewin, T. J. (1998). Patterns of current and lifetime substance abuse in schizophrenia. *Schizophr. Bull.*, **24**, 443–445.

Gearon, J. S. and Bellack, A. S. (1999). Substance abuse in people with schizophrenia: readiness to change, reasons for use, and neurocognitive functioning. *Schizophr. Res.*, **36**, 40.

Gossop, M., Darke, S., Griffiths, P. *et al.* (1995). The Severity of Dependence Scale (SDS): psychometric properties of the SDS in English and Australian samples of heroin, cocaine and amphetamine users. *Addiction*, **90**, 607–614.

Graham, H. L. (1998). The role of dysfunctional beliefs in individuals who experience psychosis and use substances: implications for cognitive therapy and medication adherence. *Behav. Cognitive Psychother.*, **26**, 193–208.

Heinssen, R. K. Jr and Glass, C. R. (1990). Social skills, social anxiety, and cognitive factors in schizophrenia. In *Handbook of Social and Evaluation Anxiety*, ed. H. Leitenberg. New York: Plenum Press.

Jackson, H. J., McGorry, P. D., Edwards, J. and Hulbert, C. (1996). Cognitively oriented psychotherapy for early psychosis (COPE). In *Early Intervention and Prevention in Mental Health*, ed. P. Cotton and H. Jackson, pp. 131–153. Victoria, Australia: Australian Psychological Society Ltd.

Johnston, L. D. and O'Malley. (1986). Why do the nation's students use drugs and alcohol? Self reported reasons from nine national surveys. *J. Drug Issues*, **16**, 29–66.

Kavanagh, D., Saunders, J., Young, R., Jenner, L. and Clair, A. (1998) *Start Over and Survive Treatment Manual. Evaluation of a Brief Intervention for Substance Abuse in Early Psychosis*. Brisbane, Australia: University of Queensland.

Kay, S. R., Opler, L. A. and Fiszbein, A. (1992). *Positive and Negative Syndrome Scale (PANSS) Manual*. Toronto: Multi-Health Systems.

Khantzian, E. (1985). The self medication hypothesis of addictive disorders: focus on heroin and cocaine dependence. *Am. J. Psychiatry*, **142**, 1259.

Khantzian, E. J. (1997). The self medication hypothesis of substance use disorders: a reconsideration and recent applications. *Harvard Rev. Psychiatry*, **4**, 231–244.

Marlatt, G. A. and Gordon, J. R. (1985). *Relapse Prevention: Maintenance Strategies in the Treatment of Addictive Behaviour.* London: Guildford Press.

Miller, W. and Rollnick, S. (1991). *Motivational Interviewing: Preparing People to Change Addictive Behaviours.* New York: Guildford.

Miller, N. S., Erikson, A. and Owley, T. (1994). Psychosis and schizophrenia in alcohol and drug dependence. *Psychiatr. Ann.,* **24**, 418–423.

Mueser, K. T., Nishith, P., Tracy, J. I., De Girolamo, J. and Molinaro, M. (1995). Expectations and motives for substance use in schizophrenia. *Schizophr. Bull.,* **21**, 367–378.

Newcomb, M. D., Chou, C., Bentler, P. M. and Huba, G. J. (1988). Cognitive motivations for drug use among adolescents: longitudinal tests of gender differences and predictors of change in drug use. *J. Counsel. Psychol.,* **35,** 426–438.

Penn, D. L., Hope, D. A., Spaulding, W. and Kucera, J. (1994). Social anxiety in schizophrenia. *Schizophr. Res.,* **11**, 274–284.

Schafer, J. and Brown, S. A. (1991). Marijuana and cocaine effect expectancies and drug use patterns. *J. Consult. Clin. Psychol.,* **59**, 558–565.

Simons, J., Correia, C. J., Carey, K. B. and Borsari, B. E. (1998). Validating a five factor marijuana motives measure: relations with use, problems and alcohol motives. *J. Counsel. Psychol.,* **45**, 265–273.

Simons, J., Correia, C. J. and Carey, K. B. (2000). A comparison of motives for marijuana and alcohol use among experienced users. *Addict. Behav.,* **25**, 153–160.

Spencer, C. R., Castle. D. and Michie, P. T. (2002). Motivations that maintain substance use among individuals with psychotic disorders. *Schizophr. Bull.,* **28**, 23–247.

Stewart S. H., Zeitlin, S. B. and Samoluk, S. B. (1996). Examination of a three-dimensional drinking motives questionaire in a young adult university sample. *Behav. Res. Ther.,* **34**, 61–67.

Strakowski, S. M., Johen, M., Flaum, M. and Amador, X. (1994). Substance use in psychotic disorders: associations with affective syndromes. *Schizophr. Res.,* **14**, 73–81.

Test, M. A., Wallisch, L. S., Allness, D. J. and Ripp, K. (1989). Substance abuse in young adults with schizophrenic disorders. *Schizophr. Bull.,* **15**, 465–476.

Warner, M. B., Taylor, D., Wright, J. *et al.* (1994). Substance use among the mentally ill: prevalence, reasons for use and effects on illness. *Am. J. Orthopsychiatry,* **64**, 30–39.

12

Addressing cannabis abuse in people with psychosis

Wynne James[1] and David J. Castle[2]

[1] Fremantle Hospital, WA, Australia
[2] University of Melbourne, Australia

As outlined in Chapter 8, cannabis use is common amongst people with schizo-phrenia and regular use, even at relatively low levels, can have a negative impact on illness course (Hall and Degenhardt, 2000). The effective management of this clinical problem is increasingly the focus of psychiatric practice and research. This chapter reviews a number of important areas that deserve consideration when developing an effective response. Aspects such as screening, assessment and models of service delivery are covered. The chapter concludes by outlining a number of psychosocial treatment interventions available for addressing cannabis use in schizophrenia and related disorders.

It must be acknowledged from the outset that there is a paucity of research evidence in terms of treatment interventions solely for cannabis use amongst people with schizophrenia. Thus, studies that have considered other drugs, and not just cannabis, are included in this review.

Screening

An awareness of any ongoing drug abuse is essential when determining psychiatric diagnosis, deciding on appropriate treatment interventions and planning future care (Zeidonis and Fisher, 1994). If undetected, drugs such as cannabis can confound the interpretation of important signs and symptoms of psychosis, possibly lead to overmanagement with psychotropic medications, as well as rendering other psychosocial treatments less effective for people with schizophrenia (Drake *et al.*, 1993b).

Unfortunately, despite such clear clinical imperatives, cannabis use often goes undiscovered and therefore unaddressed (Kavanagh, 2000). A number of factors

Marijuana and Madness: Psychiatry and Neurobiology, ed. D. Castle and R. Murray. Published by Cambridge University Press. © Cambridge University Press 2004.

have been identified that contribute to this underdetection, including: a lack of systematic screening processes to facilitate detection (Ananth *et al.*, 1989; Drake and Wallach, 1989; Milling *et al.*, 1994); an underappreciation among many clinicians of the prevalence and clinical implications of cannabis use (Drake *et al.*, 1993b); and a lack of awareness among staff regarding approaches to screening and detection (Siegfried, 1998), compounded by patients denying or minimizing their drug use, or simply considering it to be unconnected to their psychotic symptoms (Test *et al.*, 1989).

On a positive note, recent research has demonstrated that rates of detection can be significantly improved through the introduction of routine screening procedures (Appleby *et al.*, 1997). All psychiatric patients should be asked about their substance use and any related problems. This process can be facilitated by including basic screening questions about current or past drug use within admission documentation routinely used within psychiatric services (Department of Health, 2002).

The use of screening tools such as the Dartmouth Assessment of Lifestyle Inventory (DALI) (Rosenberg *et al.*, 1998), Drug Abuse Screening Test (DAST) (Skinner, 1982) or the CAGE questionnaire (Mayfield *et al.*, 1974) can also be used during intake interviews, to augment detection (RachBeisel *et al.*, 1999). These instruments have demonstrated reliability and validity within psychiatric populations (Kavanagh, 2000) and, while not designed to detect cannabis use specifically, they can be administered with respect to this substance. However, while self-report measures are useful, Weiss *et al.* (1998) caution against relying on them solely, as these instruments can prove unreliable when patients purposely deny ongoing drug use or are impaired during episodes of acute illness.

Drake *et al.* (1993b) assert that a combined approach to screening ultimately produces the highest rates of detection. Thus, they recommend that screening questions and self-report instruments should be used in conjunction with laboratory tests such as urinalysis and collateral information from family members and significant others. Urinalysis can be an effective method for detecting cannabis use, but the fact that urinary tests for cannabinoids can be positive for days to weeks after ceasing cannabis complicates the interpretation of positive results (Ashton, 2001). Collateral information is particularly useful for gaining a better understanding of changes in mental state and behaviours consistent with ongoing cannabis abuse, including signs and symptoms of intoxication or the possession of drug-using paraphernalia. Appleby *et al.* (1997) demonstrated a significant increase in the detection of substance use disorders within a public psychiatric service following the introduction of such systematic screening procedures.

In addition, consideration of findings regarding the clinical correlates of cannabis use amongst psychiatric populations should be incorporated into training curricula,

---

Box 12.1 Improving rates of detection

- Include questions addressing substance use within admission and review documentation
- Routine use of appropriate screening tools
- Laboratory findings, including urinalysis
- Collateral information from relatives and significant others
- An awareness of signs and symptoms of regular use, intoxication and withdrawal
- Clinical correlates

---

to inform clinicians about which patients should be treated with a higher index of suspicion (Box 12.1). Within this population, as within the general community, young single males with higher levels of alcohol use and poorer educational achievements are overrepresented amongst cannabis users, and as such should be assessed particularly carefully (Dixon *et al.*, 1991; Hall and Degenhardt, 2000). Zeidonis and Fisher (1994) highlight other parameters such as homelessness, legal and financial problems, violence and non-compliance with treatment as clinical clues that might indicate ongoing drug use. Attention should also be paid to any patients who remain unresponsive to conventional treatments or whose illness relapses frequently due to unexplained circumstances (Linszen *et al.*, 1994).

Assessment

While screening is concerned with case finding and triage, assessment refers to the structured collection of relevant information essential for ascertaining current need and thus determining future care. Assessing the interplay between cannabis use and mental illness and then deciding on which interventions to employ requires careful consideration of a number of complex areas, including: the nature and degree of drug use; reasons for drug use; and motivations to change drug use. Other aspects, such as impact on psychiatric illness, housing, employment and relationships, should also be ascertained (Carey and Correia, 1998).

We are not aware of any single standardized assessment instrument that encompasses all of these complex factors. As such, the components of assessment vary widely from service to service and setting to setting, depending on the information sought by clinicians. What follows are examples of specific assessment tools useful for understanding the relationship between cannabis use and mental illness, and for evaluating motivational factors such as reasons for cannabis use and readiness to change – insights deemed essential for the development of individualized care plans and for informing any subsequent treatment (Drake and Meuser, 2000).

Assessing cannabis use

Two instruments for assessing cannabis use and its impact on people with schizophrenia have recently been developed by the Dual Diagnosis Resource Centre, Australia (Rolfe *et al.*, 1999a, b). The Cannabis Amount Used and Symptom Evaluation (CAUSE) is a 10-item self-report questionnaire: six items relate to quantifying and describing the respondents' cannabis use, and four items relate to symptoms of cannabis dependence. The Cannabis Use Effect Survey (CUES) is a 25-item questionnaire. Five items relate to the circumstances of the respondents' cannabis use, such as whether they use on their own or with friends. Ten items ask about perceived beneficial effects of cannabis, for example, anxiety reduction, boredom relief and sleep assistance. A further 10 items ask about perceived negative effects of cannabis use, for example, worsening of hallucinations, suicidal ideation and amotivation. The CUES aims to identify individual reasons for use in an effort to guide the planning of interventions. It reinforces the strategy of weighing benefits against risks. The CAUSE and CUES are intended for use as self-report tools or as prompts for discussion, and can also be used for research purposes. The questionnaires are designed specifically for use by patients with a mental health problem. They can be employed cross-sectionally or to track changes in cannabis use over time. The CAUSE and CUES have been used to measure cannabis use in a 3-year follow-up study of 350 people with schizophrenia, and have proven to be well accepted by patients (Rolfe *et al.*, 1999a, b).

Broader evaluation of the nature and extent of cannabis use can be achieved by using a comprehensive assessment tool such as the Addiction Severity Index (ASI, McLellan *et al.*, 1992) or the Maudsley Addiction Profile (MAP, Marsden *et al.*, 1997). These instruments assess quantity, frequency and types of drugs used, withdrawal problems, periods of abstinence, drug use history, past treatments and other aspects such as housing, employment and relationships. They allow information to be gathered in a standardized way, thus improving the sensitivity of findings (Drake *et al.*, 1993b).

Reasons for use

Assessing underlying motives for cannabis use is an essential part of any behavioural analysis necessary to inform treatment planning (see Chapter 11). As reasons for use may predict patterns of use and also mediate the relationship between symptoms and substance dependence, they are clearly a crucial target for treatments that attempt to reduce that use. The Substance Use Scale for Psychosis (SUSP; Spencer *et al.*, 2002) is a 26-item self-report instrument that includes a number of items from the Drinking Motives Questionnaire (Cooper *et al.*, 1995) as well as additional motives specific to symptoms of severe mental illness. Its reliability and validity have recently been demonstrated among individuals with psychotic disorders (Spencer et al., 2002). The 26 items within the questionnaire relate to five subscales, viz.: social use, enhancement, coping with unpleasant affect, conformity/acceptance and coping with positive symptoms or side-effects from medication.

This information can be used to tailor individualized treatment interventions so that important motivations for cannabis use are identified and appropriate management strategies introduced. For instance, individuals who use cannabis to cope with negative affect may benefit from interventions designed to reduce or manage stress more effectively. For those who use cannabis to enhance emotional experiences, other sources of pleasure can be explored and developed.

Readiness to change

The Trans-theoretical Model (Prochasca and DiClemente, 1986) offers a useful paradigm for understanding change in relation to drug-using behaviour. This model defines five stages that reflect the preparedness and motivation individuals have to address to change their drug use. They are precontemplation, contemplation, action, maintenance and relapse. The Stage of Change Readiness and Treatment Eagerness Scale (SOCRATES) (Miller and Tonigan, 1996) is a 19-item self-report instrument useful for determining stage of change. It allocates respondents to one of three motivational groups, namely 'recognition', 'ambivalence' and 'taking steps', and has demonstrated reliability and validity within psychiatric populations (Carey et al., 2001).

Individual differences in motivation to change drug use have important implications for treatment. Strategies need to be tailored to reflect various levels of preparedness to change. For example, precontemplators may benefit from psycho-educational or motivational interventions such as motivational interviewing (MI) (Miller and Rollnick, 1991) to enhance their readiness to change, whereas those who are further along the continuum may benefit from action-oriented strategies or training in coping skills aimed at preventing relapse (Marlatt and Gordon, 1985).

As with screening instruments, the reliability of findings from any assessment tool is reliant on each patient's willingness to acknowledge and talk about his or her drug use. As such, assessors need to do as much as they can to engage patients, build rapport and develop therapeutic relationships where patients feel that disclosure about drug use may result in positive change, rather than punitive action. It is also important to acknowledge that none of the areas identified above is static: use, motives and motivation are all subject to change and may require repeated assessment over time, especially when reviewing outcomes following the implementation of specific treatment interventions (Box 12.2).

Box 12.2 Assessment

- Address current circumstances and extent of use
- History of use
- Past treatment
- Impact current use has on illness
- Motives for ongoing use
- Readiness to change
- Support

Box 12.3 Models of service delivery

- Serial: the treatment of one condition followed by treatment of the other
- Parallel: the concurrent treatment of both conditions by different services
- Integrated: the treatment of both conditions at the same time within one setting

---

Models of service delivery

Evidence supporting the design and delivery of effective treatment programs for people with serious mental illness and concomitant substance abuse is still emerging (Drake *et al.*, 2001). The literature evaluating this issue identifies three broad models: sequential, parallel and integrated (Box 12.3). Within *sequential treatment*, either psychiatric illness or substance misuse is treated before the other. An example would be addressing alcohol dependency before offering treatment for depression. This approach has been criticized for being fragmented and for placing the burden of integration with the patient (Drake and Meuser, 2000). Sequential approaches often result from psychiatric and drug services being organizationally separated and having inflexible admission criteria which prevent entry by patients with dual problems.

The *parallel model* refers to the concurrent but separate treatment of both disorders by different specialist teams (Osher and Kofoed, 1989), for example, having psychosis managed by psychiatric services, while at the same time cannabis use is addressed by drug services. The parallel model has the benefit of having both disorders treated simultaneously by experts in their field (Kavanagh, 2000). However, there are disadvantages in expecting the patient to attend two different services and engage in two different treatment styles. Treatment drop-out rates are often high with this sort of approach, and positive outcomes rely heavily on effective collaboration and communication between services.

Integrated models are currently favoured in the limited evidence base that has contrasted the three different models of service delivery (RachBeisel *et al.*, 1999).

Integrated treatment approaches have the same team of clinicians working within the same setting providing coordinated psychiatric and substance use interventions (Bellack and Gearon, 1998). These programmes originated in the USA and have a number of common elements that include case management, an assertive style of engagement, techniques of close monitoring and comprehensive services, including inpatient, day hospital and community team support, augmented by a long-term optimistic perspective (Drake *et al.*, 1993a).

While offering an innovative solution to a complex challenge, integrated models have significant resource, training and treatment delivery implications. Arguably, the lack of conclusive evidence about the effectiveness of integration makes it unclear whether such investment is justifiable (Ley *et al.*, 2001). As such, it is advisable that before making revolutionary changes, services move cautiously towards integration, while at the same time evaluating the effects these changes have on patient outcomes and the confidence and capacity of staff to manage both disorders simultaneously.

Recent guidelines for the management of dual disorders (Department of Health, 2002) acknowledge the need for integrated services and advocate a stepped approach towards achieving increased integration without resorting to immediate and radical change. The guidelines promote the development of closer links between drug and psychiatric services, supported by memoranda of understanding and agreed pathways of care. Training and supervision should be offered to mental health service personnel in treatment paradigms for substance misuse, whilst equivalent training in mental health issues should be made available to drug service staff. In addition, mental health teams should be strengthened with specialist dual-diagnosis workers who work alongside staff in helping patients with dual problems.

Treatment approaches

There is a paucity of rigorous research that has evaluated which specific treatment approaches integrated services should employ (Kavanagh *et al.*, 1998). Current practice reflects expert consensus, rather than conclusive evidence. Early treatment interventions for people with a dual diagnosis originated in the USA and utilized a stage-wise approach that relied heavily on the traditional 12-step model of drug treatment (Osher and Kofoed, 1989). The 12-step philosophy advocates total abstinence and uses confrontation as a technique to break through denial. This approach may have proven too stressful for many patients, as drop-out rates from treatment were high and other related outcomes were poor (Drake *et al.*, 2001).

Current treatment approaches to addressing cannabis use amongst this group have started to apply a combination of psychoeducation, harm reduction strategies, skills training, pharmacology and contemporary substance abuse interventions such as MI and relapse prevention (RP). Elements within these approaches are modified to accommodate the cognitive impairments associated with psychotic illnesses and can be delivered individually or in a group setting (Kavanagh *et al.*, 1998; Castle *et al.*, 2002). They acknowledge the need for patients to determine their own drug use goals and accept that change is slow and that relapse is not unusual.

Substance abuse strategies such as MI and RP have proven efficacy in the non-psychotic population for improving outcomes in relation to reducing cannabis use (Stephens *et al.*, 1994; Miller, 1996). MI is a directive, client-centred counselling style for eliciting behaviour change by helping participants explore and resolve ambivalence (Miller and Rollnick, 1991). Ambivalence reflects a state of internal conflict that can occur between two courses of action, each of which has perceived benefits and costs. RP is a behavioural self-management approach designed to teach individuals how to anticipate and cope with the problem of relapse (Marlatt and Gordon, 1985). RP combines behavioural and cognitive interventions in an overall approach that emphasizes self-management. It asserts that if an individual has an effective coping strategy to deal with a high-risk situation, the probability of relapse as an outcome decreases significantly.

Harm reduction is an umbrella term for a number of pragmatic social policies and treatment approaches that address drug-related health problems. Harm reduction strategies place high priority on reducing the negative consequences of drug use rather than on eliminating the availability of drugs or ensuring abstinence. This approach is based on the view that drug use occurs along a continuum of risk ranging from low to high. For example, a drug or alcohol abstainer is at less risk of harm than a drug or alcohol user; a moderate drinker is causing less risk of harm than a binge drinker; and a heroin smoker is causing less harm than a heroin injector. Participants are offered relevant and accurate information on high-risk activities and advice on what alternatives are available to reduce the likelihood of harm.

Treatment programmes

A number of programmes for the treatment of people with serious mental illness and drug use have started to emerge that incorporate a number of the above components within their design. Kavanagh (1995) developed an approach for addressing cannabis and alcohol use amongst people with schizophrenia. The intervention is primarily delivered on an individual basis, although supportive relatives are invited to attend certain sessions to assist in the early detection of relapse. The intervention follows a comprehensive assessment using formal measures to evaluate current levels of use, degree of dependence, psychotic symptoms, the role of cannabis in the relapse of illness, reasons for use and readiness to change.

This intervention encourages patients to determine their own goals, and objectives such as controlled use are accepted. The principles of MI and RP are strongly reflected throughout the intervention, as are aspects of psychoeduction and harm reduction. The intervention encourages adherence to antipsychotic medication to limit the role of self-medication as a possible motivation for ongoing substance use. In addition, patients are encouraged to engage in non-drug-related activities and develop alternate sources of pleasure. Research evaluating the efficacy of this approach is needed.

Bellack and DiClemente (1999) developed a treatment strategy that involves four modules that are implemented sequentially. The first module concentrates on social skills and problem-solving. The second module focuses on reasons for use, including triggers, habits and craving as well as psychoeducation regarding the dangers of drug use for people with schizophrenia. The third module contains MI strategies and goal-setting aimed at decreasing drug use. The fourth module involves training in behavioural skills for coping with urges and avoiding relapse. This treatment approach accepts drug-related goals other than abstinence, and emphasizes the learning and mastery of a few specific skills such as avoidance and refusal, rather than a number of complex cognitive strategies that may prove too challenging to implement for this group during stressful interactions. Initial results are promising and the approach is now the subject of a larger controlled clinical trial.

Barrowclough *et al.* (2001) demonstrated positive results in a randomized controlled trial comparing routine psychiatric care with a programme of routine psychiatric care augmented with a comprehensive package of MI, cognitive-behaviour therapy and family/care-giver interventions. This intervention is delivered within participants' homes over a 9-month period and requires the involvement of family or care-givers to ensure consistency of intervention. Findings suggest that integrated comprehensive care can generate significant improvements in general functioning, reduce positive symptoms and lead to an increase in days abstinent from drugs and alcohol. Cannabis was the most commonly used illicit substance amongst subjects in this study.

James *et al.* (2004) recently trialled a group-based intervention aimed at reducing substance use and improving mental health amongst cannabis users with psychosis, and also observed favourable results in several domains. The intervention was tailored to participants' motivation for drug use and preparedness to change and encompassed aspects of psychoeducation, MI, RP and harm reduction. The intervention was guided by a comprehensive treatment manual that outlined each of the weekly sessions and covered all other aspects of the 6-week programme (James *et al.*, 2002). In a pilot study, 68 subjects were enrolled and randomly allocated to either routine psychiatric care or routine care plus the group intervention. Significant improvements were observed within the intervention group regarding psychopathology, chlorpromazine equivalent doses of medication and reductions in cannabis use and polydrug use. This intervention is now the subject of a larger multisite randomized controlled trial.

Conclusions

As our understanding about the relationship between serious mental illness and cannabis use improves, the issue of how best to respond effectively to this problem becomes an ever more pertinent and important question. Deficiencies regarding the way services identify and detect cannabis use amongst psychiatric populations can be significantly improved through the introduction of routine screening and assessment procedures. Such changes can reduce the rate of non-detection and ensure that those who are using are identified and are subsequently informed about possible consequences to health. In terms of therapeutic interventions, research evidence supporting the efficacy of unintegrated paradigm has started to emerge. We are also beginning to be able to define the shape and content of specific treatment programmes. While much more work still needs to be done in this area, it would appear that an encouraging start has been made.

REFERENCES

Ananth, J., Vandewater, S., Kamal, M. *et al.* (1989). Missed diagnosis of substance abuse in psychiatric patients. *Hosp. Commun. Psychiatry*, **40**, 297–299.

Appleby, L., Dyson, V., Luchins, D. J. and Cohen, L. S. (1997). The impact of substance use screening on a public psychiatric inpatient population. *Psychiatric Serv.*, **48**, 1311–1316.

Ashton, C. H. (2001). Pharmacology and effects of cannabis: a brief review. *Br. J. Psychiatry*, **178**, 101–106.

Barrowclough, C., Haddock, G. and Tarrier, N. (2001). Randomized controlled trial of motivational interviewing, cognitive behavior therapy, and family intervention for patients with comorbid schizophrenia and substance use disorders. *Am. J. Psychiatry*, **158**, 1706–1713.

Bellack, A. S. and DiClemente, C. C. (1999). Treating substance abuse among patients with schizophrenia. *Psychiatric Serv.*, **50**, 75–80.

Bellack, A. S. and Gearon, J. S. (1998). Substance abuse treatment for people with schizophrenia. *Addict. Behav.*, **23**, 749–766.

Carey, K. B. and Correia, C. J. (1998). Severe mental illness and addictions: assessment considerations. *Addict. Behav.*, **23**, 735–748.

Carey, K. B., Maisto, S. A., Carey, M. P. *et al.* (2001) Readiness to change substance misuse among psychiatric outpatients: reliability and validity of self-report measures. *J. Studies Alcohol*, **62**, 79–88.

Castle, D., James, W., Koh, *et al.* (2002). Substance use in schizophrenia: why do people use, and what can be done about it? *Schizophr. Res.*, **53**, 223.

Cooper, M. L., Frone, M. R., Russell, M. and Mudar, P. (1995). Drinking to regulate positive and negative emotions: a motivational model of alcohol use. *J. Personal. Soc. Psycho.*, **69**, 990–1005.

Department of Health (2002). *Mental Health Policy Implementation Guide: Dual Diagnosis Good Practice Guide.* London: Department of Health.

Dixon, L., Haas, G., Weiden, P. J., Sweeney, J. and Frances, A. J. (1991). Drug abuse in schizophrenic patients: clinical correlates and reasons for use. *Am. J. Psychiatry*, **148**, 224.

Drake, R. and Meuser, K. (2000). Psychosocial approaches to dual diagnosis. *Schizophr. Bull.*, **26**, 105–118.

Drake, R. E. and Wallach, M. A. (1989). Substance abuse among the chronic mentally ill. *Hosp. Commun. Psychiatry*, **40**, 1041–1046.

Drake, R. E., Bartels, S. J., Teague, G. B., Noordsy, D. L. and Clark, R. E. (1993a). Treatment of substance abuse in severely mentally ill patients. *J. Nerv. Ment. Dis.* **24**, 589–608.

Drake, R. E., Altereman, A. I. and Rosenberg, S. R. (1993b). Detection of substance use disorders in severely mentally ill patients. *Commun. Ment. Health J.*, **29**, 175–192.

Drake, R. E., Essock, S. M., Shaner, A. *et al.* (2001). Implementing dual diagnosis services for clients with severe mental illness. *Psychiatric Serv.*, **52**, 469–476.

Hall, W. and Degenhardt, L. (2000). Cannabis use and psychosis: a review of clinical and epidemiological evidence. *Aust. NZ J. Psychiatry*, **34**, 26–34.

James, W., Koh, G., Spencer, C. *et al.* (2002). *Managing Mental Health and Drug Use.* Perth, Western Australia: Uniprint.

James, W. Preston, N., Koh, G. *et al.* (2004). A group intervention that assists patients with dual diagnosis reduce their drug and alcohol use: a randomised controlled trial. *Psychol. Med.* (in press).

Kavanagh, D. (1995). An intervention for substance abuse in schizophrenia. *Behav. Change*, **12**, 20–30.

Kavanagh, D. (2000). *Treatment of Comorbidity.* National Comorbidity Project–National Workshop Agenda Papers. Canberra. Available from Department of Psychiatry, University of Queensland.

Kavanagh, D. J. Young, R., Boyce, L. *et al.* (1998). Substance Treatment Options in Psychosis (STOP): a new intervention for dual diagnosis. *J. Men. Health*, **7**, 135–143.

Ley, A., McLaren, S. and Siegfried, N. (2001). Treatment programmes for people with both severe mental illness and substance misuse (Cochrane Review). Cochrane Library, Issue 1.

Linszen, D. H., Dingemans, P. M. and Lenior, M. E. (1994). Cannabis abuse and the course of recent-onset schizophrenic disorders. *Arch. Gen. Psychiatry*, **51**, 273–279.

Marlatt, G. and Gordon, J. (1985). *Relapse Prevention: Maintenance Strategies in the Treatment of Addictive Behaviours.* New York: Guildford Press.

Marsden, J., Gossop, M., Stewart, D. *et al.* (1997). The Maudsley Addiction Profile (MAP): a brief instrument for assessing treatment outcome. *Addiction* **93**, 1857–1868.

Mayfield, D., McLeod, G. and Hall, P. (1974). The CAGE questionnaire: validation of a new alcoholism instrument. *Am. J. Psychiatry*, **131**, 1121–1123.

McLellan, A. T., Kushner, H., Metzger, D. *et al.* (1992). The fifth edition of the Addiction Severity Index. *J. Substance Abuse Treatment*, **9**, 199–213.

Miller, W. R. (1996). Motivational interviewing: research, practice and puzzles. *Addict. Behav.*, **61**, 835–842.

Miller, W. and Rollnick, S. (1991). *Motivational Interviewing: Preparing People to Change Addictive Behaviour.* New York: Guildford Press.

Miller, W. R. and Tonigan, J. S. (1996). Assessing Drinker's motivation for change: the Stages of Change Readiness and Treatment Eagerness Scale (SOCRATES). *Psychol. Addict. Behav.*, **10**, 81–89.

Milling, R. N., Faulkner, L. R. and Craig, J. M. (1994). Problems, in the recognition and treatment of patients with dual diagnosis. *J. Substance Abuse Treatment*, **11**, 267–271.

Osher, F. C. and Kofoed, L. L. (1989). Treatment of patients with psychiatric and psychoactive substance abuse disorders. *Hosp. Commun. Psychiatry*, **40**, 1025–1030.

Prochasca, J. and DiClemente, C. (1986). Toward a comprehensive model of change. In *Treating Addictive Behaviours: Process of Change.* ed. W. R. Miller and N. Heather. New York: Plenum.

RachBeisel, J., Scott, J. and Dixon, L. (1999). Co-occurring severe mental illness and substance use disorders: a review of recent research. *Psychiatric Serv.*, **50**, 1427–1433.

Rolfe, T. J., Kulkarni, J., Fitzgerald, P. *et al.* (1999a). Cannabis use, symptom profile and quality of life in clients enrolled in the Schizophrenia Care and Assessment Program (SCAP). International Congress on Schizophrenia Research, Santa Fe, April 1999. *Schizophr. Bull.* (suppl.).

Rolfe, T. J. Williams, S., Fitzgerald, P. B. and Kulkarni, J.(1999b). Cannabis use in schizophrenia. *R Aust NZ J Psychiatry*, (supp.).

Rosenberg, S. D., Drake, R. E., Wolford, G. L. *et al* (1998). Dartmouth assessment of lifestyle instrument (DALI): a substance use disorder screen for people with severe mental illness. *Am. J. Psychiatry*, **155**, 232–238.

Siegfried, N. (1998). A review of comorbidity: major mental illness and problematic substance use. *Aust. NZ J. Psychiatry*, **32**, 707–717.

Skinner, H. A. (1982). The drug abuse screening test. *Addict. Behav.* **7**, 363–371.

Spencer, C., Castle, D. J. and Michie, P. (2002). An examination of the validity of a motivational model for understanding substance use among individuals with psychotic disorders. *Schizophr. Bull.*, **28**, 233–247.

Stephens, R. S., Roffman, R. A. and Simpson, E. E. (1994). Treating adult marijuana dependence: a test of the relapse prevention model. *J. Consult. Clin. Psychol.*, **62**, 92–99.

Test, M. A., Wallisch, L. S. and Allness, D. J. (1989). Substance use in young adults with schizophrenic disorders. *Schizophr. Bull.*, **15**, 465–476.

Weiss, R. D., Najavitis, L. M., Greenfield, S. F. *et al.* (1998). Validity of substance use self-reports in dually diagnosed outpatients. *Am. J. Psychiatry*, **155**, 127–128.

Zeidonis, D. and Fisher, W. (1994). Assessment and treatment of comorbid substance abuse in individuals with schizophrenia. *Psychiatric Ann.*, **24**, 477–483.

13

Residual cognitive effects of long-term cannabis use

Harrison G. Pope, Jr and Deborah Yurgelun-Todd

Harvard Medical School, Belmont, MA, USA

Introduction

Previous chapters of this book have addressed the question of whether cannabis can cause or potentiate frank psychiatric syndromes such as psychotic disorders. Of course, the great majority of cannabis users, including even those who have used cannabis for decades, do not appear to exhibit serious psychiatric disorders (Gruber and Pope, 1996; Johns, 2001). But what about more subtle impairments? Do long-term heavy cannabis users experience residual deficits in cognition, even if they stop using cannabis for a substantial period?

This question has proven surprisingly difficult to answer, largely because of the formidable methodological problems confronting studies in this area. Although many of these same problems have been mentioned elsewhere in this volume, it is important to review them once again here. First, there is the problem of defining a 'residual effect'. Presumably a 'residual effect' is an effect that persists after acute intoxication with cannabis has cleared. But how long an interval should be allowed between the last episode of cannabis use and the time of evaluation? Elsewhere (Pope *et al.*, 2001a), we have suggested that effects present hours or days after last cannabis use, when cannabinoids are still present in the central nervous system (CNS), should be considered separately as 'short-term residual effects'. In heavy cannabis users, such short-term effects may persist for many days or even weeks, since these individuals gradually accumulate a large burden of Δ^9-tetrahydrocannabinol (Δ^9-THC) in body fat stores, and this residue is only slowly excreted (Ashton, 2001). As a result, heavy cannabis users may display detectable cannabinoids in the urine even after many weeks of abstinence from the drug. The degree to which residues of Δ^9-THC remain in the CNS itself, and how long such residues remain psychoactive, is unknown.

Marijuana and Madness: Psychiatry and Neurobiology, ed. D. Castle and R. Murray. Published by Cambridge University Press. © Cambridge University Press 2004.

Assessment of short-term residual cognitive deficits in heavy cannabis users is further complicated by the effects of cannabis withdrawal (Jones *et al.*, 1981; Wiesbeck *et al.*, 1996; Budney *et al.*, 1999; Haney *et al.*, 1999; Kouri *et al.*, 1999; Kouri and Pope, 2000). Cannabis withdrawal is characterized by irritability, physical tension, agitation and anorexia; the symptoms typically rise to a peak several days after cannabis is stopped, and they may persist for a week or two thereafter. Withdrawal effects almost certainly impair attention and memory function, and may cause the cognitive performance of recently abstinent cannabis users to get temporarily worse before it gets better (Pope *et al.*, 2001a; b).

Given the long persistence of Δ^9-THC in the CNS, together with the problem of withdrawal effects, it would seem prudent to reserve the term 'long-term residual effects' to describe effects present a minimum of several weeks after last cannabis exposure, at a time when residual Δ^9-THC has been almost fully excreted, and when withdrawal effects have fully run their course. However, few neuropsychological studies have succeeded in examining cannabis users after such a long interval of abstinence, because of the difficulty and expense of maintaining subjects under supervised conditions for weeks at a time (Pope *et al.*, 2001a). Most studies examining residual neuropsychological deficits in cannabis users have studied subjects after only a few hours or days of abstinence, so that it is difficult to disentangle which deficits may represent relatively benign and potentially reversible short-term phenomena, as opposed to more ominous potentially irreversible long-term deficits.

A second and equally difficult methodological problem is that studies of long-term cannabis users must necessarily be naturalistic, since it would be unethical deliberately to administer large doses of cannabis over years of time to normal volunteers. Naturalistic studies, however, are subject to numerous limitations. First, recruitment of long-term cannabis users may be compromised by selection bias. For example, if cannabis produces severe cognitive deficits in some individuals, these individuals might be missed during study recruitment because they would fail to respond to advertisements for study subjects, or be too cognitively impaired to cooperate with the requirements for the study. Second, even in the absence of selection bias, results may be compromised by various forms of information bias in the subjects, since investigators must rely on the subjects' own retrospective accounts of their drug use. Some studies have suggested the drug users are reasonably accurate when reporting their histories (Rouse *et al.*, 1985; Brown *et al.*, 1992; Harrison *et al.*, 1993), but others have shown high rates of underreporting (Fendrich *et al.*, 1999; Colón *et al.*, 2001, 2002). Thus cannabis users may intentionally or unintentionally fail to disclose substantial prior exposure to drugs other than cannabis. Retrospective accounts may also omit other critical information, such as a history of a major head injury, past or present symptoms of a psychiatric disorder or current use of medications with psychoactive properties. If investigators are unaware of these exposures or fail to account for them adequately, cognitive deficits in the subjects may be falsely attributed to cannabis when they are actually due to other factors.

Perhaps the greatest problem with naturalistic studies, though, is the influence of confounding variables. Any comparison of cognitive measures in long-term cannabis users compared with control subjects is at risk for residual confounding, both from inadequate adjustment for measured confounders and from the presence of unmeasured confounders. This is because all such comparisons rest on the assumption that, after appropriate adjustments, cannabis users and comparison subjects are matched on all attributes, other than the cannabis exposure itself, that would influence the study measures. But such matching is almost impossible to achieve in real life. For example, long-term cannabis users may have lower premorbid overall cognitive abilities, or subtle deficits in psychological functioning, before they ever start using cannabis. The only way to address this problem fully would be to possess childhood cognitive testing results for groups of long-term cannabis users and control subjects, obtained when these individuals were, say, 10–12 years old, before any of them had ever tried cannabis. Then, when comparing the contemporary cognitive test scores of long-term cannabis users and controls, one could adjust for their childhood test scores in the analysis in order to control for possible differences in premorbid cognitive abilities. We are aware of only one major study that has used such a design (Block and Ghoneim, 1993). This study did find residual cognitive deficits in cannabis users even after adjustment for childhood test scores – but since users were tested after only 1 day of abstinence from cannabis, it is unclear whether the deficits represented reversible short-term effects or potentially more serious long-term effects, as discussed above.

Furthermore, even if one can adjust for childhood cognitive testing scores in cannabis users and non-users, this adjustment might not fully compensate for the effects of various conditions that affect cognitive functioning – such as conduct disorder, antisocial personality disorder, attention deficit hyperactivity disorder, depression or even subclinical psychotic disorders – all of which may be more common in long-term heavy cannabis users than in the population at large (Gruber and Pope, 1996, 2002; Gruber *et al.*, 1996). Attention deficit hyperactivity disorder (Pennington and Ozonoff, 1996; Aronowitz *et al.*, 1994; Barkley, 1997), major depressive disorder (Mialet *et al.*, 1996), a family history of schizophrenia (Williamson, 1987) and disorders associated with antisocial behaviour (Gorenstein, 1987; Lueger and Gill, 1990; Aronowitz *et al.*, 1994; Morgan and Lilienfeld, 2000) may all cause cognitive deficits in and of themselves; these deficits might then be falsely attributed to cannabis use, rather than to the underlying disorder.

Even if one can match or adjust for every one of these potentially confounding conditions, one must still allow for the effects of what we have called 'cultural divergence' (Pope *et al.*, 2003). Specifically, individuals destined to become heavy cannabis users, who may start smoking at an early age (Kandel and Davies, 1992; Chen and Kandel, 1995; Kandel and Chen, 2000; Gruber *et al.*, 2003) and who may be less motivated to pursue an education (Hammer and Vaglum, 1990; Bray *et al.*, 2000; Lynskey and Hall, 2000), are likely to diverge from the mainstream culture of their non-drug-using peers as they grow up. To take a specific example, long-term cannabis users who are chronically intoxicated during their high school classes, or erratic in class attendance, may develop a more impoverished working vocabulary than individuals who do not use drugs – even if the innate intellectual ability of both groups is identical to start with. Furthermore, the words most frequently used by long-term cannabis users in their daily speech will probably differ from the words most frequently used by non-users. If these groups are then administered a standard verbal memory test using words widely used by ordinary non-drug-users, the cannabis users may underperform simply because the words are less typical of the ones that they use in daily life.

To appreciate how profoundly cultural divergence can affect test results, consider an experience which our group has had with administering verbal memory tests to Native Americans of the Navajo tribe. We have been conducting a study comparing Navajo members of the Native American church, who use the hallucinogenic cactus, peyote, with comparison Navajos who do not use peyote. The purpose of this study was to assess whether long-term exposure to a hallucinogenic substance may create residual cognitive effects. When we compared these two groups of Navajos on verbal memory, using Buschke's Selective Reminding Test (Buschke, 1973), the peyote users recalled significantly fewer words then their non-using counterparts. Specifically, the mean (SD) total number of words recalled (out of a possible 144) was 108.4 (15.2) for the peyote users versus 116.8 (10.6) for the non-users – a highly significant difference ($P = 0.008$ by linear regression after adjustment for age and sex). This difference remained statistically significant, and almost unchanged in magnitude, even after adjusting for the subjects' years of education or for their verbal IQ as determined by the vocabulary subscale of the Wechsler Adult Intelligence Test (Wechsler, 1981). Does this mean that long-term use of peyote creates deficits in verbal memory? We wondered whether the difference between groups might simply be due to their differing familiarity with the words used on the test. Navajos who are members of the Native American church often lead a very traditional lifestyle on the Navajo reservation, have less contact with western society than many other Navajos, and hence might be less likely to use certain words in their vocabularies. Accordingly, we created a 'Navajo-friendly' version of Buschke's Selective Reminding Test

Table 13.1 Alternative versions of the Buschke Selective Reminding Test used in a study of Navajo Americans.

Conventional version (Buschke, 1973)	'Navajo-friendly' version (see text)
Bowl	Mile
Passion	Sheep
Dawn	Cough
Judgement	Fire
Grant	Snow
Bee	Coyote
Plane	School
County	Land
Choice	Sunday
Seed	Visit
Wool	Poor
Meal	Cloudy

(Table 13.1), using words that were undoubtedly familiar to all Navajos, and administered this test to the same subjects. On the Navajo-friendly version of the test, the non-peyote-users performed about the same as they did on the standard version (mean total recall 118.1 (16.1) words), whereas the peyote users improved dramatically to a score of 116.6 (14.4) words – leaving no significant difference between groups ($P = 0.71$ adjusted for age and sex). This experience shows that a subtle difference in choice of words can profoundly affect differences in test performance between groups that have different cultural exposure to those words. By analogy, long-term cannabis users might exhibit 'pseudo-deficits' on verbal memory tests simply because the standard test words are not as commonplace in their vocabularies as in the vocabularies of non-users. Interestingly, as will be seen below, verbal memory tests are the measure most frequently found to differ between long-term cannabis users and controls, even in studies where the groups are similar on other measures. Thus the possibility of 'cultural divergence' must be considered very seriously.

As one reviews the list of methodological considerations in the paragraphs above, it should be noted that most of these factors would tend to bias the findings *away from the null*. In other words, failure to account for increased levels of undisclosed substance use, neurological conditions, medical and psychiatric disorders or medication use in cannabis users; failure to adjust for lower levels of innate premorbid cognitive abilities among users; and failure to allow for test bias caused by 'cultural divergence' would all seem likely to bias the findings towards a false-positive assumption that cognitive deficits are due to cannabis use. Thus studies attributing cognitive deficits to cannabis use must be examined with particular care.

Current knowledge

Short-term residual effects

With the above considerations in mind, what can be said about the residual cognitive effects of long-term cannabis use? Currently, there appears to be reasonable agreement that cannabis users exhibit residual cognitive deficits for at least several days after discontinuing the drug. This was the consensus of most studies conducted between 1980 and 1995 in which heavy cannabis users were administered cognitive tests within 24 h of discontinuing the drug (Pope *et al.*, 1995). Several large studies since 1995 have reinforced these findings. Fletcher and colleagues (1996) administered a neuropsychological test battery to 17 very long-term cannabis users in Costa Rica (with a mean of 34 years of use) and 30 well-matched non-users. Even after a 72-h period of abstinence, the users performed significantly more poorly than non-users on memory of word lists and on selective and divided attention tasks associated with working memory. Pope and Yurgelun-Todd (1996) compared 65 college students who had smoked cannabis almost daily in the past month with 64 students who had smoked only 1 or 2 days in the past month. On testing after 1 day of supervised abstinence, heavy users performed more poorly than light users on memory of word lists and on the Wisconsin Card Sort Test, a test of mental flexibility. Croft and colleagues (2001) compared 18 heavy cannabis users, who had used the drug a mean of 8000 times, with 31 non-users. After a mean abstinence period of 67 h, heavy users performed more poorly on tests of manual dexterity, memory, learning and word fluency. Pope and colleagues (2001b, 2002) compared 77 current heavy cannabis users, who had smoked cannabis a minimum of 5000 times and a median of 18 500 times in their lives, with 87 control subjects who had smoked a median of 10 times and a maximum of 50 times in their lives. All subjects were tested on days 0, 1, 7 and 28 of a 28-day supervised period of abstinence from marijuana, monitored by daily or every-other-day observed urine samples. On days 0, 1 and 7, the heavy users performed significantly more poorly than controls on memory of word lists. By day 28, however, the scores of the two groups had converged, and few significant differences remained between groups on any of the measures of a battery of 10 neuropsychological tests. Finally, Solowij and colleagues (2002) administered a battery of nine neuropsychological tests to 102 long-term cannabis users who were seeking treatment and 33 non-using controls. Users were tested a median of 17 h after last use. Although shorter-term users showed only modest differences from controls, longer-term users showed several significant deficits, especially on a test of verbal learning.

All of these studies attempted to control for possible confounding variables such as those enumerated earlier. Although each has imperfections (Pope *et al.*, 2001a; Pope, 2002), the similarity of findings across studies argues that the short-term cognitive deficits observed are truly attributable to cannabis itself, rather than to spurious factors. The study of Pope *et al.* (2001b; 2002) particularly favours this hypothesis, because these deficits largely disappeared in the same individuals after 28 days of abstinence.

Long-term residual effects

Because of the difficulty of maintaining cannabis users drug-free for long periods, few studies have examined cognitive measures among users after prolonged abstinence. One of the few studies is that of Schwartz and colleagues (1989), who tested 10 cannabis-dependent adolescents in a treatment programme, where they had no access to drugs, after 6 weeks of supervised abstinence. In comparison to nine matched control subjects, users performed significantly more poorly on memorizing a short story and on remembering simple figure drawings. Solowij (1998) found a strong correlation between duration of cannabis use and increased processing negativity to complex irrelevant stimuli in a selective attention task in 28 cannabis ex-users, even though these individuals reported a mean of 2 years of abstinence. Lyketsos and colleagues (1999) performed serial administrations of the Mini-Mental State Examination to 1318 subjects under age 65, recruited in the course of a larger epidemiological study. These investigators found no significant differences between heavy cannabis users, light users and non-users in degree of cognitive decline over a 12-year period. Although these individuals were not necessarily tested after prolonged abstinence, the absence of differences on serial test administrations over a prolonged period argues against long-term residual effects. However, the Mini-Mental State Examination does not measure cognitive function as sensitively as a full neuropsychological test battery, and hence might miss subtle deficits. Rodgers (2000) compared 15 cannabis users, who had been smoking a mean of four times per week for a mean of 11 years, to 15 non-users matched for age and gender distribution. All users were abstinent from cannabis for at least 1 month by their own report, but they were not supervised during this period to confirm abstinence. Users performed significantly more poorly than non-users on verbal memory testing, but this comparison between groups did not adjust for potentially confounding variables. Finally, Pope *et al.* (2001b; 2002), as noted above, found no significant differences between long-term cannabis users and controls, after adjustment for verbal IQ (Wechsler, 1981), on any test measures after 28 days of supervised abstinence. Pope *et al.* (2001b) also used identical methods to examine 45 former heavy cannabis users, who had also smoked a median of 11 000 times and a minimum of 5000 times in their lives, but no more than 12 times in the 3 months prior to study entry. These subjects also exhibited no significant differences from controls on any of the tests at day 28. Finally, Bolla *et al.* (2002) examined 22 young cannabis users after approximately 28 days of abstinence on a research ward. On several neuropsychological measures, performance was negatively associated with frequency of use, despite the long washout period. Notably, however, the heaviest users in this study were smoking more than 10 joints per day – an extremely high dose that might take longer to wash out than for subjects in other studies.

In short, with the exception of the very small study of Schwartz *et al.* (1989) and Bolla *et al.* (2002), these studies suggest that heavy cannabis use does not create lasting or irreversible deficits. This impression is reinforced by a recent meta-analysis (Grant *et al.*, 2003) which examined all available neuropsychological studies of the long-term effects of chronic cannabis use that met rigorous predefined criteria for study adequacy and content. The investigators included virtually all of the studies cited above, including even those with a very short interval between last cannabis use and test administration. The meta-analysis yielded no significant evidence for cannabis-induced deficits in six of eight neuropsychological ability areas, and only small effect sizes for the remaining domains of learning and forgetting. Even the findings regarding learning and forgetting must be regarded with caution, however, since the relevant tests typically rely on word lists – and these may be particularly vulnerable to the 'cultural divergence' problem, as illustrated by our example of the Navajo subjects above.

Residual effects and lifetime duration of cannabis use

Even if cannabis users as a whole cannot be distinguished from comparison subjects in cognitive abilities, it might be that certain subgroups of users would be more conspicuously affected. One possibility is that only users with very long-term exposure will display detectable deficits. For example, as described above, Fletcher *et al.* (1996) found cognitive deficits on a number of tests administered to 17 cannabis users reporting a mean of 34 years of use. However, these same investigators failed to find comparable deficits on the same tests under identical conditions in a comparison of 37 younger users (mean of 8 years of use) and 49 matched non-users. Similarly, Solowij *et al.* (2002) found markedly greater deficits in 51 long-term near-daily cannabis users (mean 23.9 years of use) than in 51 shorter-term users (mean 10.2 years of use). Furthermore, performance measures among the 102 cannabis users as a group often correlated negatively and significantly with years of cannabis use, even after controlling for several potentially confounding variables. However, Pope *et al.* (2002), in the study described above, found no significant association between log-transformed lifetime episodes of use and performance at day

28 on any of 10 neuropsychological tests, although a few test measures approached significance in this exercise.

Residual effects and age of onset of cannabis use

Another possibility is that individuals who begin cannabis use at an early age, when the brain is still developing, may display greater cognitive deficits than those who start use when they are older. Indirect evidence for this hypothesis comes from studies showing apparently irreversible effects on brain morphology and behaviour in rats exposed to cannabinoids while still immature (Stiglick and Kalant, 1985; Landfeld *et al.*, 1988). In a study addressing this question in humans, Ehrenreich *et al.* (1999) found that 48 early-onset cannabis users (onset at age 16 or less), but not 51 late-onset users (onset after age 16), displayed significantly longer reaction times than controls in a visual scanning task. Wilson *et al.* (2000) compared 29 early-onset cannabis users, also defined as having started use at age 16 or less, with 28 late-onset users who had started use after age 16. Although these subjects were not administered cognitive tests, early-onset users were found to be lower in weight and shorter in height than late-onset users, and early-onset users also showed a lower percentage of grey matter, relative to whole-brain volume, on magnetic resonance images of the brain. Pope *et al.* (in 2003) compared test results from 69 cannabis users who had begun smoking at age 16 or before, 53 users who had begun smoking after age 16 and 87 comparison subjects with minimal cannabis exposure, drawn from their study described above (Pope *et al.*, 2001b; 2002). After 28 days of abstinence, the late-onset users showed few differences from controls on the test battery, but early-onset users performed significantly more poorly than controls on several tests, especially those requiring verbal abilities. However, after adjustment for verbal IQ, differences between early-onset users and controls generally became non-significant.

Conclusions

Although heavy cannabis use almost certainly causes some short-term residual cognitive deficits, there is little evidence to suggest that these deficits persist for prolonged periods after cannabis is discontinued. However, several studies have suggested an association between lifetime duration of cannabis use, or age of onset of use, and cognitive deficits. Such deficits cannot be explained merely by the short-term residual effects of cannabis, since this would not account for differences within samples of cannabis users who were all tested under the same conditions. Therefore, these studies continue to raise the spectre of irreversible cognitive deficits in individuals with either very long exposure and/or very early exposure to the drug.

But this possibility must be regarded with caution, as we have discussed above, because of the many factors likely to bias studies away from the null. In other words, deficits in very long-term or early-onset cannabis users might reflect a frank toxic effect of cannabis on the brain, but they might also be due to numerous possible confounding variables, such as the phenomenon of 'cultural divergence', presented earlier. At present, then, it is still uncertain whether heavy cannabis use causes long-term residual neuropsychological deficits in some individuals or under certain conditions. The effect sizes of the available studies are equally compatible with a complete absence of cannabis-induced residual cognitive effects (all effects being due to confounding factors), or with a substantial cannabis-induced effect of clinical significance. Future studies will require meticulous designs, possibly involving serial assessments of cannabis users over many years, to resolve these lingering questions.

REFERENCES

Aronowitz, B., Liebowitz, M., Hollander, E. *et al.* (1994). Neuropsychiatric and neuropsychological findings in conduct disorder and attention-deficit hyperactivity disorder. *J. Neuropsychiatry*, **6**, 245–249.

Ashton, C. H. (2001). Pharmacology and effects of cannabis: a brief review. *Br. J. Psychiatry*, **178**, 101–106.

Barkley, R. (1997). Behavioral inhibition, sustained attention, and executive functions: constructing a unifying theory of ADHD. *Psychol. Bull.*, **121**, 65–94.

Block, R. I. and Ghoneim, M. M. (1993). Effects of chronic marijuana use on human cognition. *Psychopharmacology*, **110**, 219–228.

Bolla, K. I., Brown, K., Eldreth, D., Tate, K. and Cadet, J. L. (2002). Dose-related neurocognitive effects of marijuana use. *Neurology*, **59**, 1337–1343.

Bray, J. W., Zarkin, G. A., Ringwalt, C. *et al.* (2000). The relationship between marijuana initiation and dropping out of high school. *Health Econ.*, **9**, 9–18.

Brown, J., Kranzler, H. R. and Del Boca, F. K. (1992). Self-reports by alcohol and drug abuse inpatients: factors affecting reliability and validity. *Br. J. Addict.*, **87**, 1013–1024.

Budney, A. J., Novy, P. L. and Hughes, J. R. (1999). Marijuana withdrawal among adults seeking treatment for marijuana dependence. *Addiction*, **94**, 1311–1322.

Buschke, H. (1973). Selective reminding for analyses of memory and learning. *J. Verbal Learning Verbal Behav.*, **12**, 543–550.

Chen, K. and Kandel, D. B. (1995). The natural history of drug use from adolescence to the mid-thirties in a general population sample. *Am. J. Public Health*, **85**, 41–47.

Colón, H. M., Robles, R. R. and Sahai, H. (2001). The validity of drug use responses in a household survey in Puerto Rico: comparison of survey responses of cocaine and heroin use with hair tests. *Int. J. Epidemiol.*, **30**, 1042–1049.

Colón, H. M., Robles, R. R. and Sahai, H. (2002). The validity of drug use self-reports among hard-core drug users in a household survey in Puerto Rico: comparison of survey responses of cocaine and heroin use with hair tests. *Drug Alcohol Depend.*, **67**, 269–279.

Croft, R. J., Mackay, A. J., Mills, A. T. D. and Gruzelier, J. G. H. (2001). The relative contributions of ecstasy and cannabis to cognitive impairment. *Psychopharmacology*, **153**, 373–379.

Ehrenreich, H., Rinn, T., Kunert, H. J. *et al.* (1999). Specific attentional dysfunction in adults following early start of cannabis use. *Psychopharmacology*, **142**, 295–301.

Fendrich, M., Johnson, T. P., Sudman, S., Wislar, J. S., Spiehler, V. (1999).Validity of drug use reporting in a high-risk community sample: a comparison of cocaine and heroin survey reports with hair tests. *Am. J. Epidemiol.*, **149**, 955–962.

Fletcher, J. M., Page, B., Francis, D. J. *et al.* (1996). Cognitive correlates of long-term cannabis use in Costa Rican men. *Arch. Gen. Psychiatry*, **53**, 1051–1057.

Gorenstein, E. E. (1987). Cognitive–perceptual deficit in an alcoholism spectrum disorder. *J. Studies Alcohol* **48**, 310–318.

Grant, I., Gonzalez, R., Carey, C. and Natarajan, L. (2001). Long-term neurocognitive consequences of marijuana: a meta-analytic study. Presented at National Institute on Drug Abuse Workshop on Clinical Consequences of Marijuana, Rockville, MD, 13 August 2001. Available online at http://www.nida.nih.gov/MeetSum/marijuanaabstracts.html.

Grant, I., Gonzalez, R., Carey, C., Natarajan, L. and Wolfson, T. (2003). Non-acute (residual) neurocognitive effects of cannabis: a meta-analytic study. Presented at National Institute on Drug Abuse Workshop on Clinical Consequences of Marijuana, Rockville, MD, 13 August 2001. Available online at *J. Int. Neuropsychol. Soc.*, **9**, 679–689.

Gruber, A. J. and Pope, H. G. Jr. (1994). Cannabis psychotic disorder: does it exist? *Am. J. Addict.*, **3**, 72–83.

Gruber, A. J. and Pope, H. G. Jr. (1996). Cannabis-related disorders. In *Psychiatry*, ed. A. Tasman, J. Kay and J. A. Lieberman, pp. 795–806. Philadelphia: W. B. Saunders.

Gruber, A. J. and Pope, H. G. Jr. (2002). Marijuana use in adolescents. *Pediatr. Clin. North Am.*, **49**, 389–413.

Gruber, A. J., Pope, H. G. Jr and Brown, M. E. (1996). Do patients use marijuana as an antidepressant? *Depression*, **4**, 77–80.

Gruber, A. J. Pope, H. G. Jr, Hudson, J. I. and Yurgelun-Todd, D. (2003). Attributes of long-term heavy cannabis users: a case-control study. *Psychol. Med.*, **33**, 1415–1422.

Hammer, T. and Vaglum, P. (1990). Initiation, continuation or discontinuation of cannabis use in the general population. *Br. J. Addict.*, **85**, 899–909.

Haney, M., Ward, A. S., Comer, S. D., Foltin, R. W. and Fischman, M. W. (1999). Abstinence symptoms following smoked marijuana in humans. *Psychopharmacology*, **141**, 395–404.

Harrison, E. R., Haaga, J. and Richards, T. (1993). Self-reported drug use data: what do they reveal? *Am. J. Drug Alcohol Abuse.*, **19**,423–441.

Johns, A. (2001). Psychiatric effects of cannabis. *Br. J. Psychiatry*, **178**, 116–122.

Jones, R. T., Benowitz, N. L. and Herning, R. I. (1981). Clinical relevance of cannabis tolerance and dependence. *J. Clin. Pharmacol.*, **21**, 143S–152S.

Kandel, D. B. and Chen, K. (2000). Types of marijuana users by longitudinal course. *J. Studies Alcohol*, **61**, 367–378.

Kandel, D. B. and Davies, M. (1992). Progression to regular marijuana involvement: phenomenology and risk factors for near daily use. In *Vulnerability to Drug Abuse*, ed. M. Glantz and R. Pickens, pp. 211–253. Washington, DC: American Psychological Association.

Kouri, E. M. and Pope, H. G. Jr. (2000). Abstinence symptoms during withdrawal from chronic marijuana use. *Exp. Clin. Psychopharmacol.*, **8**, 483–492.

Kouri, E. M., Pope, H. G. Jr and Lukas, S. E. (1999). Changes in aggressive behavior during withdrawal from long-term marijuana use. *Psychopharmacology*, **143**, 302–308.

Landfeld, P. W., Cadwallader, L. B. and Visant, S. (1988). Quantitative changes in hippocampal structure following long-term exposure to Δ^9-tetrahydrocannabinol: possible mediation by glucocorticoid systems. *Brain Res.*, **443**, 47–62.

Lueger, R. J. and Gill, K. J. (1990). Frontal-lobe cognitive dysfunction in conduct disorder adolescents. *J. Clin. Psychol.*, **46**, 696–706.

Lyketsos, C. G., Garrett, E., Liang, K. Y. and Anthony, J. C. (1999). Cannabis use and cognitive decline in persons under 65 years of age. *Am. J. Epidemiol.*, **149**, 794–800.

Lynskey, M. and Hall, W. (2000). The effects of adolescent cannabis use on educational attainment: a review. *Addiction*, **95**, 1621–1630.

Mialet, J.-P., Pope, H. G. Jr and Yurgelun-Todd, D. (1996). Impaired attention in depressive states: a non-specific deficit. *Psychol. Med.*, **26**, 1009–1020.

Morgan, A. B. and Lilienfeld, S. O. (2000). A meta-analytic review of the relation between antisocial behavior and neuropsychological measures of executive function. *Clin. Psychol. Rev.*, **20**, 113–136.

Pennington, B. E. and Ozonoff, S. (1996). Executive functions and developmental psychopathology. *J. Child Psychiatry Psychol.*, **37**, 51–87.

Pope, H. G. Jr. (2002). Cannabis, cognition and residual confounding. *J.A.M.A.*, **287**, 1172–1174.

Pope, H. G. Jr and Yurgelun-Todd, D. (1996). The residual cognitive effects of heavy marijuana use in college students. *J.A.M.A.*, **275**, 521–527.

Pope, H. G. Jr, Gruber, A. J., and Yurgelun-Todd, D. (1995). The residual neuropsychological effects of cannabis: the current status of research. *Drug Alcohol Depend.*, **38**, 25–34.

Pope, H. G. Jr, Gruber, A. J. and Yurgelun-Todd, D. (2001a). Residual neuropsychological effects of cannabis. *Currt. Psychiatry Rep.*, **3**, 507–512.

Pope, H. G. Jr, Gruber, A. J., Hudson, J. I., Huestis, M. A. and Yurgelun-Todd, D. (2001b). Neuropsychological performance in long-term cannabis users. *Arch. Gen. Psychiatry*, **58**, 909–915.

Pope, H. G. Jr, Gruber, A. J., Hudson, J. I., Huestis, M. A. and Yurgleun-Todd, D. (2002). Cognitive measures in long-term cannabis users. *J. Clin. Pharmacol.*, **42**, 415–475.

Pope, H. G. Jr, Gruber, A. J., Hudson, J. I., Cohane, G., Huestis, M. A. and Yurgelun-Todd, D. (2003). Early-onset cannabis use and cognitive deficits: what is the nature of the association? *Drug Alcohol Depend*, **69**, 303–310.

Rodgers J. (2000). Cognitive performance amongst recreational users of "ecstasy". *Psychopharmacology*, **151**, 19–24.

Rouse, B. A., Kozel, N. J. and Richards, L. G. (eds) (1985). *Self-Report Methods of Estimating Drug Use: Meeting Current Challenges to Validity.* NIDA research monograph 57. Washington, DC: Government Printing Office.

Schwartz, R. H., Gruenewald, P. J., Klitzner, M. *et al.* (1989). Short-term memory impairment in cannabis-dependent adolescents. *Am. J. Dis. Child.*, **143**, 1214–1219.

Solowij, N. (1998). *Cannabis and Cognitive Functioning.* Cambridge, UK: Cambridge University Press.

Solowij, N., Stephens, R. S., Roffman, R. A. *et al.* (2002). Cognitive functioning of long-term heavy cannabis users seeking treatment. *J.A.M.A.*, **287**, 1123–1131.

Stiglick, A., and Kalant, H. (1985). Residual effects of chronic cannabis treatment on behaviour in mature rats. *Psychopharmacology*, **85**, 346–349.

Wechsler, D. (1981). *Wechsler Adult Intelligence Scale – Revised Manual.* Cleveland, OH, Psychological Corporation.

Wiesbeck, G. A., Schuckit, M. A., Kalmijn, J. A. *et al.* (1996). An evaluation of the history of a marijuana withdrawal syndrome in a large population. *Addiction*, **91**, 1469–1478.

Williamson, P. (1987). Hypofrontality in schizophrenia: a review. *Can. J. Psychiatry*, **32**, 399–404.

Wilson, W., Mathew, R., Turkington, T. *et al.* (2000). Brain morphological changes and early marijuana use: a magnetic resonance and positron emission tomography study. *J. Addict. Dis.*, **19**, 1–22.

Index